GAPS, Stage

Recipes

by Becky Plotner

GAPS, Stage by Stage, With Recipes
by Becky Plotner

ISBN: 9781091590380
Published by The Dancing Rhino LLC
© 2018 Rebecca Plotner

Other titles by Becky Plotner
Probiotic Foods vs Commercial Probiotics
Joyous Song, The Proverbs 31 Woman
A Walking Tour of Lincoln Road, South Beach
Ocean Drive Guidebook, Ask a Local
The Fontainebleau, Miami & Las Vegas (Ask a Local)

I wish to thank my loving husband Kevin and my children Gage and Cooper who supported my efforts to write this book. I'd also like to thank all the practitioners and clients who have helped me in so many ways. I am grateful to you all.

Contents

It is important to have a clear answer for our clients and students.

I hope you got my new book *Gut And Physiology Syndrome*. I have covered all essential GAPS food issues in this book. Any food that is not covered in my book should be left to the discretion of the patient. It is always sensible to introduce anything new starting from a tiny amount and see how the body reacts to it. There will always be new foods and questions coming in and it is impossible to cover everything in any book.

I think that should solve this issue. GAPS patients are getting more complex and more damaged, and new issues arise all the time; and they will continue arising. You are correct: we need to have a unified policy about this without being rigid or prescriptive.

Thank you for your work! It is wonderful to have such a dedicated team of really good people!

Best wishes,
Dr Natasha

For foods that are not covered in Dr. Natasha's new book, this is my personal experience and my personal recommendations based on that experience.

Becky Plotner, BCND, traditional naturopath, CGP, D.PSc.

Forward

Becky Plotner is one of the most experienced Certified GAPS Practitioners around.

She has helped a large number of people of all ages with severe chronic health problems to regain their health and vitality. Her clinical experience is strongly enhanced by her personal journey of healing and recovery from chronic illnesses.

In her book *GAPS, Stage by Stage, With Recipes*, Becky is summarizing on her clinical experience of following the GAPS Nutritional Protocol. Every patient is a teacher for a good health practitioner!

Becky is sharing with us what she has learned from her many clients and their personal individual situations.

This book will be a valuable tool for all Certified GAPS Practitioners around the world and other people who would like to learn more about the use of the GAPS Nutritional Protocol.

I loved some recipes!

I would like to thank Becky for doing this work! I warmly recommend this book!

> Dr. Natasha Campbell-McBride, MD, MMedSci (neurology),
>   MMedSci (nutrition)
> Author of Gut and Psychology Syndrome

Chapter 1:

GAPS, Stage by Stage, With Recipes

When a person is sick with a chronic issue, it wears that person down to a state of exhaustion that is unparalleled. The desire to be healthy is all the person can think about as he or she searches the web and reads books and blogs, looking for answers. The deeper the damage in the microbiome is, the worse the situation.

To make matters worse, in a damaged microbiome situation, there are heavy metal imbalances, parasites, resident viruses, bacteria, and yeasts. These often contribute to brain fog, which can get so bad that thinking is a monumental task. Learning which protocol to do and how to follow it can be daunting. When there is brain fog, laying out a step by step plan can be helpful.

Prepping to Do GAPS

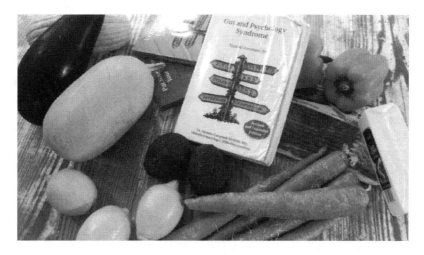

The GAPS Protocol, *Gut and Psychology Syndrome*[i] by Dr. Natasha Campbell-McBride, MD, MmedSci (neurology), MmedSci (nutrition), eliminates certain foods such as sugar, grains, conventional milk, starches, processed foods, juices, and soda, as well as others. On the protocol, foods that feed the pathogens in the microbiome are removed, and nourishing foods as well as probiotic foods are introduced to feed the good microbes in the tract. These nourishing foods are made from fresh ingredients such as meats, organ meats, fish, vegetables, nuts, seeds, beans, animal fats, fermented dairy, and other foods, including ripe fruits (for example, bananas with brown spots). Foods are cooked on the stove top or in the oven, or they are served cold. Microwave cooking is not part of the GAPS Protocol and should not be used. Cooking can be done in stainless steel, glazed, traditional clay, earthenware, and glass.

The GAPS book should be read prior to reading this book as this book is not a substitute; it is complementary.

Preparing to start the GAPS Protocol begs the desire to get started ahead of time. Early prep is not necessarily needed, but can help, if so desired. When the GAPS protocol is started, different things happen. Some kids, when starting GAPS, thrive right from day one. They progress more and more each day, showing great strides in health. Not all people progress this quickly, since the damage in their microbiome is much deeper. There is a great deal of kitchen time needed on the protocol, pulling Mom in directions she doesn't usually go.

Sometimes, for a mom, this can be torture, especially for those who are new to cooking.

There are many things on GAPS that cannot be done ahead of time. Here are some tips for some things that can.

• Meat Stock—Properly made Meat Stock is often confused with Bone Broth. It is important to know the difference since Meat Stock will cause healing and sealing of the microbiome, while Bone Broth will not. Meat Stock includes three different kinds of bones: marrow bones, joint bones, and cuts with meat on the bone. "A whole chicken, whole other poultry, a leg of lamb, neck of lamb with no meat stripped off, joints with meat on them, feet, tail, head," says Dr. Natasha.[ii] The amount of meat used depends on the person and how much they will eat, what cuts are available, as well as what the person can tolerate. Optimally, meat that is closest to the bones is the best; the farther away from the bone you go, the more fibrous the meat is, which makes it harder to digest. The meat within an inch of the bone is the gelatinous meat, which is easiest to digest. These raw pieces are cooked for a short time—1 hour for fish, 2 hours for chicken, and 3 hours for beef, minimum.[iii] The cook time is determined by the thickness of the bone. Bone broth, on the other hand, is cooked much longer—12 hours, 24 hours, and sometimes even 36 hours—and can be sourced from raw or already cooked bones.

Most GAPS Practitioners have encountered many people who have spent hours upon hours preparing stock for their GAPS journey only to find out it was Bone Broth, not Meat Stock as the protocol demands for the early stages. To make Meat Stock, which can be made ahead of time to fill the freezer, use the recipes included in the Stage One chapter. Let it cool in Mason jars or a large Pyrex bowl with a lid, and then put it in the refrigerator once it has cooled. Hot foods should not be put into the fridge as that could cause other food in the fridge to spoil. After the stock has been cooled in the refrigerator, it can be transferred to freezer bags. Do not put hot stock into plastic bags.[iv] If the stock goes directly to freezer bags for the freezer, the warmth of the stock will extract chemicals from the plastic bag and contaminate the stock. It is not a good idea to use glass in the freezer, because glass can shatter when frozen.[v] Many, many Mason jars have broken in the freezer for GAPS folks—even with ample headroom for expansion and using jars approved for the freezer.

The deeper the damage in the microbiome is, the longer the person should stay on Stage Two, which is the most healing of the GAPS stages. Some people prep early for prolonged periods on Stage Two. Dr. Natasha says, "It is best to make fresh stock every day or every few days."[vi] It's important to know that preparing stock ahead of time can also potentially lead to some trouble. There's no knowing how your child will tolerate each stock ahead of time or exactly how long the stock is to be cooked. If you spend a lot of time and money preparing chicken stock ahead of time and your child has a negative reaction with it, then your time has been wasted and you could not be more frustrated.

• Kraut Juice—Preparing probiotic foods ahead of time is wise. The older a fermented vegetable is, the easier it is tolerated for those with deeper damage. Kraut Juice is a very strong probiotic food, high in bifidobacterial and lactobacillus strains. For many, it is too strong to start with, and one drop is even too much. For these people, putting one drop in a glass of water or dropping it into hot soup will kill some of the probiotic aspects, making it more tolerable. Additionally, including other fermented vegetables is desired; this will include a variety of probiotic strains to help "heal or repair."[vii] Fermented vegetables can stay on the counter for a very long time if the temperature is correct. Most people keep fermented vegetables in the root cellar or in the basement. Some vegetables have been kept successfully for over five years, though you may find the texture or flavor a bit degraded. All vegetable ferments can be made ahead of time.

• Practice making home-brewed whey, home-brewed yogurt, home-brewed sour cream and home-brewed milk kefir (water kefir is best after the GAPS Protocol is completed, due to the remaining sugar after fermentation, as well as other undesirable traits). Fermented dairy does not have a long shelf life like fermented vegetables. If left on the shelf, fermented dairy will continue to sour to an unpalatable state. Once it is fermented, it should be refrigerated. It is good to get comfortable making fermented dairy so that it is less stressful when you get started on the protocol. The first time you do something, it's often scary, takes longer, and raises questions.

• Establish contact with local farmers for resources. If you are not aware of which local farmers are best, contact your local Weston A. Price Chapter Leader. Tell them you are on a strict GAPS Protocol and need resources for pastured eggs, meat, organ meats, milk, and Meat Stock bones. Establishing multiple sources will be a great help if you need more yolks or are burning through stock bones. I've found that stocking up on bones, chicken feet, and hooves can be the most valuable thing in terms of prep.

• Prepare detox bath products. Detox baths are a vital part of the GAPS Protocol for pulling toxins out of the skin, the largest organ in the body. Detox baths should be a nightly occurrence, rotating Epsom salts (be sure it reads USP, which means it is fit for human consumption and use on the body), baking soda, mineral salts, apple cider vinegar, and seaweed in the bathtub. The goal, as with most GAPS things, is to start slowly. Use an amount you can tolerate, and build up to a 20-minute bath containing one cup of product. One teaspoon in each bath of either vitamin C powder or bentonite clay can be added to the bath to assist in pulling the chlorine out of the water so your body doesn't absorb it.

• Purchase Lugol's Iodine Solution for iodine painting. Iodine painting is done by painting a 3 by 3-inch square of iodine on the inside of the arms, soft areas of the stomach, and inside the legs. Rotating the painted location every day is best to prevent skin irritation. Most folks paint a picture of a snake, dog, bear, or fish, because they are fun for the child. Whatever works for you is perfect.

For those who need further support that painting doesn't satisfy, Dr. Natasha recommends internal iodine.

Additional support need is determined by the absorption rate of the patch of iodine. If it disappears before the 24-hour mark, Dr. Natasha recommends taking iodine internally, starting slowly with one drop and increasing until the proper dose is achieved.[viii] [ix] Further explanation of iodine and its use is covered in the iodine section.

Bacteria, viruses, parasites, and cancer don't readily live in the presence of iodine. If you paint iodine over an area that unknowingly has any of these things under the skin, they will die. As they die, they release toxic gases which can cause die-off. Some people need to start very slowly: one drop of iodine diluted in a glass of water and painting one drop of the diluted solution. Others can just paint away with no issue. Only your body can tell you what it needs and can tolerate.

†††

There are some things to be aware of during the GAPS protocol that can negatively affect your journey. Watch for these common mistakes.

• Gelatin as a substitute for Meat Stock is not recommended or encouraged. Dr. Natasha says, "I'm not fond of hydrolyzed proteins, gelatins. It's much better to make fresh stock, fresh broth. You'll get plenty. That's where they get it from, it isn't processed."[x] Organic gelatin can be used for a rare treat, but it is not a staple. The perfect example of frequency is for a birthday celebration substitution.

• Cutting up veggies ahead of time and storing them in the fridge is not healthful, as they lose a majority of their nutrition when cut ahead of time. Frozen vegetables are GAPS approved but nowhere near as good as fresh vegetables. Dr. Natasha says that freezing changes the structure of the vegetable, making it less identifiable to the body.[xi] This can easily be seen by freezing a strawberry. After the strawberry has been frozen and then thawed, it is a totally different food than the fresh strawberry. Fresh is always best.

• Read about the sensitivity test, found on page 143 of the GAPS book.

• Digestive enzymes can be used, but are not needed by everyone. Dr. Natasha says they are for "people who belch, burp, who find that their food is not moving out, they just feel they can't digest."[xii] Seeing undigested food in the stool is just a marker showing that the microbiome is not full of good flora to process food, telling you that more time on the protocol is need.

● Often, enemas are used to clear the tract of fecal matter. GAPSters often have issues with the bowels; being prepared is optimal. If you've never done an enema, it is beneficial to watch some *how to* videos on YouTube and obtain supplies. Even if the bowels are moving daily, Dr. Natasha says, "In some situations, it's a good idea, for example, a compacted child, a child who sits on the toilet for a long period of time and says, 'I haven't finished yet.' The stool comes out kind of mushy and soft, it's squeezing between masses. So, despite the fact that the child has been to the toilet, it's still a good idea before bedtime to do an enema and keep doing them until the stools normalize and start coming out formed and looking normal, not squeezed mushy bits."[xiii]

Unfortunately, GAPS is hard, takes a lot of time, and a lot of the cooking needs to be done at each meal. Time savers exist, but preparing real food from scratch takes time. That said, before you start, if you don't own a pair of Big Girl Panties, you may want to find a pair.

The Protocol Review

The GAPS Protocol has an introduction that contains six distinct stages, then Full GAPS, and finally, Coming Off GAPS.

The Stages include:

● A full glass of mineral or filtered water first thing in the morning hydrates the body, specifically the bowel. Some people say that just drinking a quart of water first thing in the morning, before their feet even hit the ground, keeps them regular. Soda water and seltzer water are not optimal and are best after GAPS is completed. Dr. Natasha's favorite mineral water is San Pellegrino.[xiv]

● Canned foods are not optimal while on GAPS. Dr. Natasha was asked for clarification on canned fish. In the yellow book, she says canned sardines are fine and in Frequently Asked Questions it's mentioned that canned is OK if nothing else is obtainable. She says no cans, no canned goods due to the plastic lining. It's a question that comes up frequently with clients and with those on social media. Life is complicated, and folks need to do what is best and fits into their lives, while doing what is tolerated. In a perfect setting of doing GAPS, Dr. Natasha says, "No canned food!"[xv]

• Detox baths are done each day, preferably at night, to pull toxins from the skin, the largest organ of the body. Detox baths use Epsom salts, dead sea salts, baking soda, apple cider vinegar, and seaweed. The goal for the quantity is one cup in a bathtub; however, due to die-off, some must start at one teaspoon in a tub. It is fine to lean heavily on certain products. For example, if you tend toward muscle cramps or weakness, doing Epsom salt baths four nights of the week while rotating other products in the mix is fine. If eczema is an issue, leaning heavier on dead sea salt is helpful. If excessive yeast is an issue, leaning heavier on baking soda is helpful. If muscle cramps and weaknesses are an issue, leaning heavier on Epsom salts is best.

Dr. Natasha was asked, can you explain how to do baths with two kids on GAPS at the same time? Can they be in a detox bath at the same time? I've heard you answer no, they don't absorb each others' toxins and yes, they do - bathe them separately.

Her definitive answer is, "Yes, they can bathe together."[xvi]

Foot baths are easy and beneficial; they are an option in addition to the full dip in the bathtub.

"Our feet are a major detox organ; many toxins leave through the skin on the soles of the feet. Do it as often as [you] can, every time [you] sit still for a while, working, watching TV, etc.," Dr. Natasha says.[xvii]

She also says, "I recommend people do all kinds of foot baths. While they watch TV, because TV is an hour and a half, two hours. Put a tub there with hot water, half a cup of mustard, sea salt, Epsom salt, bicarbonate of soda, cider vinegar, your fermented vegetables, iodine."[xviii]

Things Dr. Natasha recommends adding to the foot bath (in a rotation cycle) are mustard powder, Epsom salt, bicarbonate of soda, apple cider vinegar, fermented vegetable brine, iodine, Bentonite clay, herbal teas, seaweed powder, and the like.[xix xx]

She goes on to say, "There are special electric foot baths on the market and stickers, which may help as well. Also having a tub with semi-precious stones/crystals under (the) desk can help (a mixture of different stones, whatever {you} can get). Keep bare feet on them every time (you) sit at the desk. Walking bare foot in the summer and swimming in lakes, rivers and sea will also help."[xxi]

Stickers that are attached to the bottom of the feet are used for pulling toxins out though the feet. They can be purchased from Purify Your Body, a company from Utah. Some people say you can smell toxins from the pads, after use, which smell like a campfire, proving the pads remove toxic campfire chemicals. This smell, however, comes from the bamboo vinegar in the pads, which off-gasses a campfire smelling aroma.

• Sunbathing is part of the foundation of the GAPS Protocol and should be done daily; it is not optional. Those with darker skin need more time in the sun so that it can penetrate the melanin. Sunscreens contain many toxic chemicals and should be avoided to reduce the body burden. Exposure to the sun, to build up tolerance, is recommended. First, spend ten to fifteen minutes in the sun one day, then increase the time by ten minutes the next day, as tolerated, and then continue to increase sun exposure daily, as tolerated. Sunlight reacts with the cholesterol level just below our skin and is part of the Vitamin D processes in the body. Once the skin properly browns, 30 minutes of sun a day is highly beneficial to Vitamin D processes. In the winter months, when the sun is not as available to some areas, cod liver oils are recommended, specifically Fermented Cod Liver Oil.[xxii]

• Cod liver oil needs are individual to each person. Many people see remarkable success taking both Fermented Cod Liver Oil and Rosita Cod

Liver Oil. Natural flavorings and other potentially pathogen feeding ingredients are to be highly avoided. The flavors of Fermented Cod Liver Oil that are best on GAPS are unflavored, orange, or mint. Many react negatively to cinnamon flavors and other natural flavorings. Most people on the protocol need supplemental marine oils in the very beginning of the protocol, but they are often not needed in the more advanced stages. The use of marine oils is bio-individual. See the section on fish oils in Stage Three for more information. Those who stay on Extended Stage Two and when folks hit Stage Three are when fish oils are introduced.

Dr. Natasha says, "People with mental illness and learning disabilities need both the cod liver oil and the fish oils. Cod liver oil is mostly used for the immune function, the immune system. So, in people whom the immune system is not working well, they are getting colds and flu and infections, I give them two teaspoons in the winter starting from September until about March, April. Then I say start sunbathing, reduce to one teaspoon. In the summer when you're in the full sunbathing season, you can stop. Then, come winter, you start again, particularly for kids."[xxiii]

• A digestive enzyme can be added; however, as soon as the kraut juice is tolerated at the level of roughly a half teaspoon with each meal, it is a desirable choice for a digestive aid. Not everyone needs this assistance but, in some occasions, clients benefit from digestive enzymes. The problem with digestive enzymes is that they contain many added ingredients that feed the problem. A proper digestive enzyme should contain enzymes, which end in -ase such as amylase, protease, lipase, as well as others, and a capsule. No other ingredients would be optimal. Additional ingredients, often listed in the ingredient section called "other ingredients," such as maltodextrin, hypromellose, microcrystalline cellulose, dextrin, citric acid, titanium dioxide, sodium benzoate, mannitol, and ingredients that are not naturally found, are not part of the GAPS Protocol.

A substitute for proper digestive support is putting two to three teaspoons of apple cider vinegar in one cup of water and drinking it 15 minutes or just before you eat. Another solution is drinking freshly juiced cabbage juice right before you eat. Both freshly juiced cabbage juice and apple cider vinegar in water act as your own hydrochloric acid in the stomach which triggers the release of enzymes from the pancreas that digest food.

Dr. Natasha comments on the minimum age that you can give HCL: "Twelve is the earliest. Before then it is best to use cabbage juice. Some parents give it to children younger than that, but I would only recommend that occasionally."[xxiv]

• Probiotics feed the good strains. This can be done in the form of GAPS approved commercial probiotics or food-based probiotics. The amount should be just below die-off levels and gradually increased as the person moves through the protocol. The goal is to be taking many different strains to create balance. It is important to remember: manufacturers are in control of what they put in their products, and they are not always required to list them on the label.

• Watch where your support information is sourced. Some of the best places to receive the most accurate, true to GAPS information are: Dr. Natasha's website GAPS.me, FAQS on GAPS.me, Dr. Natasha speaking at several conferences and radio shows linked on YouTube, and reputable GAPS sites like GAPS.me, GAPSDiet.com, GAPSAustralia.com, NourishingPlot.com, and SimplyBeingWell.com.

• Moving through the stages should be done slowly, if possible. Moving too fast can cause confusion as to intolerances, gas and bloating, or other digestive issues. If these issues appear, it is recommended to go back. Any regression in symptoms is a sign to go back, allow more repair to happen, and then progress forward later. For some, this takes a week; for others it takes months. More about this can be studied in the *Gut and Psychology Syndrome* book.

• Bakes goods, once added, are to be consumed in moderation, between meals. They are not designed to be part of every meal; the basis of a meal should be meats, fish, vegetables, and fermented foods.

• Yeast is often fed by nuts and fruits. If moving through the stages is smooth, but yeast symptoms are present, removing nuts and fruits may be necessary.

• Consuming vegetables that are raw, fermented, or cooked with meats and fish at each meal helps to balance digestive juices.

• It is recommended to eat fruit, on its own, in between meals. Eating fruits with a meal can cause fermentation in the digestive tract, causing gas and bloating, along with other symptoms. Fruits such as avocado (Stage Three) and tomato (Stage Five with spitting out the skins and eating the seeds) can be eaten with the meal, when tolerated.

• When on a budget, organic or organically grown fruits and vegetables are more important than organic meats. Animals have their own detoxification system that can neutralize some of the antibiotics and hormones.

• Canned fish of any kind, including canned sardines, canned clams, or canned salmon are not part of the protocol. In addition, canned vegetables, canned meats or any other canned foods, are not part of the protocol. Fresh food is best. Dr. Natasha says, "Nothing canned please! The plastic in the cans leaches toxins into food."[xxv]

• An abundance of natural animal fats should be part of every meal, especially in the beginning. This includes gelatinous meats which are the dark meat cuts of fowl and the meat within an inch of the bone, next to fatty portions and tendons. Meat farther away from the bone is muscle meat, more fibrous and difficult to digest. Butter, ghee, tallow, lard, lamb fat, duck fat, goose fat, chicken fat, and any other animal fats are all part of the early introduction stages. Other vegetables fats, such as cold pressed olive oil and avocado oil are introduced later in Stage Four. Coconut oil is a Stage One food and has incredible antifungal, antibacterial, and antimicrobial aspects. For this reason, it can cause die-off and should be introduced slowly.

• Meat Stock is the backbone of the GAPS Protocol and should be consumed with every meal. Some people have a difficult time digesting fat in the beginning of the protocol and may only be able to tolerate a small amount until the gallbladder begins to function more. Listening to the body is imperative.

• Fermented foods are a necessary part of the protocol. We start with fermented vegetable brine of any sort, such as kraut juice, dilly carrot juice, probiotic pickle juice, beet kvass, and others, as well as the dairy that is tolerated. Fermented drinks like kombucha can be added from Stage One, if the sugar is digested. As we progress through the stages, fermented vegetables are added, and more probiotic foods are consumed.

• Avoid all processed foods in packages and tins, including all refined carbohydrates and foods that contain preservatives, artificial colorants, chemicals, free flowing agents, added starches, and the like. Processed foods are difficult to digest and are dead foods. They have a deleterious effect on the digestive system.

Stage One consists mostly of Meat Stock meals and, for most people, is designed for one to three days. These stocks can be made with any Stage One approved vegetables, vegetable ferments or dairy ferments that are tolerated, and animal fats. Garlic and onion should be eaten in every soup, in the amount in which they are tolerated. If garlic and onion, or any other sulphur foods, are not tolerated, it is the body telling you what to do. Sulphur foods increase free thiols in the bloodstream which mobilizes mercury. If the detox systems are shut down or if too much is released, negative symptoms appear such as emotional instability, exhaustion and other adverse behaviors.

• Meats on protocol are best sourced from pastured animals or wild caught fish. Processed meats and sausages often have injected preservatives and flavorings that are not beneficial to GAPSters and should be avoided. This means no monosodium glutamate (MSG), meat glues, sodium nitrite, sulphites nitrates, sorbates, and other ingredients that are not real foods in their natural state. Usually, a good butcher can make clean sausages that contain meat and spices – nothing else. Meats close to the bone are considered gelatinous meats and are best for healing. The farther away from the bone the meat is, the more it turns into muscle meat, which is more fibrous, and thus more difficult to digest. Meat closer to the fat or marbled with fat is tastier and easier to digest. For most, when money is tight, sourcing conventional meat still shows healing.

• Organ meats are foundational to the support protocol, due to their intense nutritional profile. There is no other food consistently higher in nutrition – especially vitamin A. Eating organ meats daily, such as liver, heart, kidney, tripe, gizzards, brain, mountain oysters – whatever you can source – is vital to nourishing a GAPSter's system. If a person jumps on the GAPS Intro Diet and is hungry after eating or ravenously hungry all the time, it is usually because more organ meats are needed.

The amount of organ meat eaten weekly is up to the individual and his or her specific needs. "Making sure that your GAPS patient eats some liver on a regular basis will do immeasurably more for his or her nutritional status than the best and the most expensive supplements in the world. An anemic person should eat liver and other organ meats once a week at least. A child needs a small amount: one to two tablespoons of cooked ground liver every other day, which can be mixed with any meat dish, or a full liver meal once a week."[xxvi]

For those in a crisis, where there is chronic anemia, pale and pasty skin, tired and listless behavior, pale lips, pale gums, or pale tissue under the eyelids, liver should be eaten the size of their hand, not the palm, every day, until the needs are not so great.[xxvii]

Stage Two, Stage Three, Stage Four, Stage Five, and Stage Six keep all of the foods from the previous stages and add more foods, in order, according to their digestibility. Full GAPS consists of all meats, approved vegetables (no starches), nuts, seeds, fruits, probiotic foods, probiotic drinks, and herbal teas.

Coming Off GAPS occurs, optimally, after two years of no symptoms on Full GAPS. It is a frequent mistake to move too fast.

Off GAPS happens when the person has had no symptoms on Full GAPS for two years and has no symptoms while Coming Off GAPS.

While progressing to Coming Off GAPS and Off GAPS, it is especially important to watch for symptoms. The body speaks to you through symptoms, signs that something is not tolerated or that the pathogens have been fed. If either occurs it is best to go back a stage.

Iodine

Iodine painting or iodine consumption. Dr. Natasha recommends beginning with painting iodine, and if there is still a need, progressing to internal iodine. She says, "We live in a world full of halogens, so many people need more iodine, and this situation seems to be escalating. It does look like all the problems we are dealing with are getting worse. It was enough to just paint iodine on the skin and supplement seaweed before to help people. Today it is not enough for many, and when we start having large amounts of seaweed we have to be concerned about arsenic, mercury and other toxic metals present in seafood. The amounts of bromide in our environment are growing, and other halogens, too."[xxviii]

When working with iodine on the GAPS Protocol, it is best to work with a knowledgeable iodine practitioner. Worms, viruses, bacteria, and cancers die in the presence of iodine.[xxix][xxx] GAPSters have many resident worms, resident viruses, and resident bacterium that keep the balance of the declined microbiome.[xxxi] On iodine, the death and evacuation of these can cause extreme die-off, which should be handled slowly and appropriately.

Liquid Lugol's Iodine is the perfect balance of potassium iodide and potassium iodine needed by the body. Different cells uptake their own needed form. Dr. Natasha recommends both the liquid form of Lugol's and the tablet form, Iodoral, according to the need.[xxxii]

Painting iodine is done by painting Lugol's 5% on the soft parts of the skin; 2% should be used if the 5% burns the skin. The painted areas include the insides of the arms, the insides of the legs, and the stomach area. As more is needed, more is used. Dr. Natasha says, "Try to test yourself by painting Lugol's Solution, 5% on large parts of your body. If it absorbs in about 12 hours, you are still deficient."[xxxiii] When there is still a deficiency, we begin supplementing iodine internally.

Painted iodine oxidizes and is not always a reliable test.[xxxiv] [xxxv] It is used as a guide – not a hard and fast rule.

If you look at the periodic table of elements, column number 17 is the halides. In the halide family, we find fluoride, chloride, bromide, and astatine. If the food is deficient in iodine, the person is subsequently deficient. The cells still need iodine, so they take up what looks most like iodine – the other halides. Currently, the biggest halide that shows issues in people is bromide, which looks very similar to iodine. Bromide is used in brominated flours and is widely used as a fire retardant. That means, by law, it's in mattresses, couches, carpets, curtains, and many other household and daily use products. When we begin taking iodine, a bromide dump is common.[xxxvi] This is where a knowledgeable practitioner comes into the picture.

When taking iodine internally, it is important to precede internal iodine for two weeks with salt loading (¼ teaspoon twice daily, or ½ teaspoon once daily if loose stools are not encountered) and 200 mcg selenium. After the two weeks, these are continued while taking internal iodine. Taking mineral salt is not to be confused with taking processed salt, a foodish item that is not GAPS compliant. Celtic Grey Salt is most fitting to support the thyroid.[xxxvii] [xxxviii]

If selenium is not included in the protocol, you can give yourself Hashimoto's, a thyroid disease.[xxxix]

If mineral salt is not included in the protocol, you can give yourself Bromism.[xl]

Iodine is versatile and is a great cleansing aid. In cases of high toxicity, it can be used to help clean the bowel. This includes situations such as persistent seizures or highly toxic cases. Dr. Natasha says, "Add salt into enemas and a few drops of iodine Lugol's solution (water based); start from 1 drop per enema and see how high they can go (up to 5 drops)."[xli] Iodine is abrasive to gentle mucous membranes and can burn. For this reason, be sure the iodine is fully incorporated into the enema bag of water at no higher than a 2% solution. If any discomfort or pain occurs, stop immediately; then consider no more than half of the previous solution.

Chelation

Chelation can be used for those who have stubborn situations and when progress is stalled. There are many options for chelating; low dose chelation, as with the Andy Cutler Protocol, is the most favored.

It is often asked, "*Can you do ALA and DMSA while on GAPS?*" Yes, it just needs to be done in a way that is fitting for the protocol. When working with someone who has a high level of heavy metals, who has been on GAPS for a year, and who needs assistance with the metals, Dr. Natasha says, "Please, look into Andrew Cutler protocol for chelation. ALA has to be taken every 3 hours (day and night) on a low dose for a few days (3-7), then have a break for the same number of days. This should be done long term (for 1-2 years).

It is a good idea to add DMSA on a low dose as well taken together with ALA."[1]

The reason we wait a year is that we often see the person's flora get healthy enough that their own body starts chelating as it should. The best chelator is your own healthy gut flora. Starting earlier is not a problem.

DMSA is Dimercaptosuccinic acid and is often called succimer. It chelates lead, iron, mercury, zinc, nickel, arsenic, and cadmium and is FDA approved. It is most commonly known for lead chelation. The *Journal of Medical Toxicology* says, "Lead encephalopathy is a severe manifestation of lead poisoning that can present with altered mental status and seizures."[xlii]

DMSA and EDTA are both mentioned in the GAPS book, using the standards for DMSA and EDTA at the time the book was written, which were both as a high dose IV drip; this is not how it is used today in low dose chelation such as the Andy Cutler protocol. EDTA is not fitting for GAPS, even in low doses.

We always see heavy metals in cases such as autism, FPIES, ME, brain fog, high yeast symptoms, eczema, hives, rashes, and the like, with high, extreme sensitivity and slow progress. The toxicology world says, "It has been associated with illicit moonshine consumption,"[xliii] even though autistic children, and others, aren't known for their moonshine intake. Metals saturate our environment and are found in many places.

The National Institute of Health reports, "Researchers observed higher levels of lead in children with autism throughout development, with the greatest disparity observed during the period following birth," when studying baby teeth of twins where one had autism and the other did not.[xliv]

While doing DMSA on GAPS, small doses are given every three hours. It is finer than ALA, more of a powdered sugar consistency, so it takes a bit more attention when very low doses are tolerated. In cases where higher lead counts show, it's very important to start extremely small with the dose, just touching the DMSA with a needle or toothpick, only just making contact with the powder. Some can touch this powder to the tongue or inside the mouth, so it is absorbed through the mucous membranes. Others prefer to put the toothpick into two drops of Meat Stock and then to put that inside the mouth. Others can start with a specific measure, such as what is divided out into the measuring spoon set of drop, pinch, dab, tad, etc.

After doing DMSA for two weeks, ALA can be added to the regular dosing.

Wherever you start on your dose is where you start. Each person takes what is specifically tolerated by them; too high of a dose will be marked by flaring yeast. Working with a Certified GAPS Practitioner who is knowledgeable in these practices is always advised.

Regarding ALA while on GAPS, Dr. Natasha says, "Yes, your body makes ALA – in small frequent doses, yes."[xlv]

Alpha lipoic acid, ALA, is an antioxidant made by the body when the body is in a healthy state. ALA is different from vitamins A, C, and E in that it has a negative charge, causing it to attract heavy metals to itself; it then escorts them out of the body. This makes it a compelling chelator.

Each person is bio-individual and should be treated as such. Dr. Natasha says, "GAPS program is a journey, some people find that they get better quickly, others need more time and other interventions, such as chelation of heavy metals. Consider GAPS program as a basis for your recovery, a foundation of your health. For many people GAPS is all it takes to get well. For others, after building the foundation, they have to build other structures on top of it to get completely well."[xlvi]

Dr. Natasha says that the detox channels are opened with the GAPS Protocol, which takes time. "I do not recommend any other detox procedures for the first two years of the program, as the GAPS Nutritional Protocol will restore your own detoxification system in the body, so it starts functioning again and removing toxins naturally. However, in some cases the toxic load can be too high and still producing symptoms after two years; in these cases, I recommend natural chelating substances such as HMD™ (Heavy Metal Detox). Seaweed and probiotics are also strong chelators of toxins," she says.[xlvii]

HMD, Heavy Metal Detox, underwent a three-year double-blind placebo-controlled study involving 350 metal foundry workers. It is a natural product that contains the homeopathic remedy Chlorella Homaccord, Cilantro Leaf, and Chlorella Growth Factor. The product is recommended for three months, proceeded by a month-long maintenance round each following year. Adults are recommended to take 45 drops, three times a day. This product can be used while the person has amalgam fillings. It costs over $300 for the recommended protocol. Through discussion with the company, it was determined that they classify it as "a supplement".

As of the end of 2018, Dr. Natasha's preferred choice of chelation is low dose ALA. Using homeopathic remedies, HMD, or Nano-zeolite is not favored, not optimal.[xlviii]

Seaweed intake on GAPS can be done in many ways, including seaweed snacks, sushi wraps with GAPS approved ingredients, and soups. It is not optimal as it is known to relocate metals.

Alpha lipoic acid is another tool in the toolbox and is often chosen by GAPS people due to the small price tag and clinical effectiveness. One bottle of clean ALA (such as NutraBio ALA) is roughly $13.00 and will allow the whole family to chelate each person for their whole lifetime.

It is important to note: R-ALA is not recommended. Added ingredients such as fillers, free flowing agents, and the like, are not recommended.

Scientific World Journal says, "Alpha lipoic acid is a powerful antioxidant that regenerates other antioxidants (e.g., vitamins E and C, and reduced glutathione) and has metal-chelating activity. Both fat and water soluble, it is readily absorbed from the gut and crosses cellular and blood-brain membrane barriers. Clinical experience is that it must be used carefully as it poses particular risks of redistribution of metals."[xlix]

This can happen due to improper dosage or usage.

For folks who have damaged microbiomes, GAPS people, the use of ALA and DMSA needs to be carried out according to what supports the microbiome while chelating. The Cutler Protocol involves any form of over-the-counter ALA, along with any companion nutrients that should be supplemented while chelating, including zinc, magnesium, manganese, B vitamins, chromium, vitamin E, vitamin C, vitamin A, selenium, and sometimes others. While on GAPS, these supplements are acquired through nutrient-dense GAPS protocol foods.[l] Added ingredients are to be observed and avoided with utmost care while on GAPS, due to their potential to feed pathogens in the microbiome.

Still, many GAPSters need to add a good magnesium glycinate supplement. If they are not on at least four ounces of kraut juice a day, due to die-off, vitamin C will also be needed.

Each capsule of ALA from NutraBio is 300 mg; however, when simulating dosage of ALA similar to what the body would make, the amount the person takes is low and frequent. ALA and DMSA are taken the same way, at the same time. They can be taken with food or without food. The person does not need to be awake to take a dose. The dose is simply put somewhere in the mouth where it is absorbed into the mucous membranes. Most GAPS folks with deeper damage to the microbiome start with one speck of ALA, put on the finger and swept through the mouth every three hours. This is continued through the day and through the night for three days. This is considered a round and is repeated every week, three days on, four days off, making note of yeast flares.

Heavy metals are said by some to be encompassed with yeast, where the yeast wraps around the metal like a comforter. This yeast will not leave no matter what you do, because it is protecting the body from the heavy metals;

it is doing its job. For a person in this situation, without chelation, yeast will continue to flare, even after diligent efforts of not feeding the yeast and taking therapeutic probiotics to drown out the pathogens. When the metal is removed, the yeast that surrounded it is freed and free flowing in the body. If too many metals are removed because of too much ALA, releasing too much yeast (which cannot leave through the urine, stool, and other channels fast enough), it'll be trapped, recycling in the body. This is the dangerous redistribution of metals.

Too much yeast in the body, from too high of an ALA dose, causes yeast symptoms which is most commonly seen as off-gassing ethanol, an alcohol. These symptoms resemble a drunken person: laughing, giggling, smiling inappropriately, clinginess, "I love you Mom!!!!!", bumping into walls and doorframes, anger, snappy behavior, excessive dark circles and/or puffiness under the eyes, fits, tantrums, and erratic behavior that makes mom want to hide in her room for a break, as well as other symptoms. If this happens, the amount of ALA is too high and should be reduced until the yeast behavior is gone. If the yeasty behavior isn't seen, the amount of ALA should be increased until the yeast is seen, then reduced to just below the yeast signs. This can also redistribute metals.

It is important to be sure that the bowels are moving daily while chelating because the metals need to exit. If constipation is an issue, there are many GAPS methods described thoroughly in the GAPS book. If the person has amalgam fillings, DMSA and ALA should NOT be used as chelators as they pull the metals from the largest store in the body. Chelation is not recommended for pregnant or nursing women; it is recommended to wait 18 months after amalgam removal to get pregnant.

The amount of ALA can be increased one time during a round. Usually, folks will start at one speck, every three hours, but if there are no yeasty behaviors on day two of the round, they increase the amount. If there are no yeasty behaviors on day two after the round, they increase the amount again when starting the next round.

There is no perfect chelator; instead, they pick up the metals and then drop them according to their carbon half-life. The next dose picks up what was dropped. On day two of the round, all the metals have officially been picked up, freeing up too much yeast. On day two after the round, all of the metals have been dropped, redistributing the yeast. If the yeast symptoms flare on day two of the round or day two after the round, the amount of the chelator is too high.

Clinically, we see folks on GAPS with severe damage settle in on an amount around 5 mg every three hours, while others go a little higher. This is much lower than what many Cutler followers tolerate. If the dose is pushed too high, yeast symptoms abound. Sometimes, the amount of ALA is increased, and increased, and increased, and increased, and the parents can't figure out why the child is breaking everything in the house, not listening, loud, disruptive, difficult to control, restless, and menacing. Again, yeasty behavior is reflective of too much.

The average round looks like this:

Day one: wake up and take the first speck at six in the morning, nine, noon, three, six, nine, midnight, three in the morning, six, etc.

The round consists of all day and all night of day one, all day and all night of day two, and all day of day three with the last dose at midnight. Some folks do ALA on GAPS with their children while they are in school; so the first speck is given when they get off the bus at three on Friday and continued all day Saturday and Saturday night, all day Sunday and Sunday night, and then Monday morning until they catch the bus for school, at which point the dosing is stopped.

Setting your alarm on a cellphone for the three-hour mark is easiest to follow. Often, when people set their three-hour alarm on a microwave or oven timer, it is missed because they are in another area of the house. If a dose is missed, which will happen because humans make mistakes, the dosage can be taken up to the fourth hour, but not past the fourth hour since the metals will officially be dropped. Some people on ALA choose to use this 4-hour rule during the night so that they can get more sleep in one stretch. This is fine, but the dose should never be given over the fourth hour.

If it is past the fourth hour, the round should be stopped and resumed after 4 days have passed.

While taking ALA on GAPS, if nutrient density and proper food nutrition is taken, then the companion nutrients are satisfied through food. This includes at least three (preferably six) pastured egg yolks a day (some see great success with a dozen or more), pastured organ meat every day, lamb at least twice a week, pastured animal fat every day, kraut juice to maximum tolerance every day, and Brazil nuts (2-8 according to FDA findings).[li]

If the amount of kraut juice is microscopic, due to die-off, supplementing with vitamin C is helpful.

If muscle cramps, charlie horses, muscle spasms, weakness in the legs while climbing stairs, ADHD type behaviors, or body odor occur, supplementing with magnesium glycinate or magnesium malate may be needed as they saturate the cells with magnesium. It is important to work with a knowledgeable practitioner while chelating, for many reasons, including stress on the liver and unspeakable dangers of amalgam fillings.

The FDA says, "Dental amalgam contains elemental mercury. It releases low levels of mercury in the form of a vapor that can be inhaled and absorbed by the lungs. High levels of mercury vapor exposure are associated with adverse effects in the brain and the kidneys."[lii]

They go on to say, "Bioaccumulation refers to the build-up or steadily increasing concentration of a chemical in organs or tissues in the body. Mercury from dental amalgam and other sources is bioaccumulative. Studies of healthy subjects with amalgam fillings have shown that mercury from exposure to mercury vapor bioaccumulates in certain tissues of the body including kidneys and brain."[liii]

Poison Control, National Capital Poison Center, at Poison says, "In 2007, the National Center for Health Statistics reported that 111,000 adults said they used chelation therapy, along with 72,000 children under the age of 18. It is highly unlikely that 183,000 US residents required chelation therapy for the limited number of approved indications. Chelation therapy as a treatment for autism is based on the erroneous belief that mercury in childhood vaccines is a cause of autism."[liv]

Their summary is this: "Based on erroneous theories of disease causation, some practitioners advocate chelation therapy for such conditions as cardiovascular disease, autism, and Alzheimer's disease. There is no scientific basis for these expensive treatments, which expose patients to risks without benefit."[lv]

Andy Cutler put his findings in his well-researched book Amalgam Illness. He said, if you're planning on getting pregnant, to wait a minimum of six months if you have been chelating. He says to wait 18 months to get pregnant after having amalgams removed. These numbers are guidelines, not firm numbers, as when the time approaches, the situation should be considered. He said conception during the times when mercury is moving is often the cause for mercury damaged children.

Regarding testing metal levels to determine if you're ready to get pregnant, Cutler said that there is no real, hard-core, solid way of testing. It is simply best to wait. This is not the time for an accident. He stressed the importance of waiting so greatly that he said that if you wanted to get pregnant earlier after amalgam removal, to consider if your spouse would stick around for the support needed to handle a child with autism.

Assisting the body with removing heavy metals can be done with an infrared sauna, high dose buffered vitamin C and Liposomal C every three hours at a minimum, lots of time outside in the sunshine, sweating, and using binders such as Bentonite Clay, Food Grade Diatomaceous Earth, and Activated Charcoal, along with using GAPS foods at whatever stage tolerated (optimally Stage Two). All of these, including the sauna, can be done while on round or between rounds, according to Cutler.

Andy Cutler did not support using EDTA until after all mercury is eliminated with chelation. In addition, he absolutely did not approve of liver cleansing in any way while using chelation, including dandelion root granules. Dr. Natasha does not favor the use of EDTA while on GAPS, even in low doses."[lvi]

Chelation is started three months after the last amalgam is removed at the earliest; six months is better.

It is best to work with a knowledgeable practitioner when using low-dose chelation internally.

Dr. Natasha says, "I would not do it younger than 5."[lvii]

It is important to remember: the protocol is designed for the most damaged microbiomes. It is adjusted and adapted for each person and their situation. Please read Dr. Natasha's article "One Man's Meat is Another Man's Poison."

Food Intolerance, Die-Off, and Moving Through the Stages

Just because a food is classified on that stage, it does not mean that it will be tolerated by you. GAPS is very bio-individual; each person can tolerate foods differently. If foods on a stage are not tolerated, the person has two choices. Choice one is that they can skip the food and move forward. This option is generally reserved for the healthier person, someone who doesn't have great damage in the microbiome. Choice two is that they can stay at that stage, allow more healing to happen, and move forward slowly.

There is often a lot of fogginess on which reactions are a food intolerance and which ones are die-off. Sometimes a person should push through a reaction while other times they should back off, clouding the lines of direction. Dr. Natasha says, "There are two reasons for reacting: damaged 'leaky' gut wall and 'die-off'. Damaged gut wall allows through partially digested foods which cause reactions. If the reaction is very severe and you know which particular food you have reacted to, avoid that food for a few weeks, then try to eat a tiny amount. If you still react, again wait for a few weeks and try again."[lviii]

The backbone of the protocol, Meat Stock and probiotic brines, seals and heals the gut lining, allowing the person to reintroduce the food.

Dr. Natasha says, "As your gut wall starts healing, the food in question will get the chance to be digested properly before absorbing and the reaction will disappear. In order to heal and seal the gut lining, follow the GAPS Introduction Diet. This also applies to phenols and salicylates in food."[lix] Clinically, we see that the folks who rely heavily on animal fats in Meat Stock during this time can introduce these foods faster. The more animal fats they take in, the faster they heal.

Probiotic foods are different.

McBride says, "In the case of probiotic foods, such as yogurt and kefir, most reactions are 'die-off'. It means that the beneficial microbes in the probiotic food are killing the pathogens in your gut; when those pathogens die, they release toxins which cause unpleasant symptoms – a 'die-off reaction'. It is important to control this reaction by introducing probiotic foods gradually starting from small amounts. The introduction process is always individual: some people sail through it, others take a very long time to introduce a few teaspoonfuls of yogurt or kefir."[lx]

Moving from stage to stage, introducing foods, is bio-individual to each person. When there are food intolerances, progressing forward is best done slowly, allowing rebuilding of the foundation. Regarding moving forward,

Dr. Natasha says, "Your food intolerances are your cue (whatever symptoms they bring for you individually). If a new food causes a reaction, then you are not ready for it; go back to the previous stage and give it another 1-2 weeks before trying to move on again."

Many times, when people come to GAPS, they have a mindset of eating breakfast, lunch, and dinner. When the GAPS Protocol starts, the food is readily assimilated. This reduction of inflammation causes many different reactions, for some it's hunger. In cases like this, again, nutrient density is imperative. The most nutrient-dense foods at that time are marrow bones (6 to 10 a day), organ meats (the size of your hand every day), animal fats (a quarter cup a day), pastured yolks (8 to 14 a day) and unlimited meat close to the bone. The frequency of eating isn't not the standard breakfast, lunch or dinner schedule, on GAPS, eating happens at any time. Dr. Natasha says, "You have to eat when you're hungry."[lxi]

If a food is introduced and not tolerated, it does not mean continue. Dr. Natasha says, "If your GAPS child or adult is particularly sensitive to some food, cut it out of the diet for 4-6 weeks and then introduce it slowly, starting with tiny amounts and gradually increasing them. This way you can keep the detox reaction under control."[lxii]

Foods can be tolerated and not tolerated. At the same time, foods can feed pathogens, or feed the body, making it stronger so that it kicks out the pathogens all on its own. Navigating these waters can be confusing. Going slowly is helpful. Dr. Natasha says, "Any sign of regression in a child or an adult with GAPS would indicate that he/she may not be ready. It may be an increase in self-stimulation and worsening of eye contact, sleep disturbances and an increase in anxiety mood alterations and hyperactivity, bed wetting in a potty-trained child, eczema flare-up or worsening allergies."[lxiii]

The general rule of thumb is that if the symptoms follow a probiotic food, it's die-off. Dr. Natasha, however, says, "If new symptoms appear after introducing new food, then you are not ready for that food (your gut lining is not ready). Remove the food, work on healing your gut lining with the diet and probiotics for a few weeks, then try the new food again."[lxiv]

Some foods can cause die-off because they make the body stronger. When the body is stronger, it can kick out the pathogens all on its own. These foods include very nourishing foods such as organ meats or pastured yolks.

GAPS Is Bio-individual

Just because a food is allowed on a stage, it doesn't mean you can tolerate it at that time.

Each person has a different make-up of microbes in his or her intestinal tract. Different pathogenic overgrowth leads to different symptoms and different tolerance of foods. No one, including this book, can tell you how fast to go through the stages, which foods you can tolerate, or how much probiotic is needed. Only your body can tell you this. GAPS, as a protocol, is a general guideline for those who have deeply damaged microbiomes; however, just because a food is on a stage, it does not follow that you, specifically, will tolerate that food.

The people with the deepest damage must move through the stages most slowly. Only the body can tell you what to eat and how fast to progress. What is important is that we don't want to override what the body needs. Some people stay on Stage One for over a year, and then keep moving slowly from there. Others stay on Stage One for a day or two, then stay on Stage Two for over a year, and then progress through the other stages quickly until they hit Full GAPS. Still others do only Full GAPS and never do the Introduction Diet.

We don't want to force the body. Some people are determined to heal and after reading articles or books say to themselves, "It's time for just vegetables," or, "It's time to just do Ketogenic GAPS." This is not the goal of GAPS. The goal is to listen to what the body says it needs and to support it where needed. When you support the body correctly, it can repair itself.

Dr. Natasha says, "Your recovery process is a partnership between you and your body. So, don't try to impose anything on your body without asking it first if it agrees with that. Your body will let you know through feelings: something that is right for you will feel good. If it doesn't feel good deep inside you then don't do it even though it may seem like a good idea. Your mind is affected by many different things and can deceive you, while your body is always right."[lxv]

As people begin the protocol, sometimes the person just feels great and problems disappear one by one, day after day. Sometimes the person goes back and forth, up a stage, down a stage, up a stage, down a stage. This is called the GAPS dance – two steps forward, one step back, one step forward, one step sideways.

Sometimes, illness appears when there was none before. This happens for several reasons, mostly because the body has been working hard to keep up, masking symptoms; then when we reduce the inflammation, the body relaxes and the signs that were masked before are visible.

Sometimes, the person sees no improvement for a very long time. This can happen to anyone but often happens to those with damage so deep in the microbiome that it shuts down the detox pathways. She says, "As the detoxification system is disabled, any amount of die-off is poorly tolerated, as die-off increases toxicity in the body, and there is nobody to handle it."[lxvi]

People in this situation often have great struggles with fermented foods and deeply nourishing foods such as yolks, organ meats, and other building foods. When the pathogenic load is at a very high level, putting good into the system feeds the good, which fights the bad, which dies and releases their toxic gases. These toxic gases cause great pain. Sometimes it's bloating; other times it's gas; other times it's explosive diarrhea. The symptoms vary from person to person.

When even a drop of probiotic brine, such as kraut juice, causes excessive die-off, diluting that drop in a full glass of water, and then taking one drop of that, helps to start with less die-off. Putting the drop of kraut juice in hot soup or warm soup will kill some of the probiotics, making it easier to tolerate. It doesn't really matter which method you use if you start somewhere. Often the person looks at the greatly diluted drop of probiotic food brine, like one drop of kraut juice (then the person takes one drop of that) and thinks *it's nothing, not even worth it, I'm going to stop taking it because I'm not even taking anything.* Taking something, even in microscopic doses, is something. Something is better than nothing. The goal is to feed the good. If all you can tolerate is one drop in a glass of water, and then taking one drop of that, then it's everything to you and should be continued as your starting point.

The greater the damage to the microbiome is, the higher the load of pathogens will be, and the slower a person will need to go.

Dr. Natasha says, "That is why people with these problems have to go so slowly with increasing probiotics or fermented foods. Coconut oil has anti-microbial substances and causes some die-off. Try to modify your GAPS diet according to your personal needs: move through the stages faster or add foods which you feel will be good for you earlier, while avoiding those that are difficult for you to handle at the moment. It may be helpful for you to take digestive enzymes with your meals: stomach acid at the beginning of the meal and pancreatic enzymes at the end."[lxvii]

Sometimes, this is evident when the person cannot tolerate Stage One or Two foods and/or cannot successfully increase, or even tolerate, a drop of fermented foods. Sometimes the pathogenic load is so high that Stage One or Stage Two causes excessive illness and the person must remain on Full GAPS for years prior to trying the Introduction Diet. Only your body can tell you what it needs.

If it is difficult to introduce healing foods and probiotics, Dr. Natasha says, "Feed yourself very well with meats, fats and well-cooked vegetables for 5 days a week and then give yourself one day of rest from food—fast for 24-36 hours. For example, choose Friday as a day of fasting; so, on Thursday skip the evening meal and go to bed early. On Friday do not eat anything at all, just drink plenty of water. On Saturday have a normal breakfast and continue eating normally. Repeat this procedure every week."[lxviii]

When we eat food, our blood goes to our stomach. The attention from the body is on digestion. When we fast, the body can spend its energy on repair, including repairing the detoxification system.

She goes on to say, "By doing short 24-36 hour fasts every week you will slowly step-by-step start re-building your ability to detoxify and to produce energy. The whole process will be enhanced if you do a full coffee enema on Thursday evening or Friday morning: this procedure will unload your liver and reduce the flow of toxicity from your gut into the bloodstream. Please, look for the coffee enema procedure in the FAQs (it is important to empty your bowel fully with water enemas before doing the coffee enema)."[lxix]

Sometimes when people begin the protocol, there are unexpected symptoms such as excessive urination, bed wetting, diarrhea, bad breath, stinky feet that can be smelled when you walk in the room, body odor, foul smelling stool, toxic gases from the mouth, and more. These symptoms reflect the pathogenic overload in the body. The pathogens need to get out somehow.

Often, when someone starts the protocol, the brain fog is intense. Figuring out what to do next is like being trapped in a round room trying to find the corner. This is common. Assisting the detox pathways with things such as moving the bowels, enemas or even coffee enemas, urination, detox baths, hot soups, hot herbal teas, and just keeping on with the protocol is best. It passes. Some say that this is good confirmation that you are in the right place.

Where you start on the protocol, the time spent progressing through stages, and the specific foods eaten are all very bio-individual, specific to each person. Sunbathing for nourishment, detox baths, probiotics, and probiotic foods are all necessary and part of the protocol, in doses specific to each person. Extra perks such as dry brushing, the product used in the detox bath, chiropractic adjustments, acupuncture, essential oil therapy, herbal supplementation, metronome therapy, ABA Therapy, Occupational Therapy, Speech Therapy, and any other therapy support can all be helpful, but can also run a GAPS Mama to exhaustion, Adrenal Fatigue, and an increase in her mental stress.

Dialing down what you're doing, focusing on the food, resting, and time in the sun takes priority.

Digestive aids, if needed, are taken prior to eating by roughly 15 to 30 minutes; then the meal is eaten; then the probiotic (food or commercial) is eaten.

Some come to GAPS with issues against FODMAP foods. Those that are most applicable, especially in the early stages of GAPS, are garlic and onion. Garlic and onion are powerful foods that cause a lot of healing, meaning they can also cause a lot of die-off, causing a slower pace. Dr. Natasha says, "FODMAPS kind of agrees with GAPS in some parts, disagrees in other parts. It's too scientific. That's why the mainstream scientific community has accepted it. I would ferment the garlic. I would ferment the onion, if it's a problem. Chop them up and ferment them for a few days."[lxx] The brine is introduced first, remembering to dilute the brine if necessary.

Full GAPS is highly diverse and is where most folks camp for a long period of time. It is easier to follow as it is less restricted. However, we are seeing more and more damage in folks as of late, causing many people to go much more slowly on intro stages. Some foods are used after digestive issues, like diarrhea and constipation, have passed. This is very bio-individual. How food is treated after harvest can also make it bio-individual. Stevia is the perfect example.

When grown, the stevia plant itself grows to the size of a parsley plant or sage or basil. It'll grow more if you pick it more. It thrives in warmer climates and is delicious, albeit sweet, if you pick a leaf off the plant. Once it is picked, it is dried and then powdered. This is called green stevia. The fresh leaf is sweeter than the dried and powdered leaf. From the powdered state, it can be altered further to make it sweeter, or have other sweet boosters added, such as erythritol or xylitol, which should be avoided while on GAPS. The manufacturing process should not be trusted, as with most foods. The cleanest version of stevia would be the plant, the picked leaf, or anything close to those states.

When asked, *what stage is green stevia?* Dr. Natasha says, "I don't have a lot of experience using stevia, but I would imagine that whole leaf can be used starting from small amounts when diarrhea and other serious digestive problems are gone."[lxxi]

When asked, *is stevia that is made as a tincture OK? What stage?* She says it is "OK when diarrhea and other serious digestive problems are gone."[lxxii]

Chapter 2:
Stage One

Stage One includes:

• All animal meat that is optimally naturally sourced – conventional meats are acceptable, if tolerated. This includes pastured chicken, wild caught fish, pastured pork, grass-fed beef, hunted wild animals, and any other animal, fowl, reptile or fish prepared into Meat Stock.

• All naturally sourced animal fats such as grass-fed tallow, pastured lard, schmaltz, goose fat, duck fat, or any other animal fat. All animal fats can be added to the stock during cooking or after it has been cooked. If animal fats are added to the stock, then boiled for 20 minutes, they will incorporate into the stock. If they are added to the stock after it is cooked, they will float on top.

• Organ meats including liver, heart, tongue, or any other. Organ meats are a primary food on Stage One due to their incredibly high nutrient density.

• All animal joint bones, marrow bones, and bones with a little bit of meat on them, made into Meat Stock. Not every person can tolerate all forms of Meat Stock; the deeper the damage in the microbiome is, the less the person tolerates. Some people must start with just lamb or fish, others with just chicken, and others with only wild game. Some people respond to what the animal was fed. Only your body can tell you what you tolerate. What works for someone else may not work for you.

• Beef marrow bones, or any other animal marrow bones, all of which are cooked in stock and eaten as desired, are part of the foundation for Stage One. Often when people are on Intro, they are ravenously hungry. This is a need for organ meats, marrow bones, and animal fats. Eating seven or eight marrow bones in a ravenously hungry state will satiate the system.

• Raw meat. Dr. Natasha comments that raw meat is a Stage One food saying, "Raw meat digests better than cooked. Many people will not be that adventurous."[lxxiii] The fewer beneficial microbes in the microbiome, the more the person will enjoy raw meat. If choosing this option, only pastured animals should be used.

• Coconut oil is a Stage One food, as tolerated. Some people can add coconut oil by the scoopful; others must go very, very slowly. Coconut oil has great antifungal, antimicrobial, and antibacterial properties. The deeper the damage in the microbiome is, the slower the progression will be.

• MCT oil is Stage One approved and, some say, helpful for constipation.

• Coconut water. Dr. Natasha says, "Coconut water fermented, we can introduce from the beginning, particularly for people who are truly intolerant of dairy. Fermented coconut water, kefir, that's coconut kefir, basically."[lxxiv]

• Pork rinds, boiled in water, or other animal skins cooked the same way, are Stage One foods. Frying these foods in animal fats on the stove would be Stage Six.

• Baking soda is used in enemas but is reserved until later for cooking.[lxxv]

• Mineral water can be used from Stage One forward, if it is clean. Soda water and seltzer water are not best on GAPS and should be saved for when the person is Coming Off GAPS. One of the concerns for these items are the water source. Dr. Natasha says "No, no sodas of any kind, no seltzer, no soda water."[lxxvi] Mineral water can build mineral deficiencies. The best way to build your foundation minerals is with organ meats, the size of your hand, for a few weeks or until the levels are balanced. Some deficiency signs consist of sciatic pain on either side, or both sides, coccyx pain, low back pain, upper back pain between the shoulder blades, muscle pain, bone pain, lines under the eyes, and more.

• Fresh herbs cooked in Meat Stock and strained out or removed.

• Herbal teas

• Local honey can be added to herbal teas or whipped into butter or coconut oil. Having roughly one teaspoon a day is generally safe, but there is no real limit. Dr. Natasha says the beneficial enzymes in local honey are so beneficial that they are good, even if the quantity of honey feeds yeast. When it is mixed with fat it prevents sugar swings and more is tolerated. The quantity of honey is bio-individual. Watching for a yeast flare guides quantity.[lxxvii]

• Apple cider vinegar splashed into Meat Stock prior to cooking[lxxviii]

• Fermented dairy, as tolerated, including homemade whey, homemade yogurt, or sour cream and homemade milk kefir. Fermented dairy is very bio-individual, where some need to wait six weeks with no fermented dairy at all, to allow the body to clear commercial dairy from the system, while others can introduce it right from the start. Dr. Natasha says, "In my experience a large percentage of GAPS people can tolerate well-fermented homemade whey, yogurt or sour cream right from the beginning. However, some cannot."[lxxix]

• When introducing meats, meat close to the bone is introduced first. The farther away from the bone, the more the meat turns into muscle meat, making it more fibrous, which is more difficult to digest. Meats close to the bone are more gelatinous and easier to digest. This means, when you begin Stage One, that you should consume dark meat or meat close to the bone. White meat or muscle meats, which are farther than an inch away from the bone, are more advanced Stage One, as tolerated.

There is a condition called Alpha Gal, resulting from a tick bite. Eating meat in this condition involves great illness, vomiting, diarrhea, nausea, excruciating joint pain, as well as other normal allergy symptoms, including anaphylaxis. Alpha Gal is classified as a meat allergy, Mammalian Meat Allergy. As time goes on, new diseases develop; this is one of them. We know that when someone has Alpha Gal, there is usually some version of stock that is tolerated. For some it's wild caught fish stock; for others it's chicken stock; for others it's only Meat Stock from New Zealand lamb. Starting somewhere, wherever tolerated, and building from there is recommended.

Dr. Natasha says she thinks that the allergic reaction is just die-off. She says, "This borrelia– we probably all have it, in different forms, but it wakes up in people who have a particular toxin accumulating. Probably Glyphosate, probably something else. And it's eating it up. It's multiplying on that toxin, on that agricultural chemical, manmade chemical of some sort."[lxxx]

If Meat Stock is not tolerated due to Alpha Gal, or due to whatever depth of damage situation is present, you can start at Full GAPS and add fish stock or chicken stock into the Full GAPS rhythm, increasing as healing happens.[lxxxi]

Stage One vegetables include almost all vegetables that are not starchy or too fibrous. They should be cooked thoroughly in stock for 20-30 minutes, until soft. These vegetables include:

Artichoke (Globe Artichoke – Jerusalem Artichoke is not, as it is high starch)
Asparagus
Beet tops (Stems removed and added later as digestion heals)
Beets
Bok choy
Broccoli
Brussel sprouts
Carrots
Cauliflower
Chard (Leaves only – The stems are too fibrous and are introduced later.)

Collard leaves (Without the stem, which can be added later as digestion
   heals)
Cucumber (As with summer squashes, cucumbers are started with the
   seeds and skins removed.)
Daikon radish
Fermented vegetables like sauerkraut are added to soups or meat stock
   and cooked for 30 minutes until soft. This kills the probiotic
   properties but leaves behind a whole host of beneficial enzymes
   which aid in building microbiome foundation.
Garlic
Green onions
Kale (Leaves only – Stems are more fibrous and should be added later
   as digestion heals.)
Kohlrabi
Kohlrabi leaves
Leeks
Lettuces (Including all varieties)
Mushrooms
Mustard greens
Patty Pan Squash (A summer squash – Summer squashes should be
   started by peeling the skin and removing the seeds. Once digestion
   continues to get better, young small summer squash seeds and skin
   may be left on the vegetable while still on Stage One)
In the case of winter squash, it's very bio-individual. Some need to wait
   for Full GAPS, while most can introduce winter squashes at Stage
   One. For those that need to wait until Full GAPS, Dr. Natasha
   says, "No squashes with orange pulp, butternut, or any other winter
   squashes, the sweet ones until the Full GAPS Diet. All other not-
   sweet squashes are fine, pumpkin too."[lxxxii]
Peas
Pumpkin (Peeled with the seeds removed)
Radishes
Radish tops
Ramps – a wild harvested onion
Red onions
Rutabaga
Rutabaga leaves
Spinach
Turnips
Turnip greens
Yellow onions
Yellow crookneck squash (A summer squash)
White onions

White Scallop Squash (A summer squash)
Winter squash is bio-individual, for some it's Full GAPS, for others it
    can be added right from the beginning, depending on their
    digestions. Winter squashes include acorn squash, butternut squash,
    spaghetti squash, delicata squash, buttercup squash or kabocha
    squash, sweet dumpling squash, turban squash, carnival squash,
    hubbard squash, etc.
Zucchini (A summer squash)

Different countries have different squashes and vegetables. It would be impossible to list them all. The goal for Stage One is low fiber and low starch. Anything in the summer squash category is Stage One. Winter squash vegetables, including butternut squash, spaghetti squash, acorn squash, buttercup squash and the like, are Stage one for most people, Full GAPS for those highly sensitive, except pumpkin, which is Stage One.

In the beginning of Stage One, more fibrous parts of the vegetable like seeds and skins should be removed or peeled so that the vegetable is easier on the digestive tract. In the later parts of Stage One, "when there is no diarrhea or pain in the abdomen," Dr. Natasha says,[lxxxiii] the skins and soft seeds are left in the soups.

Sometimes, doing GAPS with no plant material is necessary, due to the lack of digestive abilities. Doing **No Plant GAPS**, means the person is eating Meat Stock soups, meats close to the bones, marrow bones, organ meats, yolks when they are tolerated, and animal fats. Garlic and onion are the only vegetables that should be in the regimen when following No Plant GAPS. Vegetables contain more fiber, and if a person has a deeply damaged microbiome, like those with Crohn's, celiac, IBD, IBS, FPIES, more advanced Autism, and the like, they will have a difficult time digesting vegetable matter. When the time comes, adding in vegetables first starts with what is easier to digest and moves to vegetables that are more advanced for digestion.

Dr. Natasha says that the first vegetables introduced after garlic and onion are "Zucchini – it is the gentlest. Pumpkins – pumpkins are great. Not winter squashes yet (if they are very sensitive and waiting for Full GAPS to introduce), because they're too sweet with the orange. But zucchini and pumpkins – that family is wonderful, very gentle. Carrot, cauliflower is great, broccoli is great, without the stalk, florets cooked well. Leek – leek is good, and [more] onion."[lxxxiv]

Slowly and gradually, more vegetables are tolerated. The slowest healing happens in the beginning. Once the foundation is laid, it goes faster.

The general rule of thumb is to avoid high starch and high fiber. Foods on the GAPS protocol should be fresh, eating what is in season.

When vegetables are started, it is best to make them as digestible as possible. This means zucchini needs to be peeled and deseeded. As digestion heals, these things can be added into the stock.

When it comes to nightshades, Dr. Natasha says, "In the first stage, I would remove the nightshades (the peppers and the eggplant and the tomatoes – nightshades). So many people react, they don't realize. I would add it later."[lxxxv]

Remember things like celery, cabbage, the stalks of broccoli, cauliflower, kale, chard, etc., are too fibrous and are introduced at Stage Five, as tolerated.

Herbal teas are also beneficial from Stage One and thereafter. Different herbal teas have different medicinal properties. Peppermint supports digestion. Stinging nettles supports drainage of the lymph. Ginger is a prokinetic and supports digestive function. Chamomile supports the bladder and lower regions. Licorice root supports the adrenals. Rooibos supports glutathione production. Dill seed is known for reducing gas, and turmeric and black pepper reduce inflammation. Chanca Piedra tea supports the body by turning gallstones and kidney stones into sludge. A full breakdown of herbal teas is later in the chapter.

On Stage One, any herbal or root seasoning can be used, such as thyme leaves or ginger, if they are tied up in an unbleached coffee filter, old piece of cotton clothing, or cheese cloth and then removed after cooking – not eaten. They can also be added to the soup but must be strained out prior to consumption.

In these initial stages, seasonings can be added to the stock pot but are difficult on digestion when the microbiome damage is deep. Seasoning on stage one includes mineral salt or apple cider vinegar, with the mother. Other seasonings, such as pepper and fresh herbs, can be added and then strained out prior to consumption. Later in the protocol, they can be eaten.

Mineral salt assists in pulling nutrients out of the bones, marrow, and joint tissues. Roughly three or four pounds of meat and bones calls for one tablespoon of mineral salt and two teaspoons to a tablespoon of apple cider vinegar. Mineral salt is any unprocessed natural salt. Generally, mineral salt has a variation of color in the salt specs. The most common mineral salts, in order of nutrient content are Celtic Grey Salt, also called Celtic Sea Salt, Baja Gold, Redmond's Real Salt, and Himalayan Pink Salt. As reported in Dr. David Brownstein's book *Salt Your Way to Health*, the mineral salt that ranks highest in nutrition is Celtic Grey Salt. Baja Gold salt ranks next to Celtic Sea Salt and is highest in magnesium. The next most nutritional salt is Redmond's Real Salt.[lxxxvi] The least ranking is Himalayan Pink Salt.

Pepper is particularly important in the early stages because it causes the digestive tract to secrete digestive juices. However, pepper is difficult to digest so it is put in the stock while cooking but removed before consuming. It is recommended to take peppercorns and crush them, then put them in the stock pot or tie them up in a cache while it's cooking, and then either strain them out after cooking or take out the cache.

Fresh herbs cooked in the stock are removed from the stock before eating. This means that bay leaves, sprigs of thyme, rosemary, or mint can be cooked in the stock pot and then removed before eating. Ginger falls into the same category and is common in Asian dishes. Be sure to put it into the stock in a large enough piece so that it can be removed before eating.[lxxxvii]

Mineral water is a great way to repopulate the body with essential minerals and hydration. A full glass of mineral water is very much part of the GAPS Protocol and should be the first thing a person drinks in the morning, even before the feet hit the ground – while still in bed. Mineral water is different from seltzer water, club soda, or soda water. Flavored waters often contain natural flavors, quinine, bitters, and other chemicals or additives, which are not a part of the GAPS Protocol.

Dr. Natasha says, "The best water is Perrier and Pellegrino (San Pellegrino). Pellegrino's my favorite. It really improves digestion. Stimulates stomach acid production. Obviously, it's more expensive. It's full of minerals."[lxxxviii]

A more economical way is to make mineral water by just putting a pinch of mineral salt and bicarbonate of soda in water.[lxxxix]

Salt on GAPS should not be processed salt, but instead, should only be mineral salt, which contains variations of color. Again the mineral salts that are most beneficial and test best in people are Celtic Grey Salt, also known as Celtic Sea Salt, Baja Gold Mineral Salt, Redmond's Real Salt, and Himalayan Pink Salt, in that order.[xc] Each person will need a different mineral structure, specific to his or her body – only your body can tell you what you need.

Fermented food brines are introduced as tolerated. For some, this means one teaspoon; for others, it's one drop. For others, it's even more diluted by putting one drop in a tablespoon of water, stirring that up, and taking one drop of that, while others have to go further diluted even in a gallon of water. Fruit kvass is added at Stage Four and does not classify as a fermented food brine here.

Dairy Introduction

The dairy introduction diet is a separate introduction schedule from the food stages. When dairy isn't tolerated, it is important to consider why. Some people have issues with casein, others with lactose, and others with commercial dairy sources. Dairy intolerances can happen for many reasons. Some people have issues with pasteurized dairy; some have issues with certain breeds of cows that are not heritage breeds. GAPS dairy is outside of these classifications.

Eating properly fermented dairy on Stage One is approved, if tolerated. GAPS dairy is best sourced from raw milk or organic milk.

Dairy is part of the GAPS Introduction Diet, introduced from Stage One, as tolerated. Many people have concerns with dairy for many reasons. It is common knowledge that people with autism should avoid casein due to the belief that they function better on gluten-free and casein-free diets. This is addressed thoroughly in the *Gut and Psychology Syndrome* book.

GAPS dairy is made from raw milk, or organic milk if raw is unavailable. GAPS dairy starts with properly fermented dairy and advances to raw milk. Your local Weston A. Price Chapter Leader is the best resource for properly sourcing unadulterated dairy. They can be found by doing a Google search for *Weston A. Price Chapter Leader*. When fermented, the lactose in milk is digested, and the casein is converted to paracasein. Some people, such as those with advanced absence of many beneficial microbes in the microbiome, see great intolerances to even properly fermented dairy. Dr. Natasha says that this should be classified as die-off due to the extreme level of pathogens. In situations like this, going very, very slowly is recommended. This is the reason for the Dairy Introduction Schedule.[xci]

Dr. Natasha says that dairy is to be introduced on Stage One, if tolerated, saying, "The only allergy we look at is anaphylactic."[xcii] There are several hundreds of documented cases where the person walks away from anaphylactic situations with GAPS. For those coming to GAPS after using commercial dairy with a hidden intolerance, it is sometimes necessary to leave GAPS fermented dairy out for four to six weeks to allow the commercial diary debris to leave the system, then GAPS diary can be started. This is very bio-individual regarding what each person tolerates. Generally, when a person is loaded with yeast, so much so that it's coming out in the skin and present in drunken like behaviors, GAPS fermented dairy is added sooner.

For some, dairy puts on weight. In these situations, Dr. Natasha says, "Dairy altogether can put weight on, particularly cream, sour cream, and butter, definitely. I think that's got to do with the person's thyroid function. Dairy is funny. Humans have used it for thousands and thousands of years. There are people who are fine with dairy, absolutely fine, but there are people [for whom] it is not quite so. They may want to just remove it."[xciii]

If starting with one drop of whey shows a lot of die-off, the choice is yours as to your direction. You could leave it out for a few weeks and reintroduce the food, or you could go slowly on the Dairy Introduction Schedule. You could go slowly on the Dairy Introduction Schedule so that it takes you years. You could go through all of the Introduction Diet without dairy and stay at Full GAPS for a couple of years, and then go back to the Introduction Diet for a second round and introduce fermented dairy at the same time. As the parent or director of your own health, you know the situation best and can choose your best plan. A properly qualified Certified GAPS Practitioner can assist you in this process.

The dairy introduction schedule starts with the following:

> Lots of animal fats
> Ghee
> Pastured butter
> Sour cream (for those with constipation), Yogurt (for those who lean towards diarrhea)

Kefir
Hard block raw cheeses
Store-bought, high quality, fermented dairy and raw milk

If a person does the GAPS Introduction Diet, then progresses to Full GAPS, and then decides to go back to Stage One and move through the stages again, they do not have to drop the fermented foods that were tolerated on Full GAPS, such as milk kefir or cheese.

Dr. Natasha says, "If you are doing intro second to third time, then you can keep all your ferments in at the amounts tolerated. But if you are doing it first time, then we need to follow the schedule, which means that cheese is introduced either later on in the intro or on the Full diet."[xciv]

Many people see remarkable success and tolerance starting with whey on their first time through the stages.

General Guidelines for Meat Stock

Meat Stock has been described with several different small variations by Dr. Natasha. In one explanation, she says to use 80 percent meat and a little bit of bone with it.[xcv] She has said to put one inch of water above the meat and has said to fill the pot up with water. There are times where you can only cook the stock for two or three hours and times when you cook it longer; as Dr. Natasha says, "The longer you cook the meat and bones, the more they will 'give out' to the stock and the more nourishing the stock will be."[xcvi]

Meat Stock can be made on the stove top or in a slow cooker. It is recommended to start Meat Stock on the stovetop before trying other methods to see how it is tolerated and to see how it tastes and looks. Dr. Natasha was asked, *In the book when you mention making Meat Stock, you give numbers for cooking in a pot (1 hour for fish, 2 hours for chicken, 3 hours for beef) and also say in a crock pot is fine. What is the equivalent time in hours for low or high temps for crock pot cooking for Meat Stock?* She said, "It depends on the setting. I would say that a good [crock pot] Meat Stock can be made in 6 hours (for chicken, 8 hours for beef). Try to experiment."[xcvii]

Another variation is that bones can be used frozen or thawed.

The important thing to remember is, with deeper damage in a person's microbiome, if you are not seeing success with the pot filled to the top with water, using frozen bones, then tighten it up a bit by using thawed bones and just covering the meat.

Soups should be made at home, as you know exactly which ingredients are in the stock and how it's made. Bouillon cubes and bone broth should not be used for healing and sealing the gut lining. When doing Meat Stock, more stock spaced out throughout the day is better. Any form is possible: a cup of clear broth, soup, or even popsicles.

Once Meat Stock is made, it should not be watered down by adding water to the soup.

Meat Stocks are bio-individual, gearing the ingredients and cook time to each individual person. It is recommended that the person eat their issue, meaning, if there is a joint issue, eating more joints in the stock is recommended. If there is a connective tissue problem, eating more connective tissues in the stock is recommended. If there is a marrow issue, or nutritional deficiencies, putting more marrow bones in the stock is recommended.

Dr. Natasha says, "Fresh herbs can be in Stage One as long as you strain them out afterwards. They're not left in the soup."[xcviii]

These recipes below are laid out as the baseline, described for the Introduction Diet, Stage One.[xcix]

Meat Stock

Meat Stock is vital to healing the damaged gut, sealing the microbiome foundation. Cooking bone broth, instead of Meat Stock, will prolong your healing time if have advanced pathogenic gut damage. Meat Stock can be made in countless different ways.

Meat Stock can be made by putting raw meaty bones in a pot and filling it up to the top with water. It can be made by filling the pot with water one, two, or three inches above the bones. It can be made by putting vegetables in the stock pot or not. It can be made by cooking a bit longer than the one hour for fish, two hours for chicken or three hours for beef size bones. It can be made and quickly frozen. It can be made as clear stock or with loads of meat, fat, and cartilage mixed into the clear stock. Sprigs of rosemary or thyme, as well as other herbs, can be added for the cooking and then removed until Stage Three when herbs and spices are introduced. It can be made on the stove top or in the crock pot overnight. Every person in their kitchen is going to put their spin on their stock, preferred by them. The choice in preparation is yours, respondent to the demands of the body.

Again, Meat Stock should be made according to each individual person's needs. If severe malnutrition is present, adding more organ meats to the stock is beneficial. If the person has issues with his or her own bone marrow, more marrow bones should be added. If the person is deeply, deeply hungry, then more organ meats, meats, and fats can be added. If the person is struggling with nausea from a sluggish gallbladder, then the fat should be skimmed off and introduced in small amounts until tolerated. If the person has an issue with his or her joints, more joints should be added to the pot.

Let's take, for example, the case of a little girl, Genevieve, who was not meeting many growth milestones, especially walking. She began standing and walking almost ten months late. She couldn't hold her weight. She pulled herself up, wobbled tremendously, and fell to the floor. Her mother and father spent tireless hours trying to teach her to walk. She visited a therapist multiple times a week. She learned to sit cross legged on the floor, then take one leg and stretch it forward, and then pull herself, scooting forward. Her leg extended and pulled herself, leg extended and pulled, leg extended and pulled. This was her mode of transport if she wasn't carried. Mom put twelve extra chicken feet in the stock and the child was standing and walking within one day of consuming the stock with more joint tissue. The more chicken feet there were in the stock pot, the easier it was for her to stand and walk.

The important thing that should be consistent with all Meat Stock batches is that the stock should be made from raw bones and meat, and should be cooked for a short period of time.

If you are cooking your Meat Stock and the person is not getting better, it may be time to consider using less water and tighten up the stock as well as cook time.

Chicken Meat Stock

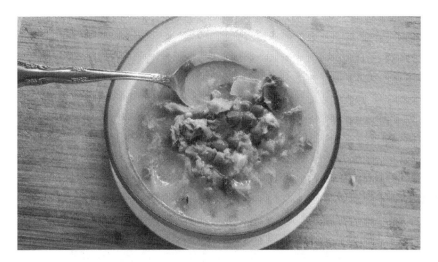

According to Dr. Natasha, chicken Meat Stock is one of the gentlest options for a sensitive system. She says, "Chicken stock is particularly gentle on the stomach and is very good to start with. The gelatinous soft tissues around the bones and the bone marrow provide some of the best healing remedies for the gut lining and the immune system; your patient needs to consume them with every meal."[c]

If the digestive system is greatly damaged, then the client needs the cleanest source of chicken. The best choice is a chicken raised on grass, bugs, and worms as it forages in an open yard. If that option is not available, sourcing an organic chicken that has "access to the outdoors" and has been fed organic feed is the next best option. Organic chickens are usually fed organic grains, even though chickens are omnivore foragers. Using Organic Chicken from Costco is a good option.

It is vital to choose a chicken that has not been given antibiotics because, if you're eating a chicken that has eaten antibiotics, you're eating antibiotics. A label on a chicken that says, "Contains up to 17% of a solution of water, less than 2% solution of..." means that it is injected with water and preservatives so that the chicken weighs more, allowing for more profit by the pound and more shelf stability. The injected solution is often potato starch, maltodextrin (which is usually derived from GMO corn), autolyzed yeast extract, torula yeast, caramelized sugar, citric acid, cream of tartar, expeller pressed canola oil, flavors, food starch, rice flour, sugar, or yeast extract – which all feed pathogens in the gut. Chickens that contain these ingredients should not be used.

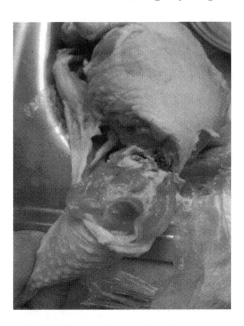

Cutting the chicken up is not vital to healing but assists in adding more nutrients and healing enzymes to the tract. Sometimes, while on GAPS, a mom needs to choose what she does in the kitchen due to time. If this is the case, cutting the chicken is not mandatory for healing; however, it is highly beneficial. Cut the chicken at the joints with a sharp knife or kitchen scissors. This can be done easily by pulling the leg or wing out and breaking it back, exposing the joint.

Do this for each leg and each wing, at each joint; opening the joints allows better accessibility to the vital nutrition contained in the joints and connective tissues. Meat Stock made from chicken is high in the amino acids proline and glycine, biotin, collagen, elastin, glucosamine, and gelatin. These are the elements that feed the enterocytes, the building blocks of the gut lining.

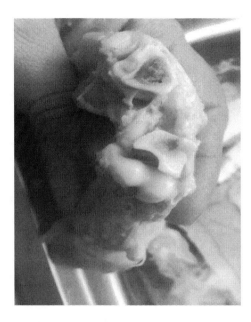

Cutting the bones half-way through the leg opens access to the marrow. Cut the bird down the breastbone and back bone. This step is not vital, but it opens the availability to further nutrition. Place the chicken pieces in a stainless-steel pot, placing them tight around each other like puzzle pieces to fit the pot. If possible, have all of the chicken pieces cover one layer so that the stock is not diluted with too much water. Cover the chicken with filtered water, one finger's width above the meat. If you have chicken feet and/or heads, adding them to the stock will greatly increase the healing nutrients.

For each average-sized, three to four pound chicken, add 1 tablespoon of mineral salt, 2-3 bay leaves, if desired, and crushed peppercorns. Optionally, you may add 2 teaspoons of apple cider vinegar, with the mother, to extract more minerals and aid in digestion. Allow the pot to rest for 20-30 minutes – this is not 100 percent necessary, but it will extract more nutrients from the bones, marrow, skin, and joints and is a very traditional method of making stock. The peppercorns can be put into the stock and strained out at the end or they can be tied up into a brown coffee filter, cheese cloth, or old scrap of cotton. Peppercorns are important to the stock because they cause the digestive tract to secrete digestive juices, which is important for repair. Peppercorns are harder to digest and are a later stage food. Turn the heat on high and bring the liquid to a rolling boil. Just before it boils, scoop off the foam that has risen to the top. Scooping the foam scoobage will give you a noticeably better tasting stock – some say this is the bones cleaning themselves. By the time you finish skimming the pot, it should be at a rolling boil.

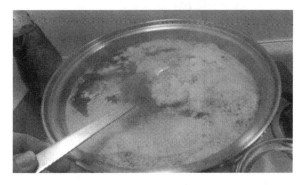

Cover and turn the heat down to a low simmer, with slight bubble activity for 1 1/2 to 2 hours. If you do not cover the pot, the stock will evaporate, and you will lose a great portion of your stock. After cooking, remove the chicken and bay leaves and scoop out the peppercorns. Allow the chicken to cool for a few minutes; then remove the skin and any other connective tissue that is soft, and add the skin back to the stock pot.[ci] With an immersion blender, mix the skin into the stock until fully combined. This aspect will add valuable nutrition to the stock; it will also make the stock taste more like a cream soup. "We need all of the natural fats in natural foods, and saturated and monounsaturated fats need to be the largest part of our fat intake," Dr. Natasha Campbell-McBride says.[cii]

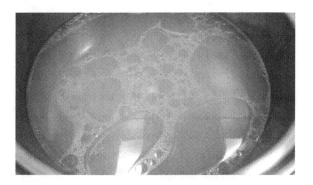

Like all Meat Stocks, chicken stock can be consumed as a clear liquid, with animal fats and meats blended back in, or as a bowl of soup. The choice is yours.

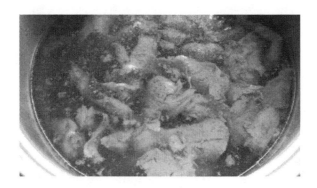

She further says, "Do not take fat out of the stock, it is important for your GAPS patient to consume the fat together with the stock."[ciii]

The only time the fat is taken out of the stock is when the gallbladder is struggling, evidenced with nausea or vomiting after eating animal fats. If this happens, we remove the fats for a few weeks, support the gallbladder with Meat Stocks, ox bile, GAPS Shakes (listed in Stage Two), coffee enemas, and dandelion root granule tea or milk thistle tea. Then we reintroduce animal fats slowly, while continuing to support the gallbladder and increase the fats as the nausea and vomiting guide.

Once the skin is blended back in, you may ladle your hot stock into Mason jars, the size of your choice, and immediately put on the lids. As the jars cool, the lids will pop down, sealing themselves slightly. This type of sealing will not make your stock shelf stable, but will allow it to remain in the refrigerator a bit longer. The length of time your stock is good in the refrigerator depends on the person and the depth of gut damage they have; it's usually a week. The most severe cases need to be consuming the freshest Meat Stock possible, sometimes in the refrigerator for only two days. These people generally say they have problems with histamine foods.

Meat Stock will naturally feed the tract if you are having histamine issues. McBride says it is important to consume many small cups of stock throughout the day, much like you would drink a glass of tea. If histamine issues are a problem, do not reheat the soup for a very long time as it cooks out the healing enzymes that calm the mast cells that cause the histamine issue.

The process I use to freeze Meat Stock is as follows. I take it off the burner and allow it to cool to warm or room temperature in the pot. Then I transfer it to a freezer-safe container and place it in the freezer. A common container used is a gallon zip-top freezer bag. This is OK, as BPAs have been reported to leach only when exposed to acidic conditions or heat.

You can also store it in freezer-safe Mason jars, filled as directed or 3/4 full. This leaves some room for the liquid to expand when freezing. They can still break, so investigate your options.

Once you have your stock in jars it is easy to pull a jar out of the refrigerator, add your desired meat and vegetables, boil for 20 to 30 minutes, and then consume.

Remove the meat from the carcass while the carcass is still warm. Some people add all the chicken meat back into the stock pot for chicken soup; others save half of it and use it for other dishes so the soup is not so meat heavy. Some people make stock out of just necks and backs so that there is less meat.

Any combination of Stage One vegetables can be used. For this recipe, we used chopped carrots, onion, garlic, and peas. Cook for 20-35 minutes, until the vegetables are soft. Add in the chicken meat and enjoy! Chicken stock is often used as a soup base. The possibilities for soup options are endless.

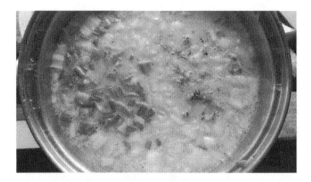

The soup recipe above is made with a quart and a half of Chicken Stock, two diced organic onions, two diced organic carrots, three chopped green onions, two shredded zucchinis, and three cloves of chopped, organic garlic.

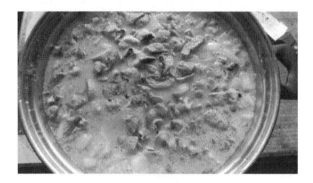

The soup above is made with one and half quarts of chicken stock, one diced organic onion, two cups of chopped mushrooms, one chopped carrot, and one cup of peas.

Beef Meat Stock

To make Meat Stock, use a mixture of raw meaty bones. Three types are best: meaty bones, bones with marrow in them, and joint bones. If hoof bones are available, they are extremely nourishing and beneficial to the protocol. Meat on the bone next to a joint will create a gelatinous stock; meat close to the bone does the same. If the stock does not gel, it's no problem. Different cuts and different animals bring different nutrients and a different outcome in the stock. Ox tail is a favorite addition to stock. Hoof bones and connective tissues (joint bones) will give you good sticky stock.

Meaty beef bones. This is an example of a minimum amount of meat.

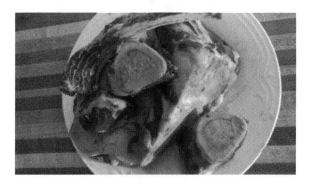

Meaty bones are the foundation of Meat Stock. Shank bones are perfect. The meat closer to the bone is easy to digest. These are considered gelatinous cuts. The farther the meat is away from the bone, the more it is considered muscle meat, not gelatinous meat. Muscle meat is more fibrous and more difficult to digest for those with the most damaged guts. Optimally, keep the meat on the bone no farther than about an inch from the bone. A solid, three-week freeze and thorough cooking will prevent any potential virus or parasite from surviving.

Put all the bones in a large stock pot; fill with filtered water no more than one inch above the bones – one finger width is optimal; add salt and mashed peppercorns. Peppercorns can be cooked in a cache so that they can be removed after cooking. The salt will pull vital nutrients out of the bones.

You can also add apple cider vinegar, with the mother, to help pull nutrients from the bones if you are working through Intro for a second or third time, or if you are on Extended Stage Two. Most people can do it from the start, Stage One, first time through. The amount of spices used is individual to each person; generally, with three to four pounds of bones, use one tablespoon mineral salt, a tablespoon of crushed peppercorns, and a tablespoon of apple cider vinegar. Five to six bay leaves and fresh sprigs of herbs can be added; however, they should be removed after cooking as they are too fibrous for Stage One.

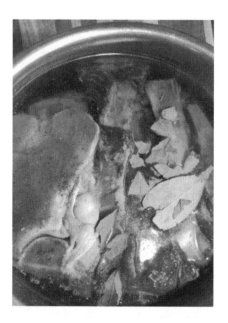

Bring the pot to a boil. Just before it is at a full boil, a foamy film, scoobage, will begin to form on top. This is the bones cleaning themselves. With a slotted spoon, scoop off the scoobage. By the time you're done scooping scoobage, it's at a full rolling boil. Turn the heat down to a low simmer, cover with a lid, and cook for 3 hours.

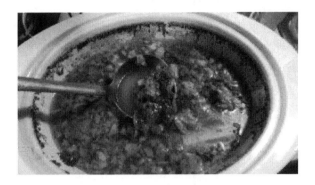

Cook time is particularly important. The longer the stock simmers, the more you cook out the two essential amino acids vital to sealing and healing the gut lining. More specifically, the longer you cook the meat bones, the more you cook out the most beneficial aspects of healing from the stock. If you cook it for too long in the pot, these beneficial healers are absent. Meat Stock is high in amino acids proline and glycine, biotin, collagen, elastin, glucosamine, and gelatin. These are the elements that feed the enterocytes, the building blocks of the gut lining. Cooking the stock for too long cooks out these amino acids, prolonging the healing process.

When the stock is done cooking, remove the bones and pick off all of the meat and connective tissues you can remove. If the connective tissue dissolves in your hands, it's perfect to add back into the soup; however, if the connective tissue is hard, it can be added to another pot to cook further with new raw bones. Remove the peppercorns and herbs from the stock; add the connective tissue back into the pot and blend it with a stick blender.

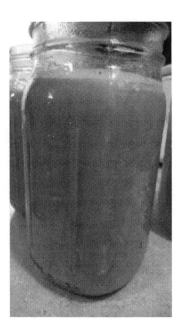

Pour the stock into Mason jars and refrigerate up to seven days. Meat Stock freezes well, but not in Mason jars.

Add whatever Stage One vegetables are desired and cook the vegetables for roughly 30 minutes, until soft, so that the remaining fiber is digestible. Garlic and onion should be added to every soup. If die-off from garlic or onion is too strong, they should be removed until more healing has happened, and then introduced in small quantities. Some people have such great sensitivities that they start with fermented garlic and onion, introducing the brine one drop at a time. When tolerated, adding garlic and onion the size of an eyelash and increasing the amount from there reintroduces the vegetables.

Bone Broth is cooked for longer periods of time; GAPS healing Meat Stock is cooked for a short period of time. The bones used for cooking Meat Stock can be used later for making Bone Broth.

For people with extreme gut damage, sensitivities arise with different stock choices. This histamine issue is difficult. Many see success with choosing wild game for stock, preferably fowl, as these are the most digestible. Wild caught fish is often well tolerated. Chicken stock is known for being gentle and tolerated by most. Lamb stock from pastured lamb is generally well tolerated, even by those with the most severe sensitivities.

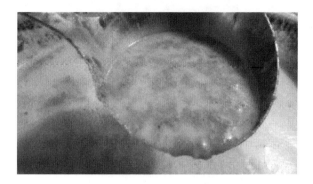

Processed meats often have additives or feed that is not tolerated in very damaged guts. Animals that ate soy often cause issues for people with a very damaged gut. Eating wild turkey and other birds removes this concern. Some farmers plant cornfields to attract deer for hunting season. Corn-fed deer often cause issues for those with deeper damage in the microbiome.

Fish Stock

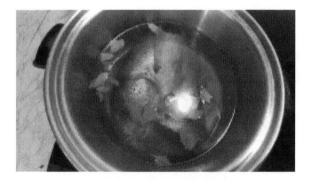

Fish stock is very gentle on the gut lining and is one of the most beneficial for damaged guts. Use fish heads, bones with some meat on them, tails and fins. Put all the fish parts in a pot.

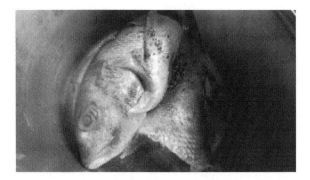

For three pounds of fish, add one tablespoon of mineral salt and crushed peppercorns. Bay leaves and other sprigs of herbs can be added for flavor. These items need to be added to a cache or removed before eating the stock.

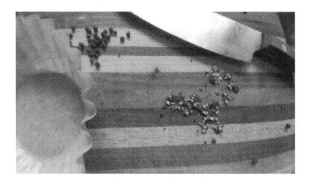

Cover the fish with filtered water until the fish is just covered.

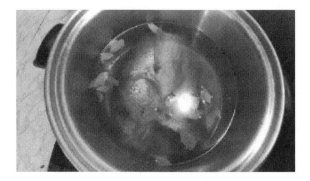

Bring the pot to a boil. As it begins to boil, a layer of foam will develop on top of the water; this is the bones cleaning themselves.

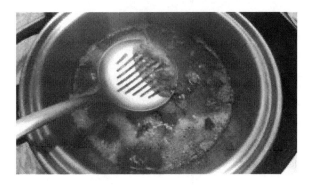

With a slotted or holey spoon, scoop off the foam and discard. Once the pot is at a full boil, and all the foam is removed, turn it down to a low simmer. Put the lid on the pot and cook for 30 minutes for small fish, or 1 hour for larger fish.

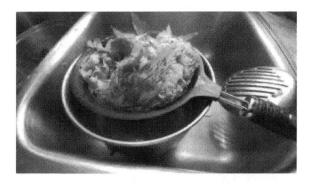

Strain out all of the bones, fins, fresh sprigs of herbs, and peppercorns. Making Fish Stock with oily fish will smell up the house; still, it's tasty! If the house does smell from cooking fish, diffusing lemon essential oil removes the smell and freshens the house wonderfully.

Any Stage One vegetable can be added to fish stock, as tolerated. This one contains three chopped onions, four cloves of chopped garlic, four chopped carrots, one cup of peas, four big leaves of chopped collards, and one cup of broccoli.

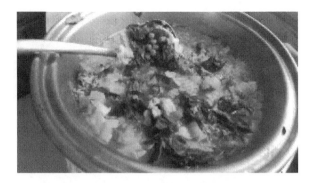

Fish stock is delicious. It's generally easier to digest and provides wonderful nutrients. It's a family favorite. Adding a cup of pastured butter to the pot while it's boiling always makes delicious Meat Stock.

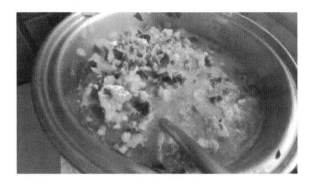

General Soup Making

Do not reheat cups of stock with the microwave as it is very damaging to the stock, killing the beneficial life-giving enzymes and nutrients that are needed for healing.

For Stage One and Stage Two of GAPS it is important to be drinking Meat Stock throughout the day continually.

Dr. Natasha says, "You can make jellies, which is set like a jelly in the fridge, soups – soup is not optional. Soup is the best food for children."[civ]

A good plan is to eat a soup for each meal and enjoy a cup of stock between meals. Add good quality, pastured animal fats to each cup.

An adult should eat a minimum of five cups of Meat Stock a day. A child should consume a minimum of three cups a day. For those in a crisis, one cup every hour is beneficial.

Any recipe can be made from these ingredients; you don't necessarily need a recipe card. Many people make Meat Stock without any vegetables and store it in Mason jars; then, when it's time to cook, they take out a quart Mason jar, add whatever approved vegetables they desire, along with fats, and bring it to a simmer until the vegetables are soft.

If you have a hankering for any vegetable, the body may need something from that vegetable, and it should be used. It is common for Mom to cook a meal, feel led to cook it with one specific vegetable and, be over the moon with how good it tastes; meanwhile the other people eating it just think it's good food, not something to swoon over – this could be due to the needs of a specific person at the time.

Most soups are divine when pastured animal fats are added. Some people add duck fat, goose fat, tallow, lard, schmaltz (chicken fat), ghee, or butter by the serving spoonful to each Dutch Oven pot. Butter, as with all animal fats, should be pastured. Optimally, cultured butter from a farmer who has cows on pasture is used; next best is butter from a farmer with pastured cows. Most people do not have access to this product. The next best thing is store-bought, cultured butter, such as Organic Pastures, and then pastured butter, such as Organic Pastures or Kerrygold. These two products are different in color and taste. Most people prefer the taste of Kerrygold; others say is it's not worth buying because 10% of the winter feed is potentially genetically modified. Sourcing what you can is best. Adding a cup of grass-fed butter to each Dutch Oven sized soup pot is so tasty, it always brings raving compliments.

Many people heal on GAPS while using conventionally raised meats and animal products. Others have to be stricter with their food sourcing. Only your body can tell you what it needs.

Cooking Meat Stock with too much water makes it too diluted. Just like you don't dilute glue, you don't dilute Meat Stock. A general rule of thumb is that three pounds of chicken has about two quarts of water in the pot. GAPS Chef Monica Corrado says, "That's why Meat Stock gels."[cv]

It's generally safe to put an inch or two of water over the meat in the pot for the Meat Stock not to be diluted. Dr. Natasha says, "maybe the same volume of water as the chicken would take – half and half."[cvi]

When discussing making stock in her GAPS book, Dr. Natasha says that the longer you cook the bones, the more nutrition you extract.[cvii] However, cooking the bones too long cooks out the three enzymes that seal the gut.

Dr. Natasha says, "Sometimes I leave it for longer, depending on what kind of meat it is, what kind of bone it is. But you want the meat not overcooked, so you can eat it, so it's nice and tasty. You want to cook it until it's nice and tender and soft, not washed out."[cviii] She allows her beef, pork, or lamb stock to cook up to six hours. For chicken, she allows it to go no more than three hours. The length of time you cook it depends on the source of the bones.

Corrado says, "Usually when you have a good chicken, it's an hour and a half."[cix] Dr. Natasha says, "If it's from the shop, but if it's a cockerel from my farm, that takes three hours. It's strong, gamey."[cx]

Meat Stock and Bone Broth Questions

The Meat Stock *vs* Bone Broth debacle is probably the most misunderstood and confused aspect for foodies today. They are both delicious and nourishing, each to be used at different points of need.

Isn't cooking Meat Stock longer better for you?

Meat Stock is cooked for a short amount of time, keeping essential elements for healing intact, whereas Bone Broth is cooked for a long time, often days. There is a lot of confusion around the difference between Meat Stock and Bone Broth. Meat Stock is for those with Intestinal Permeability, also known as Leaky Gut. Gut damage is evident through illness. Bone Broth is food, used for health maintenance. As previously stated, the three amino acids which heal and seal the microbiome are cooked out over longer periods of time. This is proven clinically with those whose digestive tracts are not working.

What do I do if I get a histamine response?

If you are experiencing histamine responses, it is a sign that you have greater intestinal imbalance in your microflora. This is good news as there is a specific protocol laid out in the GAPS book for healing this issue. Those with histamine issues are the easiest to heal because their bodies speak to them throughout the healing process, telling them what to do and what not to do. However, it often takes longer for healing to occur, especially with age.

Most histamine responses come from bones and meats that are from animals fed GMO feed, have injected preservatives or flavorings, or have been sprayed with bleach for sanitation. If you experience this situation, source cleaner animals. The easiest way to do this is contact friends who are hunters and ask them for the bones from their kill. The best option in this case is to bake cookies for the man in your area who processes deer and other in-season animals. He is most likely throwing the valuable bones away and will gladly give them to you for free.

If you feel a cold coming on, should you do Meat Stock or Bone Broth?

Meat Stock– however, we have found that it's even easier to thwart a cold by drinking kraut juice until it's gone.

Why isn't my stock sticky?

Sticky stock is best achieved through connective tissues like hooves, chicken feet, or ox tail. If you can choose bones that include a joint in the package, this makes good sticky stock; but hooves are optimal. Sticky stock stays with you, is more satisfying, and heals a leaky gut faster.

Why isn't my stock gelatinous?

Gelatin is only the result of the gelatinous tissues and joints dissolving into the stock. That has nothing to do with ACV. ACV works on the BONES to leach minerals from the bones into the stock.

If people are having trouble achieving gelatin, it is because of one or a combination of the following possible reasons:

1. too much water to meaty bones ratio (1 quart of water to 1 pound of meaty bones, or a bit more water)
2. not enough joints or connective tissue (too much meat or too many bones)
3. boiled it—cooked too high
4. cooked too low

Isn't Bone Broth healing?

Meat Stock is for healing gut issues evidenced through illnesses – from allergies to autoimmune disease. Meat Stock is for healing illness; Bone

Broth is for health maintenance. Meat Stock is what is recommended in the GAPS nutritional healing protocol.

Can I reheat my Meat Stock after the initial cooking?

Yes. Be sure to heat it on the stove top, not in the microwave. Microwave cooking kills the nutrients essential to healing. The easiest way to do Meat Stock is to prepare the stock and pour it into quart Mason jars while it's still hot. Wipe the lips with a clean towel and immediately put on the lid fingertip tight. Allow the jars to cool a bit further while they are on the countertop; refrigerate. Then, 30 minutes before it's time to eat, take out a quart jar, pour the contents in a pot, and add a chopped onion, a few chopped carrots, some grass-fed ground meat, and some peas. Cook it for roughly 25 minutes with a low boil; five minutes before it's ready, add chopped garlic. Pour soup into individual bowls; add one to two pastured yolks into each bowl of soup if you are on Stage Two and it's tolerated.

How long does Meat Stock last?

It is best to use Meat Stock within the first week of preparation. It freezes well.

Is it OK to heat up rice noodles in Meat Stock for my child with ASD (Autistic Spectrum Disorder)?

It's not beneficial for children with ASD to be eating rice noodles as the starches in rice noodles feed the pathogens in the gut. Rice, corn, wheat, grains, arrowroot powder, baking powder, garbanzo bean flour, tapioca flour, soy flour, corn starch, tapioca starch, and all starches or complex sugars feed bad bacteria in the gut. Starches are not part of the GAPS Protocol. As explained thoroughly in the GAPS book, children with autism are addicted to starches and sugars—they are feeding the pathogens.

Foods that feed pathogens cause no stomach or gut pain as the pathogen pleasure overrides the inflammation. Veggie noodles can be done with a slicer or a mandolin. After you have been eating clean, non-pathogen feeding foods for a few months, if you happen to eat something that feeds pathogens, you will feel it in your stomach or gut immediately. This happens because the masking response is gone.

Why am I not getting better on my stock?

Sometimes, it's because the stock is being improperly made. Other times, it is because the person isn't tolerating the animal used to make the Meat Stock. Other times, it just takes time. Other times, certain people need a very specifically laid out protocol of healing. A list of Certified GAPS practitioners is available on GAPS.me. Phone or Skype consultations are often available.

Why doesn't my stock taste good?

Properly made stock is so rich and yummy that even the pickiest eaters love it. That being said, my son hated stock for years. Then I found out I was making it wrong, changed my ways, and ever since he begs for stock. Even his *normal food eating friends* love it and often say things like, "You guys eat the BEST food!" Yes, I'm referring to public schooled, teenage boys who eat the traditional American diet and are also picky eaters.

Creamed Carrot Soup

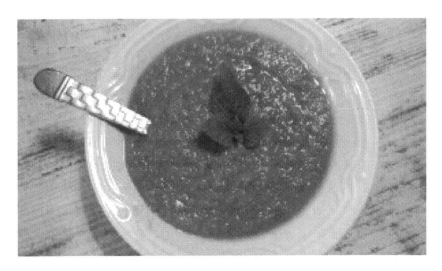

Creamed Carrot Soup is an amazing way to up your carotenoid intake, allowing your detox pathways to open and flush toxins. Any vegetable high in betacarotene is a carotenoid food. When the betacarotene is ingested, it goes to the liver where it is converted to vitamin A. All disease is a vitamin A deficiency. If the person has deeper damage, this conversion is often not being made, so the betacarotene is left floating around in the body. It has to get out somehow, so it exits through the skin, giving the skin an orange appearance. If this is the case, the way to open this pathway is to keep eating betacarotene filled foods and the conversion will eventually be made.

    3 pounds organic chopped carrots
    3 quarts properly prepared Meat Stock
    2 medium organic onions finely chopped
    2 pounds grass fed butter (as tolerated)
    9 cloves organic garlic finely chopped

Put all ingredients, except garlic, into a stock pot, and cook on medium-high for 30 minutes, or until carrots are soft. Add the garlic. Mix with a hand blender or other blending appliance until desired smoothness is achieved. Enjoy.

Turkey Chowder

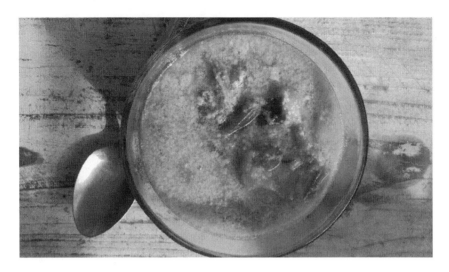

Turkey Chowder is a fine way to use leftover turkey. This is one of those dishes you may never want to stop eating. Enjoy!

This recipe is best made with stock from the turkey but can also be used with Meat Stock from beef bones; both are good.

> 2 quarts Meat Stock
> 3 tablespoons coconut oil
> 1/2 cup grass fed butter
> 11 green organic onion shoots, chopped into bite sizes
> 2 1/2 cups organic turkey
> 1 to 2 organic carrots, finely chopped
> 1 handful organic cauliflower
> 9 cloves garlic

Combine all ingredients into a stock pot, except garlic, and cook on medium-low. Cook for 25-30 minutes, until vegetables are soft. Add chopped garlic for the last 5 minutes of cooking. Remove from heat and enjoy.

Meatballs

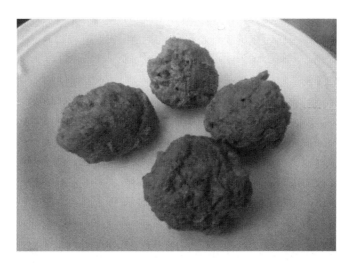

Meatballs are fun for kids and easy to make ahead of time and freeze, or to make during a time crunch. Most everyone loves meatballs, and they can be highly nutritious. If the batch is doubled, more can be made to store in the freezer for future use. Storing precooked food in the freezer reduces the nutritional value. If you have a storage container that will store the raw meatballs, this is best. Sometimes, when storing meatballs in things like a plastic zip top bag, the raw meat becomes one big blob. Those who do not have deeper damage can cook them in stock, store them in the freezer, and put them in future stock meals.

> 1/2 gallon of Meat Stock (adjust the amount as needed)
> 3 pounds of ground meat—beef, pork, venison—optionally some organ
>   meats
> 4 onions, chopped small
> A few pounds of additional Stage One tolerated vegetables, chunked
>   (optional)
> 5 large garlic cloves, finely chopped
> Salt to taste

Put the Meat Stock into a large pot over medium heat.

In a large bowl, mix together three pounds of whatever meats are available. Ground pork, ground venison, and ground pastured beef make excellent meat balls. Any ground meat can be used.

Add to the meat the chopped onions, garlic cloves, and salt to taste. For those who do not like organ meats, the organ meats can be hidden in meatballs in whatever amount tolerated, making super meat.

Roll the meat mixture into 2 inch balls.

Toss the meat balls and the tolerated Stage One chunked vegetables into the stock. Cook the meatballs and vegetables in the stock for roughly 25-30 minutes. Split a meatball and poke the veggies with a fork to see if they're cooked the way you like.

Meatballs can be made countless ways. Just ground meat rolled into balls is delicious. It doesn't have to be hard. The easiest way to make meatballs is to take a pack of firmly packed ground beef, scoop off teaspoons full, and throw the pieces in the stock pot. They don't even have to be shaped; instead, kids can find their own shapes out of them – flying carpets, triangles, stars, sleds.

Meat close to the bone, optimally within an inch of the bone, is gelatinous meat, which is easy to digest. This means the dark meat if you are using chicken or any other fowl. If using beef or any other meat, the meat within an inch of the bone is easiest to digest. The farther from the bone we get, the more it turns into muscle meat, which is more fibrous and more difficult to digest. When using ground meat, there is no telling where the meat has been sourced on the animal. Most people, even those with deep intestinal damage, tolerate ground meats at Stage One.

Beet Gel-o

By Autumn Serodino

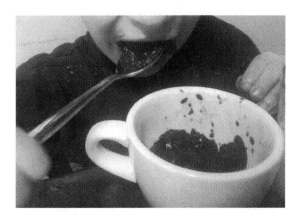

Step 1: Make some beef stock using femur marrow bones, but omit the salt. Do not exceed 1 inch of water above the bones, in order to make the stock as gelatinous as possible.

Step 2: Strain and use this unsalted beef stock to cook red or orange beets. The stock should only just cover the beets. Simmer them until just tender – approximately 25 minutes. Strain as soon as the beets are tender, and save them for other soups and meals.

Step 3: Pour the beet flavored beef stock into a baking pan or gelatin molds. Depending on the mold, the gelatin will be ready in 8-24 hours. Serve cold.

This may also be frozen into popsicle molds.

Carrots simmered for approximately 20 minutes and butternut, kabocha, or acorn squash simmered for approximately 15 minutes can also turn unsalted beef stock into a sweet and nourishing Full GAPS treat, since winter squashes are Full GAPS foods.

Ginger, chamomile, or mint, steeped for 5 minutes with a tea infuser into the beef stock, are nice additions as well.

Cauliflower Cream Soup

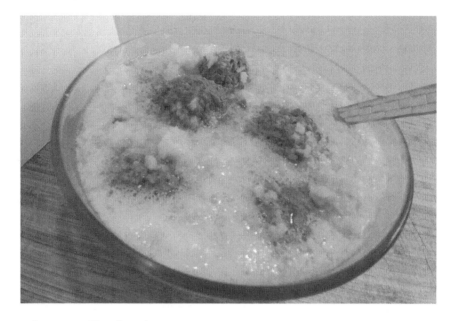

2 quarts of beef stock
2 heads of organic cauliflower florets
3 organic chopped onions
4 organic cloves of diced garlic
2 pounds of grass-fed ground beef

Put all of the ingredients into a pot; bring to a boil for 25 minutes. The cauliflower can be mashed or run through a food processor to be more of a gravy over the ground beef.

Grass-Fed Beef That Isn't Grass-Fed

"Grass-finished beef is different than grass fed beef," farmer Dudley Tapp said [cxi], showing that some farmers illegally use the term grass-fed to encompass any portion of the cattle's life feeding on grass, while saying grass-finished describes a different category.

This occurs even though, according to the USDA, grass-fed means grass-fed for the duration of the animal's life. Dudley Tapp is considered a sustainable, diversified farmer; yet, when he said that there is a difference between grass-finished and grass-fed beef, he's leading consumers astray.

"Every farm that markets this stuff has a different definition," Tapp says.[cxii]

This is where the problem lies for consumers.

"We're doing the grass-fed beef. We've experimented recently with grass-finished beef. It's different than grass-fed." Tapp reserves certain cows for milking while others are used for beef. When a cow is removed from the milking line and put on grass, she is placed there for at least 90 days. "Then we'll take her to the butcher for harvest."[cxiii]

This means that the cow is fed grain while being used as a milk cow, but if she proves not to produce adequate milk, she is moved to grass with no grain 90 days before the harvest date and is considered grass-fed, according to Tapp.[cxiv]

Dudley says that "grass-finished" is a different process altogether. In this situation, he leaves the calf with its mother for ten months, then weans the calf and puts it with the dairy herd on grass for the next 18 months. "We take them to butcher at 28 months and they are fat, similar to what you would see in a feed lot."[cxv]

He says that the major difference for these "grass-finished" beef cows is, "They've never had a bite of grain in their life."[cxvi]

According to the USDA, this is illegal labeling.

The USDA ruled in 2007, "Grass and/or forage shall be the feed source consumed for the lifetime of the ruminant animal, with the exception of milk consumed prior to weaning. The diet shall be derived solely from forage and animals cannot be fed grain or grain by-products and must have continuous access to pasture during the growing season."[cxvii cxviii]

This means that the term grass-fed means just that: the ruminant animal has only been fed grass or forage. That is the law.

Beef Magazine reported, "Researchers in Texas A&M University's Department of Animal Science have published the only two research studies that actually compared the effects of ground beef from grass-fed cattle and traditional, grain-fed cattle on risk factors for cardiovascular disease and type II diabetes in men."[cxix] They found no difference; yet, any parent with a deeply sensitive child who eats grain-fed beef will tell a different story.

This is why it is so vital that when a farmer states his meat is grass-fed, it must indeed be grass-fed, not grass-fed for a portion of the animal's life.

It is no secret that beef raised in America does not always follow these USDA guidelines.

The Chipotle restaurant chain has been recently making the switch to grass-fed beef. Founder, chairman, and co-CEO Steve Ells said, "The restaurant chain doesn't want beef that's been shot up full of hormones and antibiotics; instead it's looking for true grass-fed beef that are free from those foreign substances, and Australia is a leader in that field."[cxx cxxi]

Ells reported, "The cattle spend their entire lives grazing on pastures or rangelands, eating only grass or forages."[cxxii] Since the demand is growing, the supply should hopefully catch up with the need.

When purchasing grass-fed beef from a store, if it displays the term AGA Certified, this means they have been inspected by the American Grass-fed Association, proving "animals are fed only grass and forage from weaning until harvest."[cxxiii] Unlike the certified Organic status, the fees for AGA Certified status are minimal at $250 a year for membership dues, and then $1 a head. Following this status is more of a promise than a regularly inspected stipulation since there are no rules for farmers to maintain this feeding regimen. If a complaint is made, they are inspected another time.

The best way to know what your meat was fed is to know and trust your local farmer. Ask him questions about his herd and their daily care.

Bone Marrow

Bone marrow is powerfully nutritious and a mandatory part of the protocol. The use of bone marrow in cooking is non-negotiable for healing support. Marrow will be a natural part of Meat Stock because it is in the bones and added back into the stock. Marrow bones can be cooked in stock, removed with a fork, and eaten with a sprinkling of salt or blended back into the stock. It can be added to a cup of stock and blended into gravy. However it is added to the protocol, it should be in the protocol. People who eat marrow are often attracted to marrow bones. One bone filled with marrow is immensely satiating.

If hunger is experienced on the Introduction Diet, the intake of organ meats and marrow bones should be increased.

Marrow can be added to anything! It can be eaten independently from other foods by simply scooping out the marrow, seasoning it with some mineral salt, and enjoying.

Fats

"Fats!" says Dr. Natasha Campbell-McBride, "Very Important!"[cxxiv]

Dr. McBride hits the topic of fats thoroughly.

"What we have to understand is if you take the water away from the human body, and that's been done, about 70-75% of (the) human body is water.

The dry weight (is) about 50% protein, 50% fat. Fat is structural; it isn't optional for us," she says.[cxxv]

When the gut is deeply damaged, the nutrition isn't getting absorbed properly. When the wrong fats, toxic fats, are eaten, they poison our bodies from the inside out; causing worse damage on the cellular level. Feeding the good fats, when the damage is deep, is critical to repair.

When we eat fats that are sourced from pastured animals, which are freely ranging and basking in the sun, the nutrition from their fat is insurmountable. It is also readily absorbed by our digestive system. The body doesn't need to do any work to digest fats. The nutrition is just absorbed, sucked in for immediate use.

"Half of our structure is fat. When we analyze that fat in its chemical structure, it is similar to lamb fat, beef fat, pork fat, goose fat," McBride says. "These are the most important fats for our human physiology. They should constitute the bulk of your fat consumption."[cxxvi]

When we cook, she recommends cooking with animal fats like lamb, beef, pork, and goose. The vegetables should literally be swimming in fat; that fat should also be heaped into your GAPS Meat Stock during the introduction stage.

McBride says, "If you roast a goose for Christmas, you'll have many, many jars of beautiful fat coming out of that goose. The goose will be sitting in fat in the tray."[cxxvii]

This fat can be rendered the same as fat rendered from a cow (tallow) or fat rendered from a pig (lard). Pouring the fat, while it's still warm, through a strainer and then capping it in Mason jars is best. This fat will keep in the refrigerator for years.

McBride recommends all cooking, frying, roasting and other baking to be done with fat from these pastured animals.

"Vegetable oils are poisonous. Don't touch them; don't buy them; never cook in them," she says. "Those things sold in great big jars or great big bottles coming from the food industry—don't cook in them. These fats were known from [the] 1930s—vegetable oils and their harmful effects on the body. "cxxviii

McBride does recommend cold-pressed plant oils like cold-pressed virgin olive oil (Stage Four), coconut oil (Stage One) and palm oil (Stage Four). These oils are sensitive. The cold-pressed plant oils should be extracted in cold and preferably dark environments, but absolutely packaged in dark bottles so that they do not oxidize. Coconut oil is antimicrobial, antifungal, and antibacterial, all of which can cause die-off.

"Plants have many beneficial oils that are polyunsaturated, which means they are fragile. They are damaged by heat, by light, by oxygen, and by other influences in the world. That's why mother nature locked these fats very nicely in the cellular structure of the plants," she says. "All plants have these oils. So, when we eat lettuce, cucumber, tomatoes, fruit, vegetables, we are getting plenty of these oils in their clean, pristine, unadulterated state."cxxix

Processing is a different story.

Heat, solvents, pressure, oxygen, and chemicals all damage the fragile nature of the plant oils. This destroys the fragile polyunsaturated fatty acids. The chemical structure changes during this method of extraction and treatment, causing the plant oils to be unnatural in our bodies.

This process changes the plant oils, "turning them into many harmful things, into pollution for your bodies," McBride says. "Unfortunately, because of the commercial propaganda coming from the companies that manufacture these oils, the whole world has been convinced that this is good for us, that we should cook all our food on these oils, while butter and lard and animal fats are dangerous for us. The truth is just the opposite."cxxx

Butter from grass-fed cows is one of the healthiest fats around. The skin from a pastured chicken ranks just as high. Turkey skin is phenomenal.

McBride says that you cannot overdo it! Her clients who are most severe in their gut damage have been thriving on over 70% fat intake for years.[cxxxi]

McBride addresses the concept of cholesterol and heart damage in her book *Put Your Heart in Your Mouth*. She lays out her extensive protocol for gut healing in her GAPS book.

Butter Honey Frosting

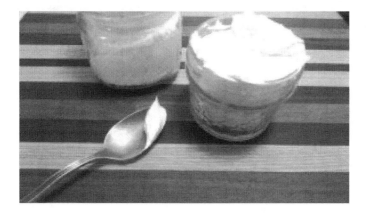

Often, when a person switches from a Standard American Diet to a healthful diet with no sugars, starches, or grains, cravings and withdrawals appear. Sugars, starches, and grains often feed yeasts, which, when not fed, get angry and exhale toxic gases. *Candida albicans*[cxxxii] is one of 250 yeasts in the body. It exhales 176 toxic gases such as methane gas, ethanol, hydrogen gas, ammonia, acetone, and more. These toxic gases have been classified as going from the intestinal tract, through the vagus nerve, to the opiate receptors of the brain, causing the desire for the foods that feed the yeast. These folks are classified as responding like drug addicts for sugars, grains, and starches, which feed the starving yeasts.[cxxxiii]

Current Opinion in Microbiology says, "Animal models argue that *Candida* colonization delays healing of inflammatory lesions and that inflammation promotes colonization. These effects may create a vicious cycle in which low-level inflammation promotes fungal colonization and fungal colonization promotes further inflammation. Both inflammatory bowel disease and gastrointestinal *Candida* colonization are associated with elevated levels of the pro-inflammatory cytokine IL-17."cxxxiv

Gut Pathogens says that those with deeper damage in the microbiome, as in those with Celiac, have excessively higher yeast counts.cxxxv

The *American Journal of Clinical Nutrition* made it clear in a study analyzing the use of saturated fat and heart disease. They found, "A meta-analysis of prospective epidemiologic studies showed that there is no significant evidence for concluding that dietary saturated fat is associated with an increased risk of coronary heart disease or cardiovascular disease."cxxxvi

Dr. Natasha says in GAPS FAQS, "Cravings for sweet things and chocolate are due to unstable blood sugar level. In order to remove your sugar cravings, you need to keep your blood sugar at a steady level. Here is what we do: make a butter / honey mixture or a coconut oil / honey mixture, put it in a glass jar and carry that jar with you everywhere. Eat 2-3 tablespoons of this mixture every 15-25 minutes all day long. Do this for a month or longer depending on the severity of your sugar cravings; in the meantime, focus on implementing the GAPS diet, which will normalize your blood sugar permanently. Once your blood sugar is normal, your cravings will be gone and at that stage you can stop carrying a jar of butter / honey mixture with you."cxxxvii

    1 cup grass-fed butter or coconut oil
    1-3 tablespoons local honey

To make the honey butter mixture, blend together in a mixer, on high, one cup of grass-fed butter (200-400 grams) and one to three tablespoons local honey. The mixture can be made with coconut oil if butter isn't desired or tolerated.[cxxxviii]

Beating the mixture for about 20 minutes, scraping down the sides to help incorporate, makes a fluffy frosting-like mixture.

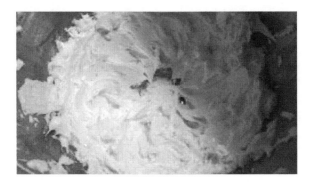

The longer you beat the mixture, the fluffier it becomes.

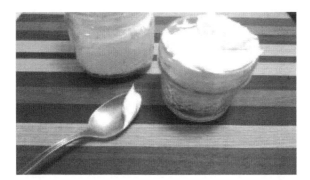

It can be stored in small glass jars and taken with you through the day. Dr. Natasha further says, "When sugar cravings are gone, you will be able to maintain your blood sugar normally between meals without having to eat anything."

Rendering Tallow or Lard

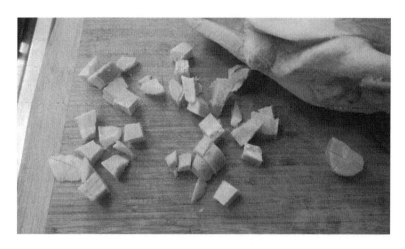

Rendering tallow and lard at home are both done in the same way. Get your slabs of beef fat (makes tallow) or pig fat (makes lard) from your local farmer, preferably grass-fed, pastured animals that have not been treated in any way with hormones or antibiotics. The fat surrounding the kidney has less flavor and is commonly used for pastry recipes. Cut the fat into small cubes; this is done most easily when it is partially frozen, not fully defrosted.

Cut the fat into small usable sections; this means, instead of cutting and rendering the whole slab, cut about a dinner plate size and fill freezer bags so that you can render only what you need at a time.

Put a portion of the cut fat into a cast iron skillet and heat on medium heat to medium-high heat.

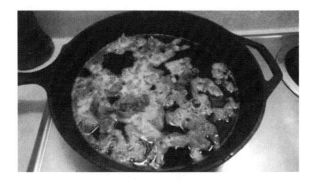

When it's done it'll look like this. The fat particles left are called cracklings which are almost the most perfect snack treat on the planet (best eaten when still warm). The fat remaining in the skillet is rendered tallow or lard. You can do your whole package of fat at once in a crock pot and store it directly to a Mason jar, straining out your cracklings. Processing it in manageable portions in the skillet gives you a specific portion of cracklings at once. Cubes of the suet can be stored in the freezer in quart-sized zip top bags so that they can be processed in manageable portions when needed; this will give you a constant supply of cracklings without it being too much.

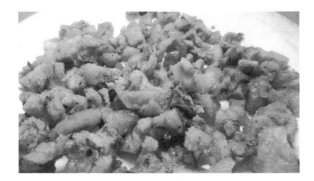

Sprinkle your cracklings with salt and enjoy.

Dr. Natasha was asked about Organic Rosemary Extract because it is now being put in grass-fed tallow, lard, duck fat, goose fat, and schmaltz here in America, by a popular company called Fat Works. It's used as a preservative. In a perfect world, we render our own; however, with an overworked mom, is it OK to use?

She answered, "It is OK."cxxxix

Lard and tallow are very stable at high heats and are good for cooking, baking, or frying. Once the fat is rendered into lard or tallow, it is considered a good fat if heated up once, twice, or three times. After it has been heated more, the molecular structure changes and it is no longer considered healthy.

Historic advertisements tell us a lot of what life was like, but they also tell us facts that have gone astray through time in the effort to sell, sell, sell. A 1920 advertisement from the Good Luck company did exactly that—it tells us how far from healthy we have strayed.

Jelke advertised a product called Good Luck, a meat fat margarine. This mixture of animal fat mixed with milk was a substitute to normal animal fats at the dinner table. It began in 1868 and developed over time into what we know today as margarine. Malnutrition presented with symptoms such a drooping posture, chronic fatigue, lack of concentration, and an abnormal desire to eat between meals. If you or your child suffered from any of the symptoms, the solution was to seek meat fats.cxl

At the time, one-third of a child's energy value came from eating animal fats. They were classified as sheer energy, 2 1/4 times more nourishing than other foods. Not getting enough was known as fat-starving.cxli

Today we are taught that low-fat choices are healthy.

In the 1920s, it was common knowledge that hunger between meals was abnormal and a result of fat starvation. It was also common knowledge that the fatty part of meat was nourishing, sustaining, and energy giving. This is very interesting information that is foreign to us today, especially at a time when so many people are obese and constantly hungry from malnutrition.

Studies today are showing us that coconut oil speeds up the metabolism and is even found to reverse Alzheimer's disease. Coconut oil is a good, healthy fat that nourishes, as are butter, tallow, lard and olive oil. This is the same information the advertisement from 1920 explained; yet we are sold the information today that low-fat diets are healthy.

Fatigue, irritability, and lack of concentration are common ailments today. People everywhere are looking for foods that provide slow-burning energy, and it was common knowledge in 1920 that nourishing energy like that came from good meat fat.

Deborah Graefer, L.Ac. M.T.O.M. and gallbladder specialist says, *"Fat*-free and low-*fat* diets can be a cause for *gallbladder problems.*"[cxlii]

The same is said about Alzheimer's disease.

In her book *Alzheimer's Disease: What If There Was A Cure?* Dr. Mary Newport, neonatologist, says, "I do have a collection now of almost 220 reports, mostly from caregivers and some from the person themselves, reporting that they saw improvement after they started taking coconut oil."[cxliii]

CBN News reported, "In patients with Alzheimer's, insulin resistance prevents their brain cells from accepting glucose, their primary fuel. Without it, the cells die. But there is an alternate fuel known as ketones, which cells easily accept. Ketones are metabolized in the liver after eating coconut oil."[cxliv]

The *European Journal of Clinical Nutrition* released a study stating, "Increasing circulating ketone bodies, via fasting or feeding a high fat low-carbohydrate diet, is effective in treating epilepsy."[cxlv] High fat low-carbohydrate diets include non-starchy vegetables and quality meats or fish.

These studies are directly proving common knowledge facts of 1920 – healthy fats nourish. We study history for information on so many topics; maybe it's time we study history for the health of our food.

Butter

Butter is big. Some folks are so madly in need of quality animal fats that they simply can't get enough butter. Moms find kids reaching for the butter or already sitting there eating a paw full of butter, eating happily. The nutritional profile of butter is rich. Dr. Natasha says, "Butter and ghee provide various fatty acids with important health-giving benefits, vitamins A, D, E, K2, beta-carotene and other nutritious substances in an easy-to-digest form."cxlvi

Sourcing the best butter possible is important. "Everyone has to do their best in their circumstances," Dr. Natasha says.cxlvii

Dr. Natasha says the best butter is bought from a farmer who makes the butter from cultured organic cream.cxlviii

She says the second-best butter is from raw organic cream, made into butter.cxlix

She says the next best is, "Organic grass-fed from shops, which is made from pasteurized cream. Then the rest, including Kerrygold."cl

Kerrygold butter is available to most, if not all, clients worldwide. Dr. Natasha says, "It is OK if there is nothing better."cli

To itemize, according to the best sourcing available to you, listing butter from the best options, down, purchased from:

1. Farmer who cultures cream and makes butter
2. Farmer who makes butter from cream
3. Organic grass-fed store-bought
4. Kerrygold and the like

Molding butter into shapes for holiday decorations adds a spark to the table that every kid enjoys. At Easter, the butter can be in the shape of a lamb, a bunny, or a cross. At Christmas, the butter can be carved into a Christmas tree, present or a lamb.

Carving the Thanksgiving bird brings on a new meaning when the butter is carved into a turkey.

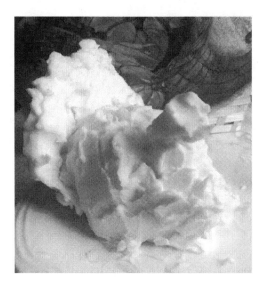

The kids love it. It's a crowd pleaser and an easy treat to take to someone else's house.

Stage One Liver Pâté

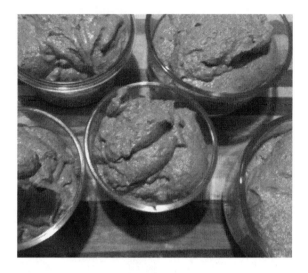

    1 pound of liver soaked in lemon juice for 4 hours
    1 pint of Meat Stock
    3 onions
    4 garlic cloves

Put all ingredients in a pan. Cook on a low simmer for 25 minutes; then run through a high-powered blender or food processor until smooth or the desired consistency is reached.

Herbal Tea

Hot or warm herbal teas are both comforting and medicinal. Using teas, according to what the body needs, can support the body in ways not found anywhere else. Different teas have various factors that support the body. Knowing what to use when can be an outstanding asset. For those rebuilding a damaged microbiome, they are quite valuable. "Herbs are generally allowed as a tea or an extract. When the diarrhea has cleared, you can start consuming them raw and dried, as by then your gut should be able to handle fiber (herbs are usually fibrous)," Dr. Natasha says.[clii]

The general rule of tea making is to steep one teaspoon of the loose-leaf tea to one cup of water. Loose leaf teas can be bought from bulk herb suppliers such as Mountain Rose Herbs, Frontier, or Starwest Botanicals. Stronger teas can use one tablespoon of the herbal remedy to one cup of water and steep much longer. Tea can be made in many ways; each person will put his or her own twist on it. You cannot steep tea too long, even though some will become bitter the longer they steep. Making tea is done by pouring boiling water over a teaspoon of herbal loose-leaf tea and letting it steep for three minutes. Tea infusions are done by pouring boiling water over the quantity of two tea bags (two teaspoons) for three to five minutes; it uses more and steeps a bit longer. Some brew it longer, even an hour. A tea decoction is powerfully strong, made by putting one ounce of herbal tea into one pint of water, in a stainless-steel pot. Heat on medium at a low simmer, without the lid, until the water reduces by a quarter in size, leaving three quarters of a pint.

Teas, while on the GAPS Protocol, should be sourced from loose leaf herbs instead of commercially manufactured teabags, due to anticaking agents and free flowing agents in the tea, as well as plastics (Abaca Plastic) used in making the tea bag. Tea can be brewed by tying up loose leaf teas in an unbleached coffee filter, securing the leaves in a stainless-steel tea ball, or using any other similar method.

Freshly squeezed lemon juice can be added to any tea, as tolerated, to add flavor and increase the medicinal effects, as lemon is an astringent.

Several teas are mucilaginous, but still have beneficial healing properties for those on GAPS. For example, marshmallow root tea is mucilaginous, but is beneficial against pathogenic species living in the stomach and tract. For situations like mucilaginous products, like marshmallow root, Dr. Natasha says, "I would do the tea."[cliii]

Other teas are high starch and should never be eaten on the GAPS Protocol, as starches are to be avoided. However, using them as tea can be highly beneficial. One example is chicory root tea. Some say that chicory root tea helps greatly with moving the bowels. Dr. Natasha says, "The tea is fine."[cliv]

Nettle Leaf: Stinging Nettles are known to have toxic substances, including stinging hairs, which are neutralized when heated. They are credited for being deeply nourishing as well as supporting lymph drainage. Sometimes drinking nettle tea drains the sinuses immediately. Dr. Natasha says, "Do not use nettles in pregnancy because it can initiate contractions. For this reason, nettle infusion has been traditionally used in the third stage of childbirth, when the baby is out, but placenta is still in and needs some encouragement to come out."[clv] Many people on GAPS use stinging nettle tea for draining the lymph, the high iron and other nutrients, as well as its ability to support the kidneys and liver. Many GAPSters find that 4 cups of nettle leaf and milk thistle seed tea help with difficulty sleeping.

Milk Thistle Seed: Milk thistle is known to support the liver, due to silymarin, the extract, flavonoids, in the seeds which work as an antioxidant that aids and assists in producing new and healthy liver cells. *Phytotherapy Research* says it "is the most well-researched plant in the treatment of liver disease. In animals, silymarin reduces liver injury caused by acetaminophen, carbon tetrachloride, radiation, iron overload, phenylhydrazine, alcohol, cold ischaemia and Amanita phalloides. Silymarin has been used to treat alcoholic liver disease, acute and chronic viral hepatitis and toxin-induced liver diseases."[clvi] Milk thistle seeds are more powerful if ground just before use.

Rooibos: Rooibos tea is credited with assisting the body in making glutathione. The *Journal of Agricultural and Food Chemistry* says, "Rooibos and Honeybush teas significantly enhanced the activity of cytosolic glutathione S-transferase alpha." They report test rats were treated with the two herbal teas showing the change in glutathione levels as significant.[clvii]

Rooibos herbal tea is harvested from a South African leguminous shrub. Due to high beneficial phenolic antioxidants, it is considered a health drink.

Chanca Piedra: The nickname of Chanca Piedra is stone breaker. When used as a tea, it is credited with turning gallstones into sludge so that the body can flush them. Flushed gallstone sludge looks like fat pudding piles floating on the top of the toilet water. The *International Brazilian Journal of Urology* says, "Phyllanthus niruri (Chanca Piedra) has been shown to interfere with many stages of stone formation, reducing crystals aggregation, modifying their structure and composition as well as altering the interaction of the crystals with tubular cells leading to reduced subsequent endocytosis."[clviii]

Pau d'Arco: Pau d'Arco is credited with reducing overgrowth of yeast. *SIDAhora* reported a study using females with vaginal yeast infections. They administered Pau d'Arco and found, "Pau d'Arco is also anti-yeast. Boil for ten to twenty minutes and take a teaspoon two or three times a day. Tea or vinegar and water can be used as a douche. Some women get relief by adding a half-cup of white vinegar to their bath."[clix]

Olive Leaf: Olive leaf is used for many reasons, including its anticancer properties, antioxidant properties and antiparasitic properties. *Nutrients* says, "Both inflammatory and cancer cell models have shown that olive leaf polyphenols are anti-inflammatory and protect against DNA damage initiated by free radicals. The various bioactive properties of olive leaf polyphenols are a plausible explanation for the inhibition of progression and development of cancers."[clx]

Licorice Root: Licorice root tea is credited with supporting the adrenals. It is ten times sweeter than sugar, adding a sweetness without the damages of sugar. The *Journal of Research in Medical Sciences* says that licorice root showed beneficial effects against normalizing Helicobacter pylori levels.[clxi] Licorice root does have the ability to raise blood pressure.

Dandelion Root Granules: Dandelion root granules are credited with supporting the liver. Most people see gallbladder by-product expelled immediately after drinking dandelion root granule tea. *The Review of Diabetic*

Studies says that it is an anti-diabetic plant because of its anti-hyperglycemic, anti-oxidative, and anti-inflammatory properties.[clxii]

Elderflower: Elderflower is credited with being supportive during flu, colds, and constipation. *Plant Foods for Human Nutrition* from Dordrecht, Netherlands published a study on elderflower tea which found, "The results of this study suggest that elder beverages could be an important dietary source of natural antioxidants for the prevention of diseases caused by oxidative stress."[clxiii]

Peppermint: Peppermint tea is credited as a digestive aid. *Phytotherapy Research* says, "Peppermint has significant antimicrobial and antiviral activities, strong antioxidant and antitumor actions, and some antiallergenic potential. Animal model studies demonstrate a relaxation effect on gastrointestinal (GI) tissue, analgesic and anesthetic effects in the central and peripheral nervous system, immunomodulating actions and chemopreventive potential."[clxiv]

Chamomile: Chamomile is credited with pulling pathogens out through the urine. The *Pakistan Journal of Pharmaceutical Sciences* says, "It has shown to be an anti-inflammatory, astringent and antioxidant especially in floral part." They further added that it could be showing results in lowering blood sugar levels.[clxv]

Rosehips: The *Iranian Journal of Public Health* says that rose hips are remarkably high in vitamin C and flavonoids. Naturally found ascorbic acid in rose hips varied due to location of growth, species, and ripeness.[clxvi]

White Pine: The *Journal of Ethnobiology and Ethnomedicine* says that pine needles are high in flavonoids, vitamin C, and antioxidants.[clxvii] White pine can be harvested outside in most regions and is recognizable by three pine needles sourced from the same follicle.

Valerian Root: Valerian Root is credited with helping people calm down for sleep. Some see extremely vivid dreams while on valerian. For those who tend toward nightmares, this can lead to vivid, extremely scary dreams. For those who tend toward happy dreams, this can lead to wonderful dreams.

Ginger: Ginger is a prokinetic, a motility agent, famous for creating function in the intestinal tract. Fresh ginger should only be used for proper medicinal properties. It is also famous for assisting in calming nausea, vomiting, stomachache, and diarrhea.

Ginger tea can be made by grating one teaspoon of fresh ginger into a cup. Pour boiling water over the ginger, and steep for 10 to 20 minutes. Enjoy as is or with freshly squeezed lemon.

Ginger tea is a highly beneficial tool to assist the microbiome function. Specifically, the aqueous extract of ginger, Zingiber Officinale, contains saponins, terpenes, phenols, flavonoids, and alkaloids. These agents cause the muscle spasms that move fecal matter through the bowel, known as peristalsis.

Peristalsis does not happen only in the intestinal tract; it begins in the throat. For this reason, many people who feel like their food gets caught in their throat find relief from drinking ginger tea.

Prokinetics can also be found in drug form.

The *International Journal of Food Sciences and Nutrition* did a study testing the ileum of guinea-pigs, mice, rats, and rabbits. They said, "The study showed that the aqueous extract of ginger exhibits species-specific spasmogenicity in gut tissues of rabbit and rat (muscarinic-type) while through an uncharacterized pathway in guinea-pig ileum, along with a dormant relaxant effect, mediated via the blockade of voltage-dependent $Ca2+$ channels."[clxviii]

The *World Journal of Gastroenterology* reported a study using ginger capsules on 11 patients with functional dyspepsia, chronic pain in the upper abdomen region without any known structural cause.[clxix]

The randomized double-blind study showed, "Gastric emptying was more rapid after ginger than placebo. There was a trend for more antral contractions. Ginger stimulated gastric emptying and antral contractions in patients with functional dyspepsia but had no impact on gastrointestinal symptoms or gut peptides."[clxx]

Functional dyspepsia is a relatively new ailment, becoming more and more prominent year after year. In the last 10 years it has become commonplace to encounter someone in a group who suffers from functional dyspepsia while the medical community remains stumped as to the cause and the resolution.

The *Journal of Association of Physicians of India* says, "Most of this symptom resolution in community subjects is likely to represent spontaneous resolution, especially since no treatment has been found to give long-term relief."[clxxi]

This is contradictory to what McBride, the front-runner in the field, has found. Dr. McBride specializes in healing the gut, reestablishing a balanced microbiome, and rebuilding the body. Her position remains: if you support the body properly with nourishing foods, the body knows how to repair itself. She says that when pathogens in the gut are imbalanced, pathogenic species can thrive. As they thrive, they live and breathe, exhaling and excreting while sloughing off dead bodies and growing new. As this happens, these pathogens release toxic gases specific to their species. These gases are what she says cause functional dyspepsia, as well as other health related issues.[clxxii]

Even though they called relief "symptom resolution," *The Journal of Association of Physicians of India* admitted, "Many episodes of symptom disappearance were due to [subjects'] changing symptoms rather than actual symptom resolution."[clxxiii]

This is reflective of the pathogens. Different pathogens release different toxic gases, causing different symptoms.

Clinically, we find that feeding the beneficial bacteria can establish a balance in the ecosystem while adding ginger to the daily regimen to activate peristalsis. When the pathogens paralyze the motion of the tract, ginger is the answer to regaining function of moving toxins from the bowel.

Hot tea is always medicinally more effective on the system than cold.

Generally, one of the signs of an overloaded liver is black and blue dark shadows under the eyes. When these individuals drink ginger tea, steeped for 10-15 minutes, they often report that the dark circles under their eyes literally recede as they drink the ginger tea.

Kraut Juice

Making kraut juice is nearly the easiest and cheapest probiotic you can make at home. Kraut juice is gentle on the stomach, which makes it easy for digestion, and is encouraged starting at the earliest stages of GAPS. Kraut juice has been shown to ease constipation and help maintain good bacteria in the microbiome.

This recipe will give you three gallons of kraut juice. Don't fret – it goes faster than you think.

Be sure to use an organic head of cabbage. Sauerkraut has 20 times more bio-available vitamin C because the fermenting process makes the nutrient from the cabbage digestible and available. The same is true for kraut juice. Vitamin C is a fantastic detoxifier, vital to GAPSters, so you want a head of cabbage with the most vitamin C possible—organic.

Take a large head of cabbage and chop it up in the Vitamix (by floating cubes of cabbage), food processor, mandolin, or simply with a sharp knife. The smaller the pieces are, the faster it will ferment. Sprinkle six tablespoons of salt (for a large, five-pound-head of cabbage) on top, and stir thoroughly. Now you have a couple of choices: pound the kraut, or ignore it and let it sit. The larger the chopped pieces are, the less it will open the cell walls if it just sits.

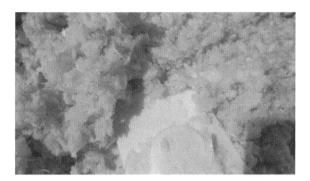

Let it sit anywhere from 20 minutes to overnight. The salt will do the work for you if your cabbage is shredded into small bits. What you're looking for is the extracted juices and limp cabbage. The salt is breaking down the cellular structure, allowing the juice of the cabbage to release.

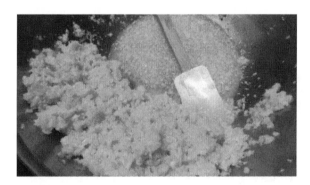

Fill your jars 1/3 of the way up with the cabbage and salt mixture. Fill the rest with filtered water.

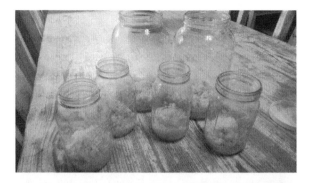

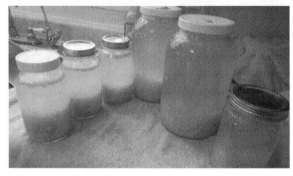

Put your lids on and let them sit on the counter for 9-12 days, preferably in a dark cool place. The amount of time for leaving out kraut juice as it brews depends on where you live – temperature is important. The other factors that make a huge difference in reference to mold growth are salt content and air. If air is accessible to your brew it will mold faster. If leaving the brew out concerns you, do a shorter brew on the counter-top and then complete the brewing process in the refrigerator. This will slow any potential mold growth. There is no absolute rule on time for brewing, as these extra factors play an important role in the process. The variables of salt, air, sinking or floating vegetables, nutrition of cabbage head, temperature, and sunlight all play a factor. You need to find what works best for you and your kitchen, as well as what is tolerable to your body. Those with the deepest gut damage to the microbiome need to allow their brew to sit for four months to a year for no histamine response.

Some stick their brewing jars under a towel in the corner of the counter-top near the air conditioning vent. Sometimes the cabbage floats; sometimes it sinks – it really doesn't matter. If the kraut juice ferments and a white yeast forms on the top (kahm yeast), just scoop it off, throw it away, and eat what's below. The product is still good.

Refrigerate and enjoy.

Beet Kvass

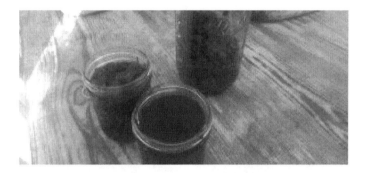

Beet kvass is a probiotic drink so common in the country of Moldova that there are kvass vending machines on city streets. You put your coin in the machine, pick your kvass flavor, and the machine squirts your flavored kvass into a glass sitting on a shelf in the middle of the machine. After the glass is filled, you drink your treat and return the glass to the shelf for the next customer.

Making beet kvass is simple. In a quart size Mason jar, fill one third of the way up with an unpeeled beet, sliced. Add a tablespoon of mineral salt and fill the jar with water, leaving one-inch headroom. Put the lid on and let it sit for 12-ish days, or until the taste is right for you. When finished, strain the kvass liquid from the jar and use the beets in the same jar to brew it again by putting in new salt and water.

The problem with kvass made this way is that it tastes like beet dirt. It is very beneficial, but not so delicious to most. Drinking it is a chore that most often involves a pair of big girl panties.

Yet, if you add a bit of sliced cabbage and onion – voila! It's a treat that you just can't stop drinking. It's smooth, fresh, crisp, and delightful.

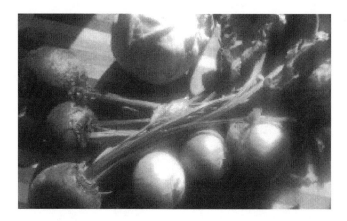

Fresh vegetables that are organic are best. The cabbage can be green or red, depending on what you prefer. To make this fantastic treat, fill your Mason jar a third of the way full of sliced and unpeeled beets, add an inch or two of chopped cabbage and then an inch or two of chopped onion. Fill the vessel with the appropriate amount of salt and water and let it sit.

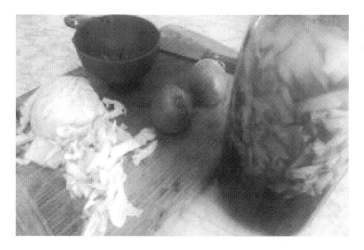

The amount of salt depends on the size of the vessel. Mineral salt is optimal as it is the natural form and loaded with minerals. The most common forms of mineral salt, in nutrient density order, are Celtic Gray Salt, also known as Celtic Sea Salt, Baja Gold Salt, Redmond's Real Salt, and Himalayan

Pink Salt. For a quart-sized Mason jar packed full of vegetables, one to two tablespoons of mineral salt are generally used. If the jar is a third full of beets with a bit of cabbage and onion, totaling around half a quart full, half a tablespoon of salt is fitting – however, the amount is up to personal preference.

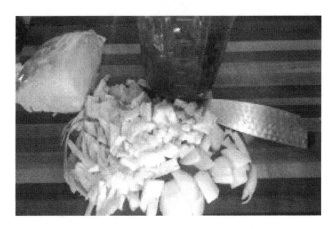

The amount of onion and cabbage used is your choice. When redoing the jar of beets for a second or third or fourth round, if the cabbage and onion were sitting on top of the sliced beets, they can be scooped off and eaten, just like you would sauerkraut. New cabbage and onion can be added on top of the beets and the ferment can be set for another round.

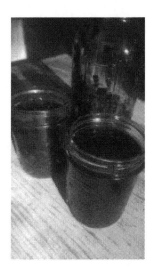

Drinking beet kvass is energizing to the liver. Traditional Russian Kvass is made with rye bread or other grains. Traditional kvass is made with fruits, filling the jar a roughly a third of the way full of fruit, adding whey and water, and then letting it sit to make a fermented beverage.

The extreme benefit of beets comes from the high number of phytonutrients reflected in their deep red color. Some beets are so beneficial to the liver, some people pass gallstones just by eating beets or drinking fermented beet beverages.

Nutrients says, "Lactofermented beetroot juices are characterized by the high anti-carcinogenic and anti-mutagenic potentials."[clxxiv]

They go on to say, "The lacto-fermented beetroot juice containing live bacteria of the genus Lactobacillus may be considered of functional foods. This product combines the biological activity of betacyanins, involved in limitation of oxidative processes in the organism, and activity of live bacteria modulating the composition and metabolic activity of intestinal microbiota."[clxxv]

Accolades for kvass were gut health, clean blood, detoxification, cancer prevention, and overall vibrant health.

Moldy Fermented Vegetables

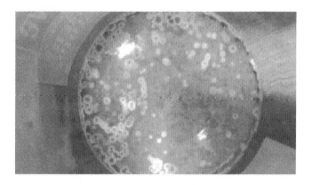

When fermenting vegetables, the vegetable pieces should be submerged underneath the brine, away from oxygen. Oxidation causes mold. Sometimes, vegetables surfacing above the brine level is inevitable, as when making kraut juice. When the vegetable is exposed to oxygen, it creates an inviting environment for growth of yeasts and mold.

Social media is filled with people saying that if your sauerkraut grows mold, you should throw it out. Sometimes this is good advice; most often, it's not. Wasting money is not the goal.

James Townsend, specialist in life practices during the 1800s, says, "If you ever find mold growing on the top of your sauerkraut, all you really need to do is scrape that moldy part off, re-submerge your sauerkraut, keep percolating. It. Will. Be. Fine."[clxxvi]

Sandor Katz, Father of Fermentation, says in his book *The Art of Fermentation*, "Surface growth is common and normal; it should be removed, but it is not cause for alarm and it does not ruin your fermenting vegetables."[clxxvii]

He goes on to say, "To get rid of surface growth, gently remove weight from the ferment. Use a wide stainless-steel spoon to get under the mold and skim it off as best you can. Sometimes it is not possible to remove all the mold, because as you attempt to remove it, the mold dissipates, and little bits are left remaining. If this happens, remove most of it, as much as you can, and don't worry. As long as mold is white, it is not harmful. If other color molds start to grow, do not eat them. Bright colors often indicate sporulation, the molds' reproductive stage. To prevent spreading the spores, gently lift the entire mold mass from your ferment."[clxxviii]

This is where some people say to throw the ferment out; however, this is not what Katz says. He would still eat it; he says, "Remove mold or other surface growth, as best you can, as soon as you notice it. After removing mold, evaluate the texture of the underlying vegetables. If the vegetables near the surface have been softened by mold growth, remove and discard."[clxxix]

Wild Ferments, a California company that specializes in fermented vegetables, says, "We often hear stories of people throwing away whole batches, because it smells or looks bad at first sight. We have found beautiful kraut under a moldy maggot-infested top layer – it was delicious. People should know that an offensive odor often decreases and sometimes even disappears once a crock is packed into jars and refrigerated."[clxxx]

Dr. Natasha agrees, saying, "I would scrape it off and eat what's below, particularly if it goes blue. You know what helps with all ferments? I find a leaf of horseradish on top, cabbage works – horseradish. When you put horseradish on top, there will be none of that film on top (just the leaf – horseradish). Grow it in the garden – it's so easy to grow!"[clxxxi]

Dr. Natasha was shown this jar of fermented vegetables that had a solid inch and a half of hairy mold growing on top. The cabbage leaf that covered the top of the kraut rose up and out of the brine and grew mold on top. The next picture is the jar from the top view.

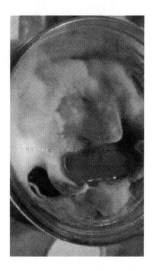

When shown this jar, Dr. Natasha said, "Oh, that needs to be removed completely."[clxxxii]

She was asked, "Removed and thrown away, and eat what's below, or throw the whole thing away?"[clxxxiii]

Dr. Natasha replied, "You can eat probably.... taste it. Scrape it off and eat what's below. You probably need to remove that much (a few inches). Because it will be slimy..."[clxxxiv]

Monica Corrado, MA, CNC, CGP said, "Whatever's slimy, throw out."[clxxxv] Corrado is a Teaching Chef to The Weston A. Price Foundation and for the GAPS Protocol.

Dr. Natasha agreed and said, "Throw it out until you get to the crunchy stuff. If it's slimy, throw it out. Get to the crunchy cabbage – if it smells good."[clxxxvi]

Monica says, "If it's crunchy, you're good. If it's slimy, throw it out."[clxxxvii]

Dr. Natasha agreed saying, "Absolutely."[clxxxviii]

The picture below is the side view of the same jar. This jar is the perfect example of the worst-case scenario, what to do when mold grows on your ferment. Looking at the jar, a cabbage leaf, which covers the vegetables to keep them submerged under the brine, is visible 3/4 of the way up the jar. The leaf is about an inch thick. On top of the leaf is another leaf which has floated up out of the brine, showing a space of air, then white mold, and then more leaves and more white mold.

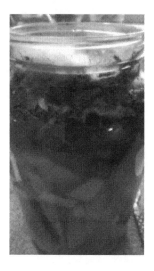

When showed the side view picture of the jar, Dr. Natasha said, "Oh my, up to here needs to be removed (just above the halfway mark, where the color is still lighter) and possibly the whole jar thrown out."[clxxxix]

This gives us a full understanding of what is acceptable for consumption.

When asked if kahm yeast on the top can be scooped off and thrown away, the answer was the same.[cxc] Kahm yeast is a white film, sometimes gray. The picture shown below, viewed from the top of the jar, has kahm yeast on top.

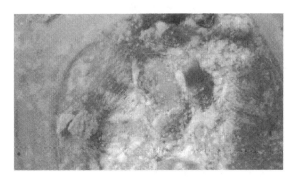

This picture below is a side view of the same jar.

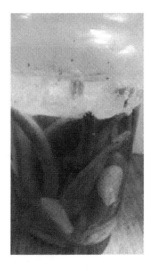

Regarding Kahm yeast like this, Dr. Natasha says, "Scoop that off and throw it away. Eat what's below. When you make all your ferments, even your pickles, put a leaf of horseradish on top."cxci

When asked, "Can you stick a rock from the garden in there?"cxcii

Dr. Natasha says, "You can. Wash it off. What I do, you see – there used to be these bread bins made out of clay with a heavy lid on top – I do my ferments in there. Then I put a leaf, and a plate on top of the leaf, and then I put an empty glass jar. I find the right size of it (a glass), put it like that; the lid goes on top. The plate is underneath; the lid pushes the whole lot down.

Even in glass jars, I put a little glass jar – a kind of shot [glass]. I put the lid on, and the lid holds it down."[cxciii]

The best way to avoid the whole issue is to seal it up, submerge it, and eliminate the oxygen as best as possible. Many folks cover the top of the vegetables with a cabbage leaf; some use a crock rock, a glass disc weight, or even just a small glass, to submerge the vegetables further. Others use air extractors in the lids. Some use fermenting weights. Some use advanced air lock systems. Some use silicone lid caps. Some use airlocks and weights together. Others just use airlocks. There are hundreds of ways to ferment – all work. It doesn't need to be expensive; it doesn't need to be complicated. It just needs to fit your lifestyle.

Fermented Dairy

It is very important that GAPS dairy is not confused with conventional dairy.

GAPS dairy builds a tolerance. If dairy isn't tolerated, GAPS dairy is designed to reestablish the foundation which is missing, allowing dairy to be part of the person's diet. Most people come to GAPS with a dairy intolerance. Fermented GAPS dairy is optimally made from a heritage breed cow's fresh, raw milk, which is then fermented. The fermentation process on the GAPS protocol should be 24 to 27 hours long; this is so that the lactose is digested and the casein is converted to paracasein, making it easier to digest. Dairy that is from cows that are not from heritage breeds are not as identifiable to the body. The more damaged the microbiome, the more identifiable the food should be. If raw is not available, for whatever reason, organic milk from the store is the next best choice.

Dr. Natasha was asked, "If you have your own cow and you have a lot of raw milk, is it better to take your milk and put it in the freezer, then take that frozen, raw milk, thaw it, and make yogurt and kefir? Or is it better to get store-bought organic milk? Which is better?"[cxciv]

She answered, "Frozen, raw milk."[cxcv]

When asked, "Which is better: a cow eating candy (literally candy) from a candy factory around the corner, or organic milk from the store?"[cxcvi]

Dr. Natasha answered, "Organic milk from the store. Those poor animals."[cxcvii]

To rebuild, the GAPS dairy intro starts with adding lots of pastured animal fats to your soup protocol, shooting for an intake of over a quarter of a cup a day. Once that's tolerated, ghee is introduced slowly. Some must do this introduction with the toothpick method, where they take a toothpick, touch the ghee, and then touch their soup. When that's tolerated, they take the toothpick and put it deeper in the ghee and then touch the soup. When that's tolerated, the toothpick goes deeper in the ghee, then in the soup. When that's tolerated, the toothpick scoops a tiny bit of ghee and then touches the soup. The quantity is built up slowly, while on GAPS probiotic foods, until the food is tolerated. After ghee is tolerated, move to grass-fed butter. Then move to whey, made from properly fermented GAPS dairy. Once whey is tolerated, move to yogurt (for those with diarrhea) or sour cream (for those who are constipated). Once that is tolerated, move to milk kefir, and then move to raw block cheeses.

The GAPS dairy introduction is done with real milk that is first fermented. Conventional dairy, unless organic, is not part of the GAPS protocol. Dairy intolerances are most often due to conventional dairy as its molecular structure is not easily identified/tolerated by the body. When taking dairy and fermenting it on the GAPS protocol, the casein is converted to paracasein and the lactose is digested. This makes GAPS fermented dairy more tolerable.

The GAPS book says that some foods to avoid are cream cheese and cottage cheese, as well as some other dairy. When fermented properly, at home, they are perfect for the GAPS Protocol. Dr. Natasha says, "Not the shop-bought, but the homemade [cream cheese and] cottage cheese [are] fine."[cxcviii]

GAPS dairy is fermented. Dr. Natasha says, "Only fermented!"[cxcix] Raw milk can be consumed when Coming Off GAPS.

Whey

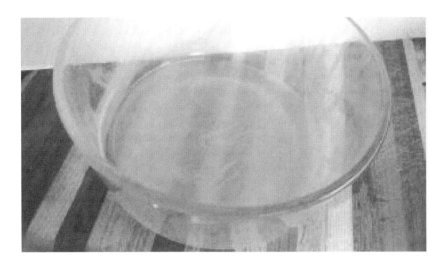

Whey is a very gentle probiotic food, making it an easy starting point for those with deep damage in the microbiome. On GAPS, homemade whey is one of the earlier ways to introduce dairy when building up from a dairy intolerance.

To make whey, first make GAPS-approved yogurt, sour cream, or kefir. While fermenting any of these options, turning the heat up a bit, to 115 or 120, will create more whey and less yogurt, or the like.

GAPS dairy is fermented for 24 to 27 hours so that the lactose is digested and the casein is converted to paracasein. After fermenting, take a medium-sized bowl and lay cheese cloth (folded over multiple times) on top. An old cotton t-shirt or cloth can also be used, as shown. Pour the yogurt, or the like, over the cloth, into the bowl; tie up the cloth with a tie or rubber band, and hang it from a cabinet knob. This one shown is tied up to a KitchenAid mixer. The whey, which is a clear, protein liquid, will drip into the bowl.

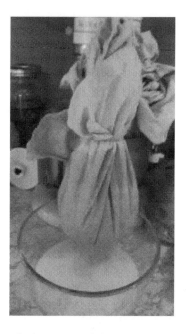

If there is a hole in the cloth, more of the yogurt, or whatever you use, will also drip through, as shown in the above picture.

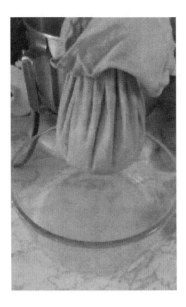

If rebuilding a dairy intolerance, it is important to start with clear whey. Some can begin with a teaspoon; some must start with a drop. Others must start with one drop in a teaspoon of water, stirring it up and taking one drop of that. Others still must put the one drop in a tablespoon of water or a quarter cup of water or a whole glass of water and take one drop of that – wherever you start, you start. Only your body can tell you where to start.

Whey is smooth, delicious, and satisfying. It lasts in the refrigerator for a very long time; the length of time it lasts depends on the time of fermentation and the specific milk. It usually lasts in the refrigerator safely for a few weeks. Bad whey usually has a pink film on top or tastes off in a bad way. Whey can be consumed by drinking it straight, using it to speed up lacto-fermentation of vegetables, or using it in smoothies.

Yogurt

There are two types of milk used to make GAPS-compliant yogurt.

One method uses store-bought, organic milk; the other uses raw, unpasteurized milk.

When using store-bought, organic milk, heat the milk up the 180 degrees.

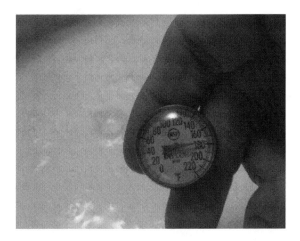

Cool it down to 120 degrees.

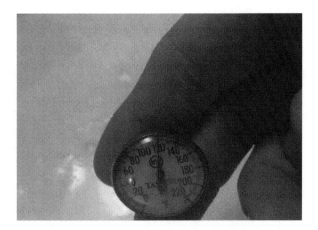

In a pint of raw milk, stir in two to four heaping tablespoons of quality, full-fat yogurt from the store, or use your previous batch of yogurt. Lower quality yogurts are often started with powdered culture and do not yield a good quality yogurt, batch after batch, if the yogurt is made and is used as the starter culture for the next batch. Low quality yogurt from the store is not GAPS-approved as a starter. Different starters, including yogurt from the store, a farmer's yogurt, starter packets, and probiotic capsules used as a starter, are all GAPS-approved, with each creating a different product. For this reason, any and all of them should be used and rotated. For store-bought milk, which has been heated, only two teaspoons per gallon are needed since the beneficial microbes are gone.

Whisk until combined thoroughly.

Pour the mixed milk mixture into Mason jars.

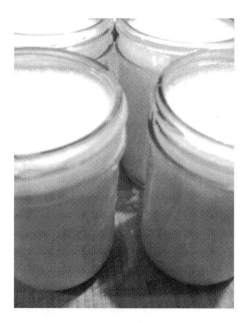

For Making Yogurt Using an Instant Pot:

Put jars filled with milk and yogurt starter into Instant Pot, click on "yogurt," and then immediately press "+" until the clock reads 24:00 or higher, but not more than 27:00. If this button isn't pressed immediately, the machine will automatically default to an 8-hour yogurt brew. The machine will start itself. GAPS yogurt is left to ferment 24 to 27 hours as this ensures that the lactose is consumed by the bacteria, leaving the yogurt lactose-free. This brew time also ensures that all the casein, the protein in milk, has been converted to paracasein, an easy to digest molecule.

For Making Yogurt Using Other Methods:

If you do not have an Instant Pot, put jars in the oven with the light on for the same 24 to 27 hours, on a heating pad with a towel over top of the jars, on top of an old refrigerator where heat emits, or in the dehydrator set between 95-110 degrees. Note: most dehydrators run roughly five degrees high which will be too hot if the dehydrator is set at 110.

***** If you are trying to make more whey, due to a dairy intolerance, where you wish to rebuild the precursor enzymes, set the dehydrator a bit higher. Temperatures at 115 degrees or just higher will yield more whey, less yogurt.

To make **_raw milk yogurt_**, put three heaping tablespoons of your yogurt starter or previous batch of yogurt into a pint-sized Mason jar. Pour raw milk on top, leaving an inch of headroom. Stir the yogurt into the milk until thoroughly combined. Raw milk yogurt does not need to be heated prior to making yogurt. Raw milk yogurt requires more starter due to the high number of enzymes in the yogurt. The good in the milk fights the starter a bit, so more is required to get it started. Raw milk yogurt is teaming with more beneficial strains.

Put jars in the Instant Pot, click on "yogurt," and then immediately press "+" until the clock reads between 24:00 and 27:00. The machine will start itself. GAPS yogurt is left to ferment 24 to 27 hours as this ensures that the lactose is consumed by the bacteria, leaving the yogurt lactose-free. This brew time also ensures that the casein, the protein in milk, has been converted to paracasein, an easy to digest molecule.

If you do not have an Instant Pot, put jars in the oven with the light on for the same 24-27 hours, on a heating pad with a towel over top of the jars, or in the dehydrator between 95-110 degrees.

Some people add gelatin to their yogurt to make it thicker. Yogurt made with the proper amount of starter has the same consistency as store-bought yogurt, after refrigerated. Gelatin is not necessary. Adding gelatin instead of more starter robs you of a higher probiotic quantity in the yogurt. It's better to make the yogurt properly instead of adding other ingredients.

A few years ago, a popular food blogger said yogurt that is over a certain age is useless as the colony collapses. Dr. Natasha says, "No, the colony does not collapse. If yogurt was made with a commercial starter, the microbes there can be quite weak, so some of them can disappear. But if yogurt was made with kefir or just with microbes naturally present in the fresh raw milk, these microbes persist for more than a month in the fridge."[cc]

Sour Cream

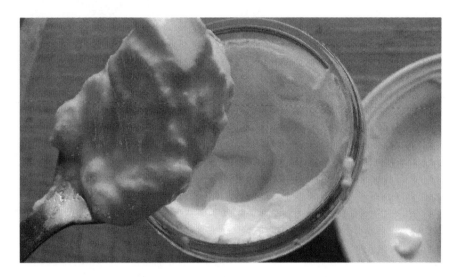

Home-brewed sour cream is one of the healthiest home brews you can eat because it carries a negative charge. Sour cream is made the same way that yogurt is made. Sour cream is made with cream; yogurt is made with milk.

"Sour cream is a very healthy food because it has both the fat and the lactate. Lactate is very, very interesting fuel because it's not sugar, and sugar has a lot of bad issues, and it carries a negative charge," says Dr. Stephanie Seneff, the leading expert on sulfur and how it functions in the body. She is an electrical engineer, a computer science specialist who then converted into the biological sciences with a biology degree as well as food and nutrition specialty.[cci]

Dr. Seneff adds, "It's very interesting that lactate carries the negative charge. Negative charge particles in the blood are very, very important to the blood's colloidal stability. This is a crucial thing that is happening to people as they get older: they lose the colloidal stability in the blood and they start to get into blood clots and hemorrhages."[ccii]

Dr. Joseph Mercola refers to it this way: "It's kind of an electron deficiency syndrome."[cciii]

The hardest thing about making your own sour cream is obtaining the raw cream. Organic cream from the store can be used, but it's not optimal.

To make sour cream, take one quart of raw cream, add 3 tablespoons of raw yogurt, and stir to combine. Be sure to leave one inch of headroom (space on top of the cream between the cream and the lid). Put the lid on top, and leave it on the counter for 2-3 days, shaking twice a day. After you put the jar in the refrigerator, it will get even thicker.

Making Milk Kefir

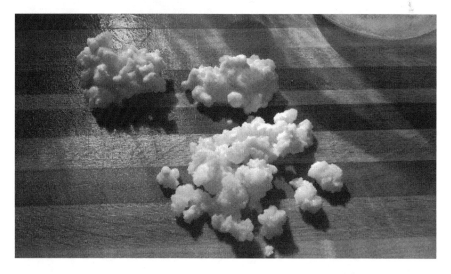

Making milk kefir is easier than it looks. As one of the strongest food-based probiotics, learning to make milk kefir at home will pay you back a million times more than the effort. The first step is to acquire kefir grains, which can be done by ordering them from Amazon, getting them from a friend, or contacting your local Weston A. Price chapter leader. Kefir grains look and feel like white gelatinous mini-cauliflowers. As the grains grow, they can invert themselves, expand, and explode much like popcorn. This leaves a flatter, more stretched out kefir grain.

When asked if the milk needs to be heated prior to making milk kefir, Dr. Natasha said, "You don't have to, but many people do."[cciv]

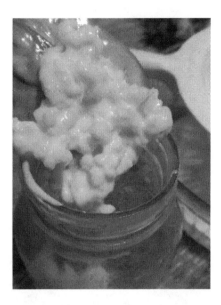

Put the kefir grains into a glass jar, and cover with milk (preferably raw milk). The general ratio of grains to milk is one tablespoon of grains per one cup of milk to brew in 24 hours; however, this is not a solid rule. Fewer grains will still ferment the kefir; it'll just be slower. More grains will ferment the milk into kefir faster. Put a lid on the kefir as it is anaerobic. Fermenting milk kefir isn't as concerning as fermenting vegetables in terms of keeping the grains submerged below the milk line.

Shake the bottle once or twice throughout the day to relocate the grains. Kefir grains only ferment what they are touching so relocating the grains creates a tastier and more even-keeled product. Once the milk is fully fermented, the lactose will be digested, the casein will be converted to paracasein, and it will be more solid in form, much like yogurt. As in the picture below, the kefir will stay in more of a solid shape. It can also be liquid, not thick, depending on what is happening in the milk and grains at the time; both are normal. Kefir is known as the Champagne of Milk, filled with bubbles and effervescent.

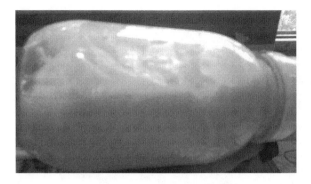

The longer the kefir ferments longer, a whey break line will appear about 2/3 of the way down the jar. This means that the lactose has been digested and the casein has been converted to paracasein. Most people like kefir best just before the whey break line breaks.

When you open the lid, the kefir will be thicker than milk and will stick to the sides of the jar. If it doesn't stick to the sides of the jar, it's fine. Every time you brew kefir it will look a tiny bit different – sometimes more curd-like, others more liquid.

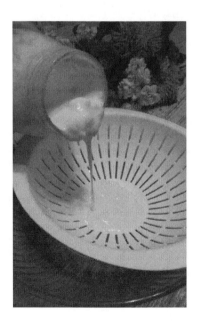

Use a stainless-steel strainer or plastic colander, spoon or spatula, and glass bowl. Place the strainer over the bowl and pour the contents of the brewing milk kefir jar into the strainer.

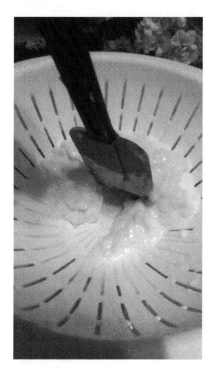

Push the milk back and forth. The fermented kefir will fall through the strainer, and the kefir grains will remain in the strainer.

The more you brew milk kefir, the more the grains will multiply. Propagating grains are healthy grains. They will all be different shapes and sizes, depending on their age.

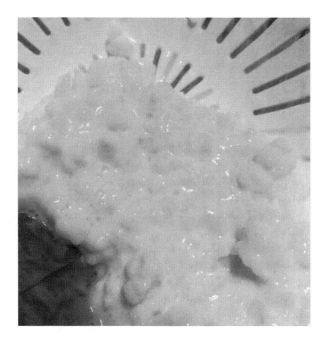

Put the kefir grains back in the same jar where they were previously brewed; there is no need to wash this jar every time you brew kefir. In fact, using the same jar will provide more grains as the tiny dots stuck to the side wall are new grains forming. Some folks keep using the same jar until it smells sour on the top; then they switch to a clean jar. Pour new milk over the kefir grains. Put a lid on the jar, and let it sit another 24 hours.

The milk kefir in the bowl is ready to drink. Many folks like it plain, while others like it mixed with vanilla and honey. A second ferment can be done using fruit. To do this, just pour the strained milk kefir into a new jar (without grains) and add fruit. Put a lid on the jar and let it ferment longer, until the fruit has colored the milk kefir. The thinner you slice the fruit, the more completely it may be digested in the second ferment.

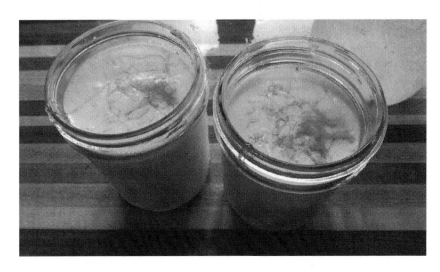

The brewing kefir can sit on the countertop or in a cabinet. There is a lot of forgiveness when making milk kefir. Some people just stick their hands into the jar to pull out the grains, then stick the grains into a new jar and pour new milk over top, and then drink the original jar.

As your kefir grains make new baby kefir grains, you'll be overrun. They can be mailed by putting a tablespoon or two of grains in a snack pack zip top bag, double bagged, and then put in an envelope.

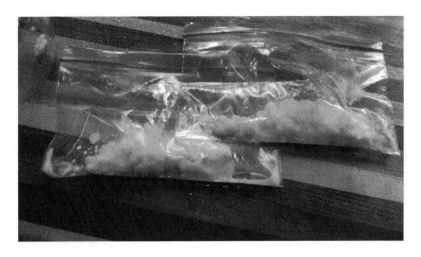

The more grains there are in the envelope, the more stamps you will need. Mailing them on a day that has consecutive mail delivery is best so that the grains don't sit in the heat or mail office for more days than necessary.

Milk kefir is specific to drowning out pathogenic yeast strains, drowning out streptococcus strains that cause tics, and drowning out pathogenic strains that cause eczema.

Fermented Coconut Water

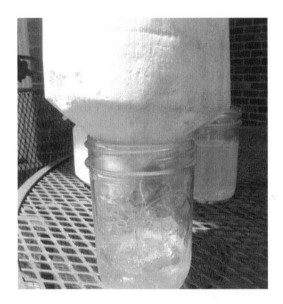

Fermented coconut water is one of the easiest probiotic drinks to make. It's also one of the best candida fighters on the market. If you're not up to the adventure, or if you just want to see how much money you're going to save, you can order fermented coconut water online.

Start by buying a fresh coconut for coconut water. The best option would be to pick a coconut from the tree yourself. Store-bought coconuts are sometimes sprayed with a layer of formaldehyde to keep the coconut from spoiling while shipping. This is by no means acceptable; formaldehyde will not nourish your body in any way.

You are drilling a hole through this layer. Watch for sensitivities, and consider this fact if reactions other than die-off exist.

In the past, GAPS has followed the protocol of NOT using prepared, packaged coconut water as it is pasteurized and dead food. If you don't have access to real coconut water, Dr. Natasha has recently said that using packaged coconut water with no added ingredients can be used. It is not optimal but can be used. If using a coconut, use a fresh coconut. Coconuts grow as small green balls that advance in size until they are fully grown. As full-grown green coconuts, they are filled with coconut water and a thin layer of "coconut pudding" on the side wall of the nut. As the coconut matures the outer copra turns brown, while the water inside the coconut turns into coconut meat. This meat is shredded, creating coconut flakes, which we buy in bags at the store. Left to further grow, all the water inside the coconut goes toward growing a tree by creating a spongey layer on the side of the coconut meat. this sponge layer is a delicacy. When this happens, roots sprout out of two of the eyes on the nut, while a sprout grows from the third eye. This sprout will become a new palm tree.

Remove the plastic wrap coating, if it has one. Drill two holes into the top of the coconut.

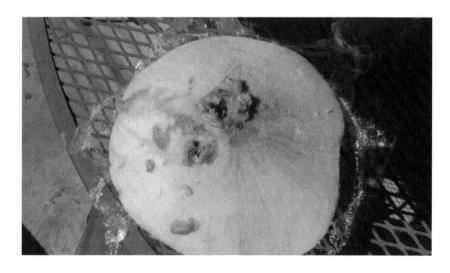

Invert the coconut over a glass to drain.

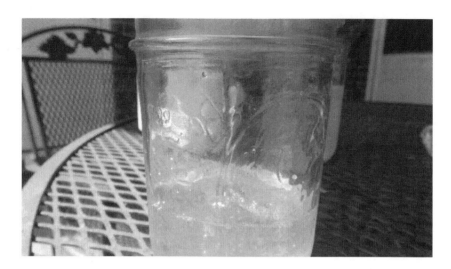

Some particles of coconut will fall into the glass, which is not concerning.

Open one of your favorite probiotic capsules and add it to the coconut water. Stir and let it sit on the counter for 3-12 days, depending on the temperature in your room, or until your desired fermented flavor is achieved. Kefir grains added to the coconut water create different strains that are also highly beneficial.

Fermented coconut water can be made by using a probiotic capsule or by using kefir grains. Both work well, each with different probiotic strains.

Kombucha

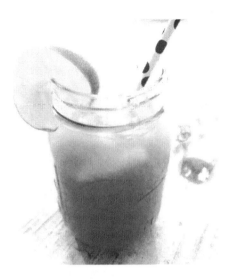

Kombucha is often tolerated on Stage One but is very bio-individual and needs to wait for others until Full GAPS. It's important to remember that we ferment Kombucha much longer on GAPS, until the sugars are digested. As it ferments it gets less sweet, then tastes tart. If over brewed, it tastes like apple cider vinegar, which we don't want as it can alter stomach acid production. The brew time depends on your location and temperature. For where this author it's roughly three weeks.

Central Laboratory for Analysis at the University of Science, Vietnam National University ran a study on Kombucha trying to find if it was more effective using added beneficial probiotic strains in the ferment.

"(Kombucha) is considered a health drink in many countries because it is a rich source of vitamins and may have other health benefits. It has previously been reported that adding lactic acid bacteria (Lactobacillus) strains to Kombucha can enhance its biological functions, but in that study only lactic acid bacteria isolated from kefir grains were tested," says *Springer Plus*.[ccv]

The three main biological functions of Kombucha are glucuronic acid production, antibacterial activity, and antioxidant ability.

The study desired to show *Lactobacillus casei* and *Lactobacillus plantarum* from kefir and pickled cabbage, seeing if it would enhance Kombucha's bioactivity. The kefir, pickled cabbage, and Kombucha were obtained from a market in Ho Chi Minh City, Vietnam.

The kefir in the study was made from defatted homogeneous milk.

It showed that the antibacterial and antioxidant activities of the Kombucha were improved.

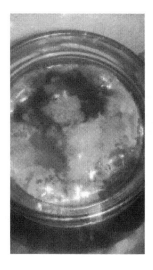

They found, "On the fifth day of fermentation, the combination of strain *lac5* and the [Kombucha] layer produced 39.6% more GlcUA (glucuronic acid) than the original culture (42.3a mg/L compared with 30.3b mg/L). Thus, strain *lac5* was more effective at stimulating GlcUA production than the other LAB strains studied."[ccvi]

The *Cancer Letters* says Glucuronic acid is known to be effective against cancer.[ccvii]

In another study, Kombucha was tested to determine its wound healing effects. It was tested on mice against an antibacterial ointment, Nitrofurazone, a wound and hoof care ointment used for bacterial infections of wounds, burns, and cutaneous ulcers.[ccviii]

Food-producing animals are protected by federal law against the use of Nitrofurazone, prohibiting the use of this product in food-producing animals. It stands to reason that a natural product that accomplishes the same results, if not better, would be optimal.

They said, "The clinical findings indicated that the Kombucha fungus resulted in precipitating healing [better] than Nitrofurazone; however, it was not significant (p > 0.05). In order to [perform a] pathological comparing of wound healing process, several wound biopsies were taken on 4, 8, 12, 16 and 20th days."[ccix]

They further reported, "Additionally, the histopathological results demonstrated that there was inflammation in Nitrofurazone group through twelfth day, somehow the epithelium was formed, and abundant vessels were visible. Although on 16th day and the previous days the healing condition of Kombucha fungus was considered as minimal rate, revealing it is similar to Nitrofurazone group on 20th day."[ccx]

Acta Periodica Technologica says, "Acetic acid, Kombucha samples and heat-denatured Kombucha showed significant antimicrobial activity against bacteria. However, there was no activity against yeasts and molds. Kombucha showed higher antioxidant activity than tea sample for all applied sample volumes."[ccxi]

Springer Plus published a study saying, "The bacterial component of [Kombucha] cultures has not been extensively studied but is known to comprise several species, including acetic acid bacteria. The antioxidant properties of Kambucha may be high because vitamin C, vitamin B and DSL are synthesized during fermentation. The antioxidant properties of [Kombucha] may be high because vitamin C, vitamin B and DSL (D-saccharic acid 1,4 lactone) are synthesized during fermentation."[ccxii]

Medline Plus says, "There is some concern that Kombucha tea might decrease niacin absorption. But this needs to be studied more."[ccxiii]

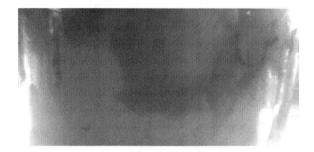

The Mayo Clinic says that Kombucha "contains vinegar, B vitamins and a number of other chemical compounds."[ccxiv]

They go on to say, "In short, there isn't good evidence that Kombucha tea delivers on its health claims. At the same time, several cases of harm have been reported. Therefore, the prudent approach is to avoid Kombucha tea until more definitive information is available."[ccxv]

Kombucha contains Butyric acid which assists in cellular membrane health. The glucuronic acid found in Kombucha is known to strengthen the walls of the intestinal tract.[ccxvi]

In November of 2017, Dr. Natasha made an official statement that Kombucha is a Stage One food.[ccxvii] There are many ways to make Kombucha; each person will put his or her own twist on the process. The determining factor of when it is ready, for a GAPS person, depends on the digested sugar.

Kombucha can be made using one Kombucha SCOBY (Symbiotic Culture of Bacteria and Yeast), one cup of sugar, one cup of starter, and 6-8 tea bags brewed into tea. Put all the ingredients – not the tea bags – into a glass gallon jar; then fill the rest of the gallon with water. If the sugar is stirred into the tea when it is hot, it dissolves easier and is easier for the culture to consume. Do not put hot tea into the starter cup or the SCOBY, as it kills the live strains.

The top needs to breathe; this is one of the few fermented foods that is aerobic, meaning that it uses oxygen. Put a thin towel or unbleached coffee filter over the top of the jar, and hold it securely with a rubber band. Kombucha likes to brew in a dark place, so wrapping it in a towel or putting it in a cabinet or closet that is opened frequently is best. The time that it takes for Kombucha to brew depends on the temperature of your location – the warmer it is, the faster it will brew.

Hannah Crum from Kombucha Kamp says, "The sugar in Kombucha is for the culture to consume, not for you. When done fermenting, there will be about 2-6 grams per 8-ounce glass of unflavored Kombucha. By contrast, an 8-ounce glass of orange juice has about 24 grams of sugar. Natural carrot juices have 13 grams per 8 ounces. If fermented longer, say for 3 weeks or longer, sugar levels in Kombucha may be even lower – *Recommended for diabetics and others with low sugar tolerance.* Without sugar, Kombucha cannot ferment."[ccxviii]

Crum also says that the more SCOBYs there are in the ferment bottle, the faster the brew will ferment.[ccxix]

She goes on to say, "The culture consumes the sugar and converts it into healthful acids."

If you want to test the sugar content in your Kombucha, you can use a refractometer, which costs about $30 online, or Accuvin Residual Sugar Test Strips, which are roughly $3 for each test strip.

The goal for Kombucha, when it is done brewing, is that it doesn't taste sweet, and it doesn't taste like apple cider vinegar, but is right in the middle.

Flavoring Kombucha can be done with a variety of flavors. If using things that are not sweet, it ferments faster. Flavors which fall into this category are things such as ginger, lemon ginger, grapefruit, lemon basil, lemon, lime, etc. If flavors such as grape juice or strawberry kiwi juice are used, the jar should be sealed and left to sit longer to consume the sugars. The more juice that is used and the sweeter that juice is, the longer it should sit. If the jar is filled a third of the way full of grape juice, and the rest of the way full of Kombucha, it should sit for roughly an extra week. This will make a very strong-flavored Kombucha, which makes for an easy step for those going from a Standard American Diet of over-the-counter juice to flavored Kombucha.

Dr. Natasha says, "We have a lot of berries on our farm. We have two, three freezers full of berries. What I do, I make like a compote where I have a big pan – 6 liters. Berries go in there – blackberries, loganberries, usually. Fill it up with water, bring it up to boil; don't boil – just bring it up to boil. Then it cools down. I strain it; add honey to taste, so it tastes nice, not too sweet, but nice. Then I have a jug with a SCOBY sitting there. I take probably half of the liquid out of there and replace that with this compote. My Kombucha lives on honey and berry juice, this compote. A day and that goes fizzy it's fantastic. It's delicious; it's fizzy. It's the best refreshing drink. People say you can't make Kombucha with honey – nonsense."[ccxx]

Making A SCOBY From A Store-Bought Bottle of Kombucha

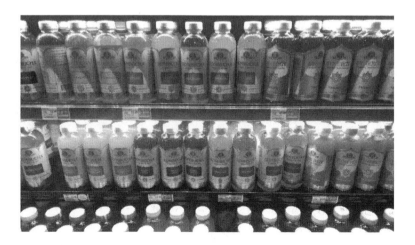

Kombucha is a favored probiotic that is both refreshing and health promoting. Store bought Kombucha runs from $2.50 to $7.00 for roughly 12 ounces. Meanwhile 128 ounces, in a gallon, costs roughly $1.50 to make. That's equal to buy one, get nine free if you're making it yourself. That's math even a tired mom can calculate. Making Kombucha is so easy, it's laughable. Make it one time and you'll wish you had done it earlier.

A Kombucha SCOBY can be gifted from a friend, purchased online, or gotten by using a store-bought bottle of Kombucha. All three options are equally good. If you are choosing to make a SCOBY from a store-bought bottle, choose an unflavored bottle with the most particulates in the bottle. If flavored Kombucha is the only option, it's fine. If a bottle with no particulate is the only option, it's fine.

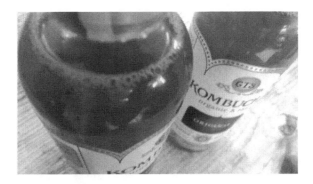

In a stainless-steel pot, heat up one cup of water and three to four organic black tea bags or loose-leaf black tea, the equivalent of 3 to 4 teaspoons. Steep the tea for 3 to 5 minutes or longer if you like. Herbal teas can be added to the mix. Herbal teas with medicinal qualities that are brewed into Kombucha are amplified in their medicinal qualities.

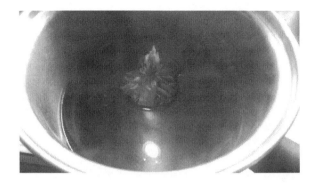

Pour 1/2 of a cup of organic sugar into the hot tea. This sugar is consumed in the fermentation process. If you are too busy, and the tea is already cooled, the sugar can be added to the tea; it will still be consumed – it just may not fully dissolve, which is fine. Organic sugar should be used to ensure the optimal nutritional quality of the tea.

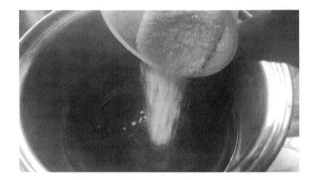

Pour the cooled sweet tea into a quart Mason jar or glass jar. When the tea is room temperature, meaning you can stick your finger in the sweet tea and stir it around for ten seconds without it being too hot or too cold, add the bottled Kombucha from the store to the quart Mason jar. If the tea is hot at this time, the beneficial aspects of the Kombucha will be killed by the heat and impede the process.

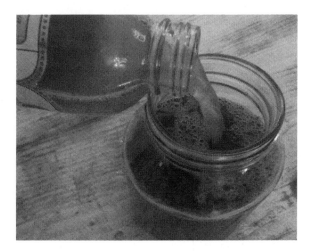

Once the sweet tea and store-bought Kombucha have been added to the Mason jar, fill the jar to one inch from the top with filtered water.

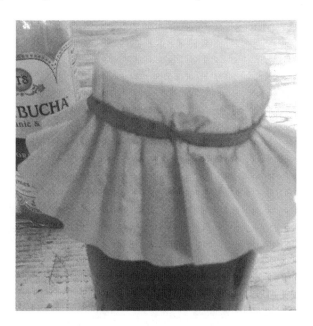

Top the jar with a coffee filter or cloth and secure it in place with a rubber band. If the liquid in the jar is too high, it will cause the SCOBY to bulge to the top of the vessel and attract fruit flies to lay their eggs on top of the coffee filter, which will then leach into the brew.

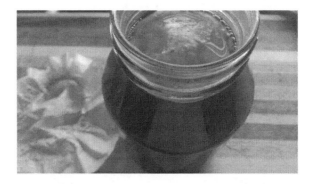

A new SCOBY will form on top of the liquid. The SCOBY will grow to the size of the vessel as it is sealing the tea, preserving it from contamination. If you use a very wide mouth vessel, you will have a very wide SCOBY. On the contrary, if you have a very narrow vessel, you will have a very narrow and small SCOBY.

Writing the date with a marker on top of the coffee filter enables you to know the time the SCOBY is formed. The time depends on the temperature of your house, as well as the air flow where the vessel is placed. It usually takes anywhere from a week to three weeks for the SCOBY to form. It will start out as a thin pancake and get thicker as it brews. The thin pancake is just as beneficial as the thick one.

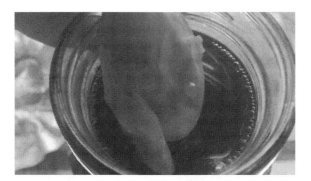

The coffee filter can be removed to check the status of the SCOBY. This SCOBY is very durable and can be touched, picked up with your fingers, removed with a utensil, or poked. Do not allow the SCOBY to meet freezing temperatures, very hot environments like boiling liquid, direct sunlight, or metal utensils (stainless steel, plastic, or wooden are all fine to use with the SCOBY and Kombucha).

During the brewing process, the Kombucha consumes the caffeine in the tea, as well as the sugar. Brewing Kombucha for the first time can be a bit scary and you're not sure what the SCOBY should look like—it is very common to feel the SCOBY has gone moldy.

Sometimes the SCOBY will have different colors within the SCOBY itself. There may also be particulate pieces surrounding the SCOBY or falling from the bottom of the SCOBY. All of these are fine. Pour the liquid out of the Mason jar into another glass, being sure to leave one cup of the Kombucha as the starter for the next batch. Once you have a SCOBY made, a gallon vessel can be used to allow more Kombucha in the end. If brewing a gallon of Kombucha, add one cup of organic sugar and one cup of the previous batch of Kombucha, as well as the sweet tea (six to twelve tea bags) to the gallon. The rest of the vessel is filled with filtered or spring water to one-inch headroom.

Flavoring Kombucha

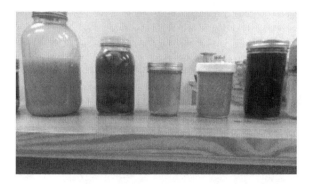

Kombucha can be flavored with any and every flavor imaginable. From left to right, these Kombucha flavors include mango, strawberry banana, ginger, unflavored, and grape. If you are using a flavored juice to flavor your Kombucha, be sure the ingredients are clean and do not contain any food colors, agave syrup, or other fake and unnatural sweeteners and chemicals.

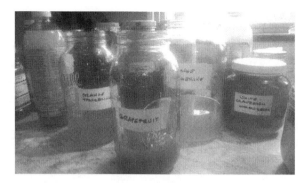

Fill the jar a third of the way full, or less, with the juice; then fill to the top with the freshly brewed Kombucha. If ginger is chosen as a flavor, juice fresh ginger in a juicer and fill the bottom of the jar with the ginger juice. More ginger than what fills the bottom of the jar will contain a lot of heat. Frozen fruit can be used for flavoring. Fruit used to flavor Kombucha is also a probiotic treat.

Electrolyte Drink

When a person gets sick with vomiting and diarrhea, the electrolytes can take a dive, causing further depletion. Electrolytes are minerals in the body, consisting primarily of sodium, calcium, potassium, chlorine, phosphate, and magnesium. These minerals contain an electrical charge essential to bodily functions. Illness, strenuous exercise, heat, altitude, and dry air can easily offset our electrolytes, which then need to be replaced.

The principle electrolytes are sodium, potassium, and chloride.

Electrolytes are generally acquired from water.

Many over-the-counter drinks are sold as electrolyte replenishing essentials, but their health value is depleting to overall function. This is not the goal. Finding the answer through supportive food is always best, especially when it works.

The GAPS rebuilding protocol is specific to laying balance in the foundation of the microbiome. Sometimes, while on protocol, the body will purge a virus or parasites. This can deplete electrolytes. The worst thing that can be done at this time is to choose a man-made, chemical-laden, sugar-filled drink.

There are three primary options, while on GAPS.

1. Any fermented vegetable brine is optimal. This includes kvass, vegetable medley, kraut juice, fermented garlic, kimchi, and probiotic pickles, which are generally favored, even by children.

2. Dr. Natasha says, "Some people drink a solution of a teaspoon of natural salt in a glass of water and find it helpful for their health. Meat Stock and Bone Broth have salt added and are rich in minerals and can be an electrolyte solution."[ccxxi] Natural salt is any salt with a color to it, such as Himalayan Pink Salt, Redmond's Real Salt, or Celtic Grey Salt.

3. Meat Stock is the third option; it is rich in minerals and can be made in a few hours.

Some folks use Gatorade for electrolyte support; however, it contains two forms of sugar, citric acid (which is a black mold converted from sugar), and monopotassium phosphate (which is used as a fertilizer, a food additive and a fungicide). It also contains brominated vegetable oils which displace iodine, a valuable nutrient to every cell of the body, including the thyroid gland.

The Natural Flu Shot

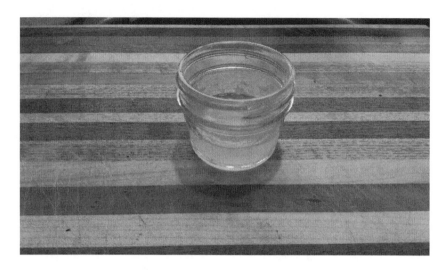

The flu shot is known publicly as "the most defective vaccine ever made."[ccxxii]

Vincent J. Matanoski, Deputy Director, Torts Branch, from The Department of Justice, released a report in March of 2016 divulging statistics of The Total Petitions Filed in The United States Court of Federal Claims during a three-month period starting at the end of 2015. This is vaccine injury court, where those who can prove they have been directly injured go to claim compensation for their loss. The claims from children totaled 28; the claims from adults totaled 100. Of these, 52 were given compensation for their injuries, 27 of which were damaged from the flu vaccine. Again, that's 27 provable claims from flu shot damage in three months' time.[ccxxiii] [ccxxiv]

The damages from the flu vaccine included: Guillain-Barré syndrome (where the immune system attacks the nerves), transverse myelitis (acute swelling of both sides of the spinal cord which causes loss of spinal cord function), Bell's Palsy (paralysis or weakness in the muscles of one side of your face), and neurological demyelinating injury (damage to the myelin sheath in the brain and spinal cord), just to name a few.[ccxxv]

This means that 21 people got a flu shot and now have great difficulty walking or can't walk at all.

Moreover, the effectivity of the flu vaccine is still under debate. A recent study analyzed health care workers, flu shots, and illnesses or deaths. They concluded, "Current scientific data are inadequate to support the ethical implementation of enforced healthcare worker influenza vaccination."[ccxxvi]

It's not uncommon for people to have a fear that a virus is lurking, seeking to devour them.

Meanwhile, *Bioresource Technology* reported a study determining the stability of probiotic cabbage juice including the presence of *Lactobacillus plantarum C3*, *Lactobacillus casei A4*, and *Lactobacillus delbrueckii D7*. They concluded, "Fermented cabbage juice could serve as a healthy beverage for vegetarians and lactose-allergic consumers."[ccxxvii]

It has been shown to shut down a virus by drowning out the pathogens.

Biotechnology Research International says, "Lactobacillus is proposed as potential probiotics due to its potential therapeutic and prophylactic attributes. *L. paracasei*, *L. rhamnosus*, and *L. casei* belong to the group of Lactobacillus which are commonly found in food and feed as well as common inhabitants of the animal/human gastrointestinal tract."[ccxxviii]

When a person is sick, coming down with the flu or a cold, replacing these missing probiotic strains is what is believed to prevent the pathogenic viral overgrowth that leads to cold and flu like symptoms. This highly effective method of preventing the flu has not been studied; however, individuals are doing it across the world with enormous effectiveness.

Enormous effectiveness.

People are finding that when they take the maximum tolerated levels of kraut juice daily, the illness comes to a screeching halt; they don't get sick.

Each person's maximum tolerated level is specific to that person, the amount just before die-off is seen. Others are reporting that if they begin to feel sick, even to the point of skin crawling, diarrhea, and vomiting, taking kraut juice to their maximum levels makes the feeling go away. It is important to note that if a person takes a quarter of a cup of kraut juice on a regular day, if illness appears, they will have to take more than the normal quarter of a cup – often closer to a full pint. The quantity is determined by die-off signs.

Research in Microbiology says probiotics are defined as "living microorganisms which, when [administered] in adequate amounts, confer health benefit on the host."[ccxxix]

The Journal of Nutrition and Metabolism says, "There is growing scientific evidence to support the concept that the maintenance of healthy gut microbiota may provide protection against gastrointestinal disorders, such as gastrointestinal infections and inflammatory bowel diseases. The use of probiotic bacterial cultures may stimulate the growth of preferred microorganisms, crowd out potentially harmful bacteria, and reinforce the body's natural defense mechanisms."[ccxxx]

Stevia

Stevia is used as a no-calorie sweetener that supposedly doesn't negatively impact blood glucose levels; however, stevia has been shown to be detrimental on reproduction function and is used in South America as birth control. Other areas of the world use stevia medicinally. For people who currently suffer from health issues indicative of microbiome issues, the use of stevia is potentially harmful.

Specifically, stevia showed over a 50 percent effectiveness when used as birth control. Of course, the amounts used are much greater than any human would ingest. This is an example of using an herbal for medicinal purposes as opposed to using the herbal as food.

Science magazine published a study showing, "A water decoction of the plant Stevia rebaudiana Bertoni reduces fertility in adult female rats of proven fertility. The decoction continues to decrease fertility for at least 50 to 60 days after intake is stopped."[ccxxxi]

Making a decoction is done by using a pint of filtered water to 1-ounce herb, bringing to a simmer over medium heat and allowing the mixture to cook down, without the lid, until it reduces by 1/3 in size.

The study said that Matto Grosso Indians tested dry powdered stevia leaves and stems used as oral contraceptive with albino rats. Their 6-day mating period was monitored with the powdered decoction administered before, during, and after. The male rats were not treated with the stevia – only the females were. The experiment was repeated three times with a 50-60-day rest period between tests where no therapy was administered.[ccxxxii]

They found, "Fertility was reduced 57-79% in rats drinking the decoction as compared with controls. A reduction of 50-57% in fertility was still present at 50-60 days after intake of the decoction. In the 1st experiment 11 of the young, belonging to different litters, lost their tails without apparent cause at ages of 12-15 days. This did not occur in the other experiments."[ccxxxiii]

Healthline says, "A highly refined form of stevia called rebaudioside A (marketed as Rebiana) is approved by the U.S. Food and Drug Administration (FDA) as a food additive." The FDA has strict guidelines and believes raw stevia leaves or minimally processed leaves "can damage heart and reproductive health, and might do harm to the liver."[ccxxxiv]

Stevia is a plant, grown naturally, which is claimed to be anywhere from 20 to 200 times sweeter than table sugar. The leaves are green. When dried, they are still green. When pulverized they are still green. Stevia purchased in the store is white. Manufacturing processes alter the plant from its whole food form. Green Stevia tastes less sweet than processed Stevia, remarkably. Unprocessed green Stevia is used on GAPS; processed Stevia is not.

Business Wire says, "The human body does not metabolize the sweet glycosides (they pass right through the normal elimination channels)."[ccxxxv]

The glycosides contained in stevia are Steviosides, Rebaudiosides, and a Dulcoside. *Total Health Secrets* says, "Refined Steviosides & Rebaudiosides are the sweetest form of Stevia and may be purchased in a semi-white powder form (usually referred to as an extract) or in a clear liquid made by adding the powder to water and a preservative."[ccxxxvi]

Healthy Shopping Network says, "Although Stevioside is a desirable sweetener it does not have the extraordinary health benefits of the Stevia leaf or products made from whole leaf Stevia concentrate."[ccxxxvii]

One placebo-controlled, double-blind study published in the *British Journal of Clinical Pharmacology* on Stevioside showed no difference with human test subjects in comparison to the placebo.[ccxxxviii]

Stevia processing involves drying the plant with the use of the sun, heat, or microwave, depending on the manufacturer.[ccxxxix]

Truvia is an artificial sweetener derived from Stevia. It is highly processed even further and compromised from the original Stevia state.

Stevia is considered a medicinal compound due to the plant chemical structure with over 100 phytochemicals found including: Apigenin-4'-o-beta-d-glucoside, austroinulin, avicularin, beta-sitosterol, caffeic acid, campesterol, caryophyllene, centaureidin, chlorogenic acid, chlorophyll, cosmosiin, cynaroside, daucosterol, diterpene glycosides, dulcosides A-B, foeniculin, formic acid, gibberellic acid, gibberellin, indole-3-acetonitrile, isoquercitrin, isosteviol, jhanol, kaempferol-3-o-rhamnoside, kaurene, lupeol, luteolin-7-o-glucoside, polystachoside, quercetin, quercitrin, rebaudioside A-F, scopoletin, sterebin A-H, steviol, steviolbioside, steviolmonoside, stevioside, stevioside a-3, stigmasterol, umbelliferone, and xanthophyll.[ccxl]

Interestingly, researchers found anti-tumor properties from stevia compounds saying, "The anti-inflammatory effect of steviol glycosides, stevioside, rebaudiosides A and C and dulcoside A against TPA-induced inflammation and found these compounds to possess a marked inhibitory effect."[ccxli]

Medicinally, stevia is used in Brazil, Paraguay, and South America for several reasons, including cavities, depression, diabetes, fatigue, heart support, hypertension, hyperglycemia, infections, obesity, sweet cravings, tonic, urinary insufficiency, wounds, diabetes, hypertension, infections, obesity, vasodilation, and as a sweetener.

The concern for the product is the amount of processing. The human body is made to digest food in its whole food form, complete with all the accompanying components and health benefits. Food processing has been shown to degrade and compromise the beneficial aspects. If Stevia is your sweetener of choice, it is best to have a plant of your own and use the leaves as your chosen sweetener instead of purchasing the manufactured product. If a purchased one is your option, finding one that the least processed with no added ingredients is best.

Dr. Natasha says the healthiest sweetener known today is still local honey from bees pollinating their local flowers, not fed sugar water.

Soap

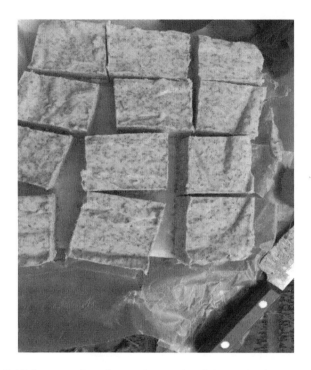

When on GAPS, removing the toxic overload from the body is essential to flushing out the pathogens that cause GAPS illnesses. Dr. Natasha recommends dropping lotions and potions, as she calls it, from the daily regimen to reduce the chemical overload. She recommends not using chemically filled soaps as the skin is the largest organ, absorbing chemicals readily. The less the body must process, the more it can spend its energy on healing.

The skin has natural oils and flora. Washing it off is not ideal or recommended. For those who just can't go without using soap, it is best to use soap made from clean ingredients instead of adding more chemicals to the body. For those who exercise, live in hot climates, and need to wash their private areas, soap is non-negotiable. For those who live in colder climates, soap isn't as needed.

Again, optimally, we don't use soap, as it alters the natural oils found on the skin.

In reality, some cannot do without it.

Medical Doctors and pharmaceutical companies are becoming more and more aware of the ability of the skin to absorb pharmaceutical medicines topically though patches. The nicotine patch, hormone patches, motion sickness patches, angina patches, birth control patches, and even pain killer patches are populating pharmacies. Poison Control says, "Even after taking the patch off, some drug remains in the body." The skin is an excellent avenue to absorb whatever is applied topically.[ccxlii]

Avoiding chemicals reduces the toxic overload processed by the body.

Making soap at home allows the person to use clean ingredients – even ones they would eat. Soap is made by using oils, liquid, and lye. Through the process of saponification, the ingredients go through a chemical transformation, turning the oil and lye into a salt.

Using lye is scary for some folks. If you add the liquid, whether it be goat's milk or water, to the lye, it can explode. It is said, "Water to lye and you may die." But, adding the lye to the liquid is perfectly safe. This is the most dangerous and difficult part of soap making. If you can remember to put the water or goat's milk in a bowl, and then sprinkle the lye on top of it, you're good.

Lye is caustic. This means that if you pour it on your skin, it'll burn your skin. For this reason, wearing a long sleeve shirt, gloves, a bandanna over your mouth and neck area, and protective eye wear is recommended. If lye happens to be splashed on your skin, it can be relieved by spraying white vinegar on the spot. Flushing it with water is also effective. Many people first make soap protecting every inch of their body with a spray bottle of vinegar within arm's reach. As they keep making soap, the protective gear is often exchanged for an open window and a water faucet.

Homemade Soap

Using stainless steel or glass utensils and bowls is recommended so that there is no adverse chemical response.

A scale is important to soap making. Exact measures are important, sometimes down to the hundredth of the gram. This recipe has a lot of forgiveness. When measuring ingredients for soap, put the bowl for measuring ingredients on the scale. Zero out the scale; then add the ingredient into the bowl until it meets the appropriate measure.

Prepare your soap mold before making the mixture. Specific molds can be purchased. You can make a rectangle box out of wood for a mold. You can also use an almond milk container or something similar since it already has a wax coating. A cardboard box lined with wax or parchment paper works perfectly. A smaller box makes a thicker bar that needs to be sliced lengthwise like a loaf of bread. A flatter box will make one layer of soap that will eventually be cut into bars looking like brownies.

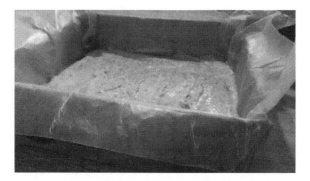

First—Put a bowl on the scale; then zero out the scale.

Then add 430 grams of frozen goat's milk (or water) into a stainless steel or glass bowl. Lye added to liquid causes heat. This combination can get very hot. Using frozen goat's milk keeps the temperature tolerable and manageable. Measuring out the goat's milk into zip top bags and freezing them keeps the temperature from getting too hot. When they are pulled from the freezer, put in the bowl, and chopped into smaller bits, then add the lye – the heat balances out as it melts the frozen milk. This keeps the temperature manageable. Goat's milk makes the soap more luxurious and nourishing to the skin.

Here's the breakdown:

Chop the frozen goat milk into small pieces.

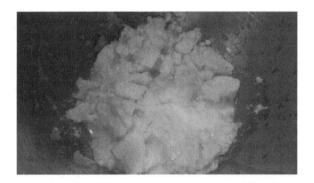

Place a plate on the scale. Zero out the scale. Measure 170 grams of lye onto a plate. Making soap is a chemical reaction, exact measurements are important.

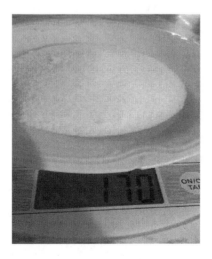

Pour the 170 grams of lye onto the frozen goat's milk.

When the lye is added to the goat's milk, it will transform into a hot combination. Stir the mixture with a wooden, plastic, or stainless-steel spoon immediately after combining or it can burn. The orange bit in this picture is a burning response. If the hot spot is left too long before mixing, it will burn into a chunk that can't be broken down into the mixture. This is not desired as it unbalances the measure. This mixture is going to be added to the oil mixture. Both mixtures should be roughly the same temperature when combined. This does not need to be exact; again, this recipe offers a lot of forgiveness—not all do. If this bowl gets too hot for your comfort (a rare thing), fill a sink with cold water and set it in the sink to cool.

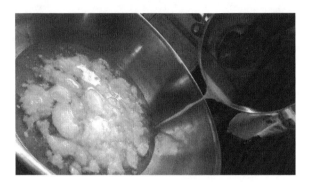

In a separate bowl, add an equal mixture of coconut oil and olive oil (any oil can be used; coconut oil gives lather to the bar) until the mixture totals 1134 grams. If you want a harder bar with less lather, 100 percent of the oil can be olive oil. Remember, essential oils displace oils. If you add two ounces of essential oils, subtract two ounces of olive oil or coconut oil. Some add coconut oil until it is almost half the measure on the scale and then pour in the olive oil until it totals 1134 grams.

Once the two oils are combined, pour the lye and goat's milk into the bowl. Essential oils can be added at this time.

Use a stick blender to mix the ingredients. This takes longer than you think; time depends on your blending appliance and the oil. The stick blender will get hot. It can get very hot. Continue to mix the ingredients until trace appears. Trace is where you move the stick blender through the mixture and it leaves a line like it would if you had dragged it through pudding. Historically, they didn't have stick blenders and made soap without blending for so long. If it's not mixed until trace happens, the soap will still be fine for use.

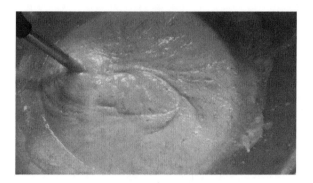

Added soap bling can be introduced at this point, stirring in with a rubber spatula. We like dried lemon zest added to lemongrass essential oil soap. Nutmeg and cinnamon are good with clove essential oil. Note: lemon or other citrus essential oils do not retain their aroma long. Lavender essential oil used with lard or tallow soaps smells like gentle refreshing lemon after curing.

Once all of the soap bling is combined, pour the mixture into the prepared box.

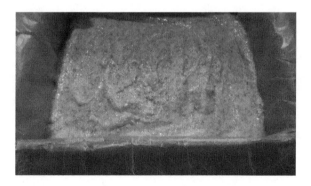

Leave your soap box on the counter or table.

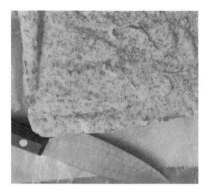

After 24 hours, or just less, turn the block out onto a cutting board and remove the parchment or wax paper if there is any.

With a large kitchen knife cut the soap into bars of the desired size.

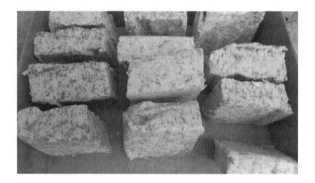

The soap bars need to cure for 6 weeks before use. The bars can be set side by side in a box or stacked up on each other, tip resting on tip, with lots of room to breathe, and then put in a closet for the 6-week curing time.

Hand Soap

Rebuilding the body often includes removing all chemical overload intake. For some, this means no soap at all. Using homemade soap, made from natural ingredients, can sometimes be the only option.

If you choose to use a foaming soap dispenser, reduce the Dr. Bronner's soap ingredient by 1/4 cup so the soap is not too foamy.

The base of the recipe is Dr. Bronner's Pure Castile Soap and jojoba oils. The head of Dr. Bronner's Magic Soaps, David Bronner, has been a key player in Oregon in the effort to label genetically modified organisms. The soap is made from a collection of organic oils and vitamin E with saponification.

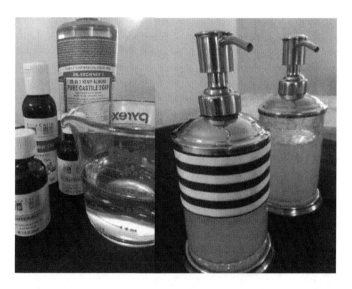

To make hand soap, just add your favorite essential oils to the castile liquid soap. The quantity is your choice; usually 2 cups of Dr. Bronner's Castile soap to 2 teaspoons of essential oil is a good balance. Tea tree oil will make the soap antibacterial. Lower grade essential oils are usually used in soap making. If you like thinner soap, add water.

To GMO or Not to GMO

"If there's a single industry author on a paper, you will not find any intelligent or adverse effect of a genetically engineered product," says Dr. Michael Hansen, Senior Scientist with Consumers Union (CU)[ccxliii ccxliv], the publisher of *Consumer Reports* who works on food safety issues specifically connected to GMO products. His work with CU has a heavy focus on labeling of genetically engineered food.

Dr. Hansen says this because there was a study published in *Food Policy* in 2011 where the authors, Deals, et. al., described how three independent scientists scoured the genetically engineered industry.

The first scientist scoured a PubMed and Scopus database searching for feeding studies or nutritional quality studies of engineered foods. He collected 97 papers.[ccxlv]

The second scientist took the 97 papers and determined if the genetically engineered foods caused a problem.[ccxlvi]

The third scientist analyzed each of the 97 papers looking for a financial or professional conflict. He flagged every paper that had someone working in the industry of genetically engineering of food.[ccxlvii]

All three scientists worked independently of each other, without knowledge of what each was doing.

Dr. Hansen said, "What they found was there were not enough studies without funding, 7 out of 95. There was an extremely highly significant difference when it came to professional conflict. They found 41 papers where at least one of the authors came from industry. In every single one of those cases the paper found no problems. There were 51 papers where none of the authors came from industry, 39 of them found no problems, 12 of them did indeed find adverse health effects."[ccxlviii]

The FAO (Food and Agriculture Organization of the United Nations) did a survey of almost 80 countries and found three countries responsible for the vast bulk of the problem: the US, Canada (because of the Canadian rape seed), and China.[ccxlix]

Dr. Hansen said, "China is actually a problem because they haven't approved BT rice and it's being planted. It's being caught going into the European Union."[ccl]

On March 20-21 of 2014, there was a meeting on the low-level presence of GM material in both food and feed. At this meeting Dr. Hansen said, "We don't require safety assessments for engineered crops. Our US Department of Agriculture does not require sequence information or reference material for any of the engineered crops that are in field trials, which means they have no way of telling if there's been contamination. If you're not given the sequences of what to look for, you can't look for it."[ccli]

The response came from Michael Schechtman, Office of Pest Management Policy, Biotechnology Coordinator. Hansen said Schechtman's response was, "It's true they don't require sequencing information or reference materials for experimental planning because there's thousands of them. They only require sequencing for those that will seek approval."[cclii]

That's protocol. However, this protocol doesn't work and is proven by current genetically engineered contamination.[ccliii]

Dr. Hansen says, "LL601, Liberty Link 601 rice, in 2006 ended up contaminating over half the US rice exports, costing over a billion dollars to rice farmers, being the worst rice incidence in our history. That was from a rice variety that was only tested experimentally. They stopped the experimental test in 2001. Five years later in 2006, it ends up contaminating half of our long grain rice exports."[ccliv]

Currently, 55 countries have a zero-tolerance policy on contamination – even low-level contamination. Food products must pass their own tests, not only the tests from another country.

The Transpacific Partnership (TTP) is a free trade agreement that apparently isn't transparent or about free trade at all. Dr. Hansen says, "This is not just about trade, it's about financial mechanisms and other things. I believe there are 600 industry lobbyists who have access to the documents, and the vast majority of folks in Congress have not been able to see these documents, even in the Senate, people on the committees."[cclv]

Dr. Hansen goes on to say, "This raises concern that business interests may be trumping one of the most upsetting aspects of the TTIP (the free trade agreement with Europe) and the TPP. If they think they're impacting their own bottom line, the companies themselves will get a dispute panel to challenge a country's laws. That dispute panel would have 3 judges on it that rotate off from the industry. This is a potentially horrendous process by which companies could help get rid of environmental and other regulations they don't like in any of the signatory countries."[cclvi]

One example is the European Union, which has denied imports from US factory farms using growth hormones in the beef. Companies are using the TTIP and TPP to open these trade routes.

The countries blocking these products want the labels to say things like "Product Contains Growth Hormones". The US is refusing.

Currently, it's considered unethical and illegal in the EU to give animals medicines if they aren't sick – this includes antibiotics, growth hormones, and others.

Scientists are beginning to speak out against misinformation on GMOs. In fact, over 300 of them are putting their jobs on the line to get the facts straight.

"This notion on GMO safety (among scientists) is just not true. There was this controversial feeding study by a French scientist, Gilles-Eric Seralini from CRIIGEN, published in *Food and Chemical Toxicology* 2012 and was withdrawn in November 2013. The study showed rats fed GMO corn died sooner and developed more tumors than the control group of rats. The retraction of that study has been condemned," says Dr. Michael Hansen,

Senior Scientist with Consumers Union, the publisher of Consumer Reports.[cclvii]

Ten rats were used in the study, which is a small number; however, it was the same size sample used when Monsanto did the study and published in the same journal, Food and Chemical Toxicology.[cclviii] The only difference in the two studies was that Monsanto's study lasted 90 days, and the French scientist study lasted 2 years.

The breed of rat was also shown to be the reason for pulling the study, as this breed of rat is prone to tumors. However, the French scientist used the same rat that Monsanto used to get their product approved originally. If he had used a different rat, the study would have been rejected due to lack of control. In addition, that same rat breed, same strain, is the exact rat used by National Institute of Health in long-term cancer rat studies.[cclix]

When retracted, the Editor in Chief of Food and Chemical Toxicology said they "found no evidence of fraud or international misrepresentation of the data." He stated that the reason for pulling the study was for inconclusive size (10 rats being too small) and the strain of rat, even though the study used the same number of rats and the same breed of rats.[cclx]

The publisher of Food and Chemical Toxicology is a member of The COPE (The Committee on Publications Ethics). The COPE says that only 4 reasons exist to retract a scientific article: 1) honest error or scientific misconduct, 2) prior publication, 3) plagiarism, and 4) unethical research.[cclxi]

The editor said that none of these reasons were used in the decision to pull the study.[cclxii]

More than 150 scientists subsequently signed a statement condemning the retraction, saying it was an attack on scientific integrity.

Even more importantly, in February of 2014, Environmental Health Perspectives, a publication associated with the NIH printed an editorial, signed by Lynn

Goldman, assistant administrator at the EPA, currently working at Johns Hopkins. It said, "Efforts to suppress scientific findings, or the appearance of such, erode the scientific integrity upon which the public trust relies. We feel the decision to retract a published scientific work by an editor against the desires of the authors because it is 'inconclusive based on a post hock [*sic*] analysis' represents a dangerous erosion of the underpinnings of the peer review process. [The publisher] should carefully reconsider this decision."[cclxiii]

Dr. Hansen says, "That suggests perhaps the reason it was retracted was because the Editor in Chief brought in a new editor to deal with issues like biotechnology, and that new editor is someone who used to work for and has gotten a fair amount of money from Monsanto and the other biotech seed companies."[cclxiv]

The European Union made an announcement in July of 2013 that they are starting a 2-year cancer feeding study, spending $4 million US dollars to investigate Roundup Ready corn, NK603, the same product Gilles-Eric Seralini exposed.[cclxv]

In October 2013, "There's No Scientific Consensus on GMO Safety" was released. This global document was signed by over 300 academics, scientists, physicians, and individuals representing the legality of safety and social aspect of GMOs. The document expresses strong rejections of claims by developers, saying that there is a scientific consensus on GMO safety.[cclxvi]

John Francis Queeny named his new business Monsanto in 1901 after his wife, Olga Mendez Monsanto. Monsanto has become symbolic, not for just greed, but for arrogance, scandal, and hardball business practices. Monsanto was heavily involved in the creation of the first nuclear bomb for the Manhattan Project during WWII in Dayton, Ohio.[cclxvii]

For the fiscal year of 2010, Monsanto reported $10.5 billion in sales with 27,600 employees.[cclxviii]

In recent years, they have received resistance. Monsanto withdrew its GM wheat in 2004 after receiving worldwide opposition.

A great deal of the opposition against GM wheat came from the canola crops in Canada that were being pollinated by Roundup Ready canola crops involuntarily. The Canadian Wheat Board was recently presented a report saying Monsanto has apparently changed its mind and again is attempting to commence cultivation of GM wheat. "'We're encouraged,' says Monsanto's Trish Jordan. 'There may be some opportunity for us to re-enter the wheat space'."[cclxix]

Most of our current food sources are in danger. Every single cell is like a spray bottle of insecticide, treating the environment that is our bodies. A bug bites into the food, causing intestinal permeability, and the toxin leaks into the bug's system and kills the bug. BT toxin comes from soil bacteria where it washes off and biodegrades. They take that gene and put it in the seed, says Jeffrey Smith, author of *Genetic Roulette, The Documented Health Risk of Genetically Engineered Foods* and *Seeds of Deception*.[cclxx]

Smith influenced US laws regulating GMO use, and is widely known as the "leading world expert on GMOs." He is the Executive Director at the Institute for Responsible Technology and the source behind the films *Hidden Dangers in Kids' Meals* and *Milk on Drugs, Just Say No.*

Smith goes on to say, "When it gets out of the intestinal walls it becomes pathogenic."[cclxxi]

Some say it is an area of great concern.

"Wheat is currently not genetically modified or genetically engineered[;] it is selectively bred to bring out certain traits," Smith says. Selective breeding makes our breads lighter and makes them rise higher.

Yet Monsanto is currently in the process of preparing wheat as a Roundup ready crop. "We believe they are changing the physiology in such a way that people become more reactive," leading to gluten sensitivities and allergies, Smith says.[cclxxii]

This will be added to the current GM crops of corn, soy, sugar beets, and alfalfa.

The Journal of Toxicology published a study in 2012 that proved that **BT toxin pokes holes in the human intestinal tracts and causes intestinal permeability**. Monsanto says that our digestive process negates the BT toxin and that it is not harmful to humans.[cclxxiii]

However, Sherbrooke University Hospital studied patients and found that **93% of pregnant women had BT toxin in their bloodstream and in the cord blood as well as the fetus. They found BT toxin in 2/3 of the non-pregnant women.**[cclxxiv]

It is no surprise to those in the natural clinical field that we are now seeing abdominal areas that are called Swiss Cheese where hernias are bulging through many holey areas. It is no surprise that hernias are on the rise overall. It is no shock that stomach acid imbalance is at an all-time high, that ulcers in the stomach have increased, that Ulcerative Colitis and so on, and so on, have escalated to record numbers.

Gastrointestinal disorders are being linked to GMOs causing intestinal permeability, known as Leaky Gut. The BT toxin is being blamed for poking holes into the intestines. Smith says, "If you eat a corn chip that has the gene that produces the toxin in the corn, if that gene ends up in your gut bacteria, transferring into the gut bacteria inside your intestines, that means it's producing BT toxin while inside your blood stream."[cclxxv]

Smith is saying that the current theory for people suffering with Leaky Gut is, "Their own gut bacteria [is] producing the BT toxin."[cclxxvi]

Another theory is that BT toxin present in the bloodstream is coming from the livestock eating the GM corn and soybeans. If we eat the livestock, we eat the toxin. The toxin enters our intestinal tract where it passes through intestinal ulcerations for patients with Leaky Gut, enters the blood stream, and goes directly to the umbilical cord where it is being detected.

Smith sites that 18% of celiac children have unidentified bacteria in their intestines. These bacteria are not supposed to be in the intestines. Even more shocking is that most of the bacteria has never been seen before.[cclxxvii]

This bad bacteria overgrowth is related to Leaky Gut and is blamed for causing celiac disease and autism. Bad bacteria overgrowth is dominating the good bacteria, which normally overrides the pathogens. When the good bacteria are killed off by pesticides within our food, the pathogens become prolific.

Butyrate is the fuel that builds a new lining on your intestines every 3 to 7 days. Butyrate is built by the fiber on vegetables. Studies have shown that low butyrate levels develop colon cancer.[cclxxviii]

"[There are] very few studies on GMOs in terms of health and safety. The FDA said no safety studies are necessary. This was because the person in charge of policy at the FDA when the policy was created completely lied about the studies on GMOs. Scientists where demanding more studies[,] saying it was different and dangerous[,] but Michael Taylor lied and sold it to the FDA as safe. He was a lawyer for Monsanto, the Vice President of Monsanto and [then went on to be] the Food Safety Czar at the FDA," Smith says.[cclxxix]

Taylor left his position during the following presidency in 2016.

Yet we still struggle with food that keeps us healthy. Livestock are consistently suffering illnesses in their intestinal tracts and respiratory systems, and are dying from GMO feed. "Livestock taken off GMOs [show] life threatening diarrhea disappears in two days[;] ulcers that were killing animals disappeared immediately," Smith remarks.[cclxxx]

To learn more about avoiding GMOs, go to Responsibletechnology.org to see the shopping guide that explains the 9 foods to avoid, or download the free app *shopnoGMO*.

Grass-fed cattle that can range freely on open pastures do not carry this risk. The safest meat to eat is grass-fed, grass-finished livestock. Currently, the law that accepts the label "grass-fed" allows the animal to be fed grass 50% of the time. The remainder of the time it can be GMO feed and still be labeled "grass-fed". To ensure the safest food, buy your "grass-fed, grass-finished" beef from a farmer you know and trust.

Hidden Toxicity

Toxicity is hidden in countless areas. It's important to study the things happening around you when illness just won't leave. The truth is, people are getting sick and some fingers are pointing at mold hidden in walls, perfumes, ice machines, added ingredients in foods that aren't listed on the label (including real food such as cuts of meat or coatings on vegetables), and preservatives. It's important to be aware so that toxicity can be managed. Doing your best is where we start. If healing isn't happening, looking for hidden toxicity may be necessary.

Since looking for hidden toxicity can drive a person over the edge, it's important to keep this information as important, but don't let it own you. Again, we generally only look for hidden toxicity when a person is on GAPS and doesn't begin to get well. The most common hidden toxicity is mold and heavy metal exposure. Mold can be found in the home or outside the home. Heavy metal exposure can be found in our food, air, water, and even our own mouths. Navigating these factors can be expensive, scary and emotionally traumatizing.

There are many factors we encounter daily that often aren't considered.

Ice

The Ice Man Cleaning Machine Services says, "Microbial growth can cause biofilm or 'slime' buildup inside commercial ice-making machines. Bacterial growth includes pathogens like Salmonella, Listeria, *E. coli*, Shigella, and the Norwalk virus."[cclxxxi]

The Joint Institute for Food Safety and Applied Nutrition says, "Once microbes grow into well-developed biofilms, cleaning and sanitation become[s] much more difficult. Biofilms have a shielding effect on the bacterial cells within them, and normal cleaning and sanitizing methods may not eliminate them."[cclxxxii]

Food regulation covers food contact surfaces.

Ice cubes are consumable and therefore need to come from a clean source.

"Clean and sanitize the ice machine every six months for efficient operation," says the Manitowoc Ice Machine Manual where they cover cleaning the machines over 8 lengthy pages of instructions. They further say, "The ice machine must be taken apart for cleaning and sanitizing."[cclxxxiii]

The Ice-O-Matic Manual also recommends cleaning every 6 months.[cclxxxiv]

Food Service Warehouse says, "Many commercial ice machines have antimicrobial protection built into the plastic used in the food-zone areas of ice production and are guaranteed to inhibit the growth of slime and mold for the life of the machine." Yet they also say that all machines should be cleaned every 6 months.[cclxxxv]

The Houston Department of Health and Human Services says that the culprit in ice machines is slime, "a type of mold or fungus that accumulates from bacterial growth on surfaces that are constantly exposed to clinging water droplets and warm temperatures."[cclxxxvi]

They go on to say, "If the residuals are left exposed and not wiped clean or the machine is not sanitized regularly, you will then see bacteria and mold growths in the moist, cool environment of your ice machine. Most times, slime will take on a pinkish tone; if left untreated, the pink will turn to red, green, brown and even black ropes of slime hanging from the freezer panels inside the machine."[cclxxxvii]

Consumerist.com recommends that restaurants should clean their ice machines twice weekly, a drastically different schedule than the manuals. They say, "Sanitize the interior and the lines using quaternary ammonium (QAC) at 200 parts per million. Wipe the condensation from the ice machine surfaces. Take a clean cloth, moisten it with sanitizer, wring it so it won't drip then wipe down the surface."[cclxxxviii]

The list of questions you ask your waiter is now getting longer: Is there MSG in this? Do you use high fructose corn syrup in that? Is there wheat in the ingredients? Now we should ask, "When was the last time you cleaned your ice machine?"

Consumers can and should demand a standard of clean food. Cleanliness is important to healthy eating as well as drinking. Cleaning an ice machine can be as simple as running a sanitizing solution through the cycle and then running two cycles of ice that you toss before running ice for ingesting.

This is also true for ice machines that live in your home freezer.

Ice is not the only victim. Any item manufactured in a machine that chills can fall subject to slimy mold growth. This includes Italian Ice, popsicles, and yogurt.

New York Daily News reported in December of 2013, "A U.S. Food and Drug Administration report says the Idaho State Department of Agriculture detected abnormalities in yogurt at a Chobani facility two months before the company issued a recall, but state officials say that's not true. "Over 300 customers reported getting sick from the yogurt." More than one Chobani recall has been made over the past five years.[cclxxxix]

Rely on your taste buds and your sense of smell. They are wonderful markers. The safest food is the food prepared in your own kitchen.

Dimethylpolysiloxane

Dimethylsiloxane is used in food as an anticaking agent, which keeps food from clumping. It is also used as an emulsifier, which assists in forming food together that normally wouldn't mix, like oil and water. Dimethylpolysiloxane also works in assisting foam formation.

Dimethylsiloxane is commonly used in adhesives, caulk, lubricants, sealants, anti-foaming agents, cosmetics, and food. It is a common ingredient in fast food.

In 1993, the FDA ordered testing of Dimethylsiloxane as it was proposed for use in testicular implants. No tests have been performed for using Dimethylsiloxane in food.

Propylene Glycol

Propylene glycol is used in food for many reasons. It is used to keep packaged foods moist (as a preservative), to keep ice cream soft enough to scoop, as lubrication in spice concentrates, and to blend foods that don't mix well with water.

The FDA has banned the use of propylene glycol in cat food, saying, "Propylene glycol in or on cat food has not been shown by adequate scientific data to be safe for use."[ccxc] It is still used in human foods.

Formaldehyde

Formaldehyde is used as a preservative and as a bleaching agent in food. It is commonly used with hydrated foods, vermicelli, chicken feet, and dried bean curd.

The Center for Food Safety, a Hong Kong Special Administrative Region, calls the use of formaldehyde in food "abuse".[ccxci]

Food scientist Dr. Woodrow Monte, in his book *While Science Sleeps, A Sweetener Kills*, refers to cancer as the hallmark of formaldehyde exposure. He says aspartame is "an artificial sweetener, containing methanol which is metabolized into deadly formaldehyde within the brain and sinew of all who consume it."[ccxcii]

Sodium Benzoate

Sodium benzoate is an inexpensive preservative that inhibits yeast, bacteria, and mold growth. It is commonly used in food manufacturing because it is the least expensive preservative available.

Sodium benzoate is a chemical preservative. When added to ascorbic acid (vitamin C), it forms benzene, which is a carcinogen.[ccxciii ccxciv ccxcv]

The Lancet reported a clinical trial registered with Current Controlled Trials (registration number ISRCTN74481308) which says, "Artificial colors or a sodium benzoate preservative (or both) in the diet result in increased hyperactivity."[ccxcvi]

Ironically, this chemical preservative is being used to treat autism.[ccxcvii]

Eating a diet filled with nutrient-dense foods is the goal. We are not designed to crave sugar, caffeine, or bread products. We are designed to be simply hungry. Craving these types of foods is a sign of nutrient deficiencies, cured by a nutrient-dense diet.

Transglutaminase

Meat glue, a product linked to ADHD behaviors, dementia, and other diseases, is known to many chefs and meat processors as a common ingredient used to take lesser cuts of meats and glue them together for resale as a higher cut of meat.[ccxcviii] Briefly put, transglutaminase, or meat glue, bonds any food containing protein. It is currently used in meats (including chicken and beef), fish, dairy products, and bakery items.

Currently, there is a part per million (ppm) allowance for transglutaminase for processed cheese, hard cheese, cream cheese, yogurt, frozen desserts, vegetable protein dishes, and meat substitutes. This is in addition to meat and seafood items.

Correspondence with the Office of Premarket Approval at the FDA says that the approved amount of transglutaminase for "Eaters Only" was categorized for the sum total consumption as 12 mg/person/day (12 milligrams per person per day).

The process of using meat glue is simple: take otherwise discarded meat pieces, coat them with meat glue, mix together well, roll the meat product in a sheet of cling wrap, and refrigerate overnight. The result is a new cut of meat made from lesser cuts of meat that is unrecognizable as an impostor. When you pull on the meat, it does not separate and responds as a normal piece of muscle tissue. When cut, the meat responds exactly like a piece of meat not using meat glue. In fact, the meat-glued product looks, feels, responds, cooks, and tastes exactly like the cut of meat it is pretending to be—the difference goes unnoticed even to professional chefs.

Transglutaminase (TG) is legally referred to as a protein cross-linking agent. Meat glue is described as a naturally occurring enzyme in plants, animals, and bacteria. Use of the product is considered normal, just as any enzyme in cooking is normal, like starches to brew beer or rennet to make cheese.[ccxcix]

C & P Additives, producer of transglutaminase, lists on their website the benefits of using TSG in food products as:

Texture improvement
Meat bonding
Elasticity increase and improvement
Standard size quality
Yield increasing
Cost reduction (ingredients)
Creation of new products[ccc]

Transglutaminase is also produced as Biobond by Shanghai Kinry Food Ingredients Co., Ltd.

In the '60s, transglutaminase was extracted from the livers of guinea pigs. In 1989, Ajinomoto, a Japanese company famous for producing MSG, took transglutaminase through further testing and commercialized transglutaminase for human consumption as Activa. Today, transglutaminase comes from pig or cow blood but can also be plant-based. It can be purchased through Amazon by anyone and added to any food.

Nils Norén, the Vice President of Culinary and Pastry Arts at the International Culinary Center says, "Some studies have shown that stomach enzymes have difficulty breaking down proteins after they have been bonded by TG."[ccci]

He goes on to say, "When TG-ases are improperly regulated in the body, they are associated with plaques in the brains of Alzheimer's, Parkinson's, and Huntington's patients as well as in the development of cataracts in the eyes, arteriosclerosis (hardening of the arteries), various skin disorders, etc."[cccii]

With this information, Norén does not associate these issues with the consumption of transglutaminase but sees it as a problem with the body not regulating the transglutaminase it manufactures itself.[ccciii]

The FDA considers transglutaminase a GRAS (Generally Recognized as Safe) status.

Interestingly, when the meat glue is bonding it produces a molecule of ammonia.

This ammonia is seen in the cooking world as an aid. Different forms of transglutaminase have an unrefrigerated shelf life. The rule of thumb for chefs for testing to see if your meat glue is still good to use is to glue a few pieces of meat together and smell the meat while it is still moist. If the meat smells like a wet wool sweater or wet dog, it is still good. This smell comes from the ammonia.[ccciv] [cccv]

The New York State Department of Health, in a document describing ammonia under the subheading of "Chemical Terrorism" says, "Ammonia is also produced naturally from decomposition of organic matter, including plants, animals and animal wastes." Chefs are encouraged by Cookingissues.com to use plastic wrap as "the plastic wrap technique is great because there are no rules regulating its use, and it is simple, fast and cheap; foods can be cooked in water directly in the plastic wrap."[cccvi]

Meat glue cooking kits can be bought through mail order for under $40 and contain enough meat glue to adhere 36-40 pounds of meat.

Transglutaminase is also used as a tenderizer.

Ideas in Food, a book about transglutaminase with recipes, says, "Efficiency can be improved with the addition of gelatin, caseinate, potassium chloride, and fiber, and these ingredients are sometimes added to transglutaminase blends to facilitate the bonding process. Salt and phosphates also increase the effectiveness of transglutaminase by increasing the availability of salt-soluble proteins."[cccvii]

The addition of caseinate is highly concerning as many people today suffer from casein intolerance; celiac patients and children with autism are primary victims. The difficulty in avoiding casein is navigable through the elimination of milk products such as cheese, ice cream, or yogurt. When products such as medicine gel caps are added to the product list containing casein, the puzzle gets more complicated. Now, knowing that meat and fish also contain casein, the puzzle is not only mind boggling – it's disheartening.[cccviii]

Researchers are finding large amounts of transglutaminase, meat glue, in diseased tissues within the body. This is especially true with cataracts, rashes, and herpetiformis, a highly itchy, chronic rash composed of bumps and blisters that last a long time, according to Medline Plus.[cccix]

Homeopaths often say that this is the body's way of responding during detox. The body is trying to push out the toxic substance forming these responses.

Transglutaminase must be noted as an ingredient on a food label. It can be listed in many forms including: transglutaminase, TG enzyme, enzyme, or TGP enzyme. If a product uses meat glue, the label should also read *formed* or *reformed*, saying things like "formed beef tenderloin". The challenge for the average consumer is that a formed beef tenderloin with enzyme in the ingredient list can easily be read over as safe, even by foodies.

Meat glue underwent some drastic criticism from consumers, most specifically from consumers with celiac disease. The same issues affecting celiac patients affect some children with hyperactivity or other behavioral issues. The manufacturer of meat glue, Ajinomoto, responded by saying that eating meat glue is the same as eating compounds occurring naturally from cooking meat or fish. They added that transglutaminase is a safe product for people diagnosed with celiac disease.

The Truth in Labeling Campaign stepped forward and began researching and testing. They found that many people who have celiac disease have intestinal issues with MSG. Some protease enzymes produce MSG as they break down proteins. Ajinomoto is the founder of MSG. Celiac patients also have issues with Maltodextrin and Sodium Caseinate, which are both ingredients in some of the meat glue products that can contain MSG, even though MSG is not on the ingredient list.

Again, as an ingredient, it can simply read: enzyme.[cccx]

This generates one massive issue in organism growth. The outside cut of meat comes in contact with many surfaces, grabbing hold of potential bacteria. Those outer sides of meat are formed together and are now in the inner slice of the meat after being formed with meat glue. If that cut of meat is not fully cooked on the inside, leaving the inside more tender, the now prolific bacteria are eaten. This could be a possible invitation to E. coli as well as other bacteria.

The University of Rochester Medical Center says, "Tissue transglutaminase is an enzyme that repairs damage in the body. People with celiac disease often make antibodies that attack tissue transglutaminase. They are called anti-tissue transglutaminase antibodies, or immunoglobin A (IgA) antibodies. Therefore, a blood test that shows higher levels of anti-tissue transglutaminase antibodies can help your doctor figure out if you have celiac disease."[cccxi]

This poses the question of why people with celiac disease are having issues with meat glue if it is an enzyme that repairs damage in the body.

Transglutaminase also appears to affect the gliadin process, which is the stretchy aspect of wheat flours. This specifically would cause damage to a person with celiac.[cccxii]

Feldhues, a company from western Germany that now operates out of Ireland, specializes in children's character meat with fun shapes like clowns, trains, bunnies, bright suns, and happy bears. Fun food for children is not the goal.

The human intestinal tract normally contains tissue transglutaminase, which is part of the transglutaminase enzyme family. The challenge is that the form of transglutaminase found in meat glue is different from the transglutaminase found in the human intestinal tract. "In celiac disease, our systems make antibodies to our own tissue transglutaminase enzyme, causing our immune systems to attack our intestinal linings," says Jane Anderson, a guide on celiac and gluten sensitivities.[cccxiii]

An article entitled "Transglutaminase treatment of wool fabrics lead to resistance to detergent damage," and published in the *Journal of Biotechnology*, Volume 116, Issue 4, 6 April 2005, Pages 379–386, discussed damage to and rehabilitation of wool fabrics. They used transglutaminase not for food, not for transforming food, but for "distinct biochemical properties, for their ability to protect wool fabrics from the chemical and enzymic damage caused by common household detergents."[cccxiv]

Eating meat sourced from a local farmer raising grass-fed cattle is best. Preparing fresh food at home is optimal.

Chapter 3:

Stage Two

Stage Two, like all stages, keeps the previous foods, but adds more advanced foods. Adding foods creates variety and adds nutrition. The more foods a person eats, the less likely they are to go off protocol, as they don't feel deprived. Stage Two is the most detoxing stage. Some people stay on Stage Two for a few days; others stay for a year, or a bit longer.

In Stage Two we add:

• Pastured eggs, starting with the yolks first in Stage Two, and then going to the egg white in Stage Two, for those who show great sensitivity to the white it can be added at Stage Three.[cccxv] Yolks are most nutritious eaten raw, added to warm soup. When whites are added, they are soft boiled so that they are cooked. For many folks egg whites can be an issue, often due to heavy metals in the body. Be mindful of reactions when adding the whites.

• Food probiotic brine and commercial probiotics are increased in dosage on Stage Two.

• Green beans are added. String beans have a very fibrous string that is difficult to digest and not GAPS-approved. Green beans are extremely easy to grow at home in pots or in a small patch of soil.

• Freshly picked herbs.

• Celery root is added, cooked in soups.[cccxvi]

• Lemon juice is added at Stage Two. Dr. Natasha says, "That's all right with the lemon, that's OK. I would not do it from Stage One, I would do it from Stage Two. Just juice, lemon juice, squeezed from fresh lemon."[cccxvii]

• Nutritional yeast can be added in Stage Two.[cccxviii] It adds a cheesy taste but is not tolerated by all. When introducing nutritional yeast, watch for adverse symptoms, which are often yeast related in nature. This can include the flaring of skin rashes or yeast infections. Nutritional yeast is what Dr. Natasha recommends when B6 and magnesium are needed, saying, "I would do it from Stage Two. I find it's the best B12, B vitamin group supplement. And Kombucha, of course, and liver."[cccxix]

• Ginger cooked in soups and eaten, as tolerated, can be added.[cccxx]

• Italian Casserole is a more advanced form of cooking introduced in Stage Two. The recipe for Italian Casserole is listed in the GAPS book recipe section. Italian Casserole is cooked by putting any raw meat or joint pieces with any Stage One vegetable into a casserole pan, add water to fill the pan 2/3 of the way full, add salt, peppercorns, and sprigs of fresh herbs, if desired. Put the lid on the dish and cook it in the oven with the lid on. Cook at roughly 300 degrees for five to six hours. Vegetables can be added in the last 40 minutes of cooking if preferred. This can make a Turkey Casserole, Pigeon Casserole, Venison Casserole, Chicken Casserole, or any other meat casserole.

Dr. Natasha says Italian Casseroles cooked in the oven "can be either, with a lid or not. Without the lid the top of the meat will be brown, give those bits to somebody else in the family, but a person on the 2nd stage should not eat browned meat yet."[cccxxi] Cooking without the lid should only be tried after cooking in the oven with the lid.

• Meat stews are also added to the rotation of food.

• Animal fat intake should be increased. Ghee should be added if it has not been already. Properly fermented whey, yogurt, sour cream, or kefir should be increased, as tolerated.

• Gravlax and other homemade fermented fishes are also added in Stage Two.

- In Stage Two, we can begin cooking liver pate by cooking liver in a pan, swimming in butter or ghee, with onions, garlic, and lemon juice.[cccxxii]

- GAPS Shakes are also added on Stage Two.[cccxxiii] GAPS Shakes help to lubricate the bowel through increased bile flow. They are reported to gently massage the gallbladder while opening the bile ducts. "Fat in stools means that not enough bile is being released from the gallbladder to emulsify fats. The most common reason in GAPS patients is gallstones. A gallstone is a clump of infection or a fragment of a worm, coated by bile: this is a defense reaction the liver has, when pathogens get into the bile ducts," Dr. Natasha says.[cccxxiv]

Fat in the stool is often recognized by noting stools that float. This is not a point of concern as it adjusts in time as the microbiome repairs.

Parasites can also cause a struggling gallbladder.

A struggling gallbladder can cause a person to feel nauseous or vomit when they eat more fat than the gallbladder can process. Feeling nauseous or vomiting after eating fats is just the body's way of telling you to support the gallbladder and work on gallstones.

McBride goes on to say, "[When] the liver does not get enough stimulation to empty the bile into the duodenum, the bile stones stay in the bile ducts too long and become calcified. As the stones accumulate calcium salts on their surface, they get larger and their surface becomes hard and rough, so they cannot be easily passed through the bile ducts."[cccxxv]

These stones build and grow in the liver and gallbladder. As they grow, they block the bile ducts and bile is not passed through into the intestines. This leads to inadequate digestion of fats.

A GAPS shake is fresh-pressed juice from a juicer (discussed further in the Stage Four section) with a large dollop or two of home-brewed sour cream and one or two yolks from pastured chicken eggs. The juice should be comprised of 50% organic green apple as the malic acid in the apple assists in softening gallstones. The remainder of the juice should be organic greens and 5% organic beet, according to Dr. Natasha's recommendation.

Dr. Natasha says the reason for a small portion of beet is "because beet is too powerful. It can make you nauseous if you put too much. It can make you vomit. It can really make you feel sick because it really cleanses – very powerful."cccxxvi

If you don't have the nausea or the vomiting, Dr. Natasha says, "I would build it up gradually. You can have up to one beet root per one quart of juice."cccxxvii

This author's favorite juice is 50% organic kale, one organic lemon and two small organic green apples with one or two dollops of home brewed sour cream and one or two pastured yolks.

If you cannot do GAPS shakes due to the sour cream, coconut oil is recommended as a substitute.

Drink the juice within 30 minutes of juicing as it loses its nutritional value quickly. The sooner you drink after juicing, the more nutrition is retained.

Yolks

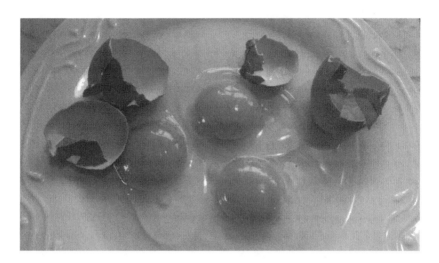

Organic eggs, vegetarian-fed eggs, free-range eggs, cage-free eggs, and pastured eggs are all very different products.

Organic eggs come from chickens that are fed organic grains. These chickens are raised in a chicken house, without sunlight or fresh air. They are often stacked in cages with enough chickens in each cage to fill the space.

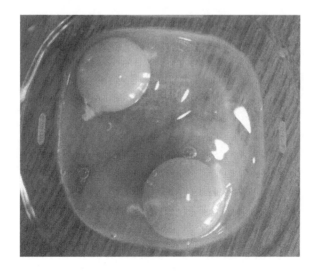

Vegetarian eggs are in the same situation; however, they are fed high starch vegetables such as corn and soy. The above picture is from chickens on pasture, fed vegetarian feed.

Free-range eggs mean that the chickens are in the same situation but have free range of an appendage.

Cage-free chicken eggs come from chickens that are kept in a chicken house, but they are not kept in cages; instead they are all tightly packed into the space.

Chickens in these situations often die due to the conditions. They are frequently kicked by workers to move them about and, when they pass away, are often ground into food to be fed to other chickens or tossed into the dumpster.

Pastured chicken eggs come from chickens that roam outside on green grass where they eat grass and bugs. This is the diet chickens would have in the wild. These chickens often die due to predators such as coyotes, raccoons, opossum, or hawks. Farmers often raise companion animals that protect chickens from predators. Pasture-raised chicken eggs are the most natural and most highly praised.

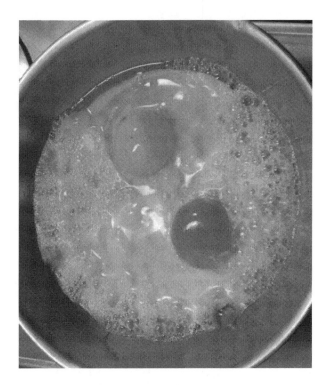

The above eggs are from chickens on pasture. The lighter colored yolk is from chickens that are not supplemented with additional feed; the darker orange yolk is from chickens supplemented with raw organ meat. Pastured chickens, eating bugs, worms, and grass, will always have varying colors because some chickens eat different food, according to what they locate; some find tick nests, and others find different worms.

Building an Egg Tolerance

As with all GAPS-approved food, doing a sensitivity test, as described in the GAPS book, is advised on protocol. This sensitivity test is described in the book and includes putting some of the food on the wrist and watching for a negative response.

Some people have issues with egg intolerance. The sensitivity test should be used in this case. For many people with an egg intolerance, switching the egg source to a cleaner egg, one that eats bugs and worms out on grass all day, is all that is needed. For others, they need to get more extreme. A lot of people who have an intolerance to eggs actually have an intolerance to the white, not the yolk.

Egg Introductory Schedule

If clean, pastured chicken yolks are not tolerated, it is recommended to back up to duck eggs. If they are not tolerated, it is recommended to back up to quail eggs. When testing, it is recommended to start with the toothpick method, sticking the toothpick into the center of the yolk, away from the white. Once you can touch the center of the yolk with the toothpick and touch your soup with no negative symptoms, you're ready to stay steady and continue. Slow and steady wins the race.

Egg yolks are referred to as the most nutrient-dense food known to man; they are also easily absorbable, next to human breast milk. They are off-the-charts nourishing and high in vitamin A, vitamin D, choline, zinc, and others. Since they are so nourishing, they will nourish the body, making it stronger. This will allow the body to kick out the toxins all on its own. For this reason, there can very well be die-off with yolks. Going slowly is important for some.

There is no need to limit the number of yolks on Stage Two if they are fully tolerated. The more yolks that are eaten, the more nutrition will be delivered to the body. The more nutrition delivered to the body, the stronger the body will be. The stronger the body is, the faster it heals.

Acupuncturist Kenneth Moorhead read the book Factory Farming when he was seven years old. It profoundly moved him. He said, "One of the things it describes is there's only one-twelfth the nutrition in a store egg than there was in a country egg."[cccxxviii]

Low nutrition and unnatural foods cause inflammation.

"When you're in chronic inflammation you're in chronic toxin retention," says Christopher Shade, PhD of Quicksilver Scientific, LLC. in his presentation "The Human Detoxification System," aired by the Silicon Valley Health Institute.[cccxxix]

Shade received his PhD in mercury.

Shade says that when a person gets a pronounced Herxheimer Effect or die-off, it's because the detoxification system is broken.[cccxxx]

The body has two main ways to detox: cellular detoxification and drainage. Cellular detoxification is where toxins are taken from the cell and delivered on the exit train, the lymph system and the blood. Drainage comes from the blood and lymph through the kidney, liver, intestinal tract, and skin.[cccxxxi]

Shade says detoxification and inflammation are sort of a teeter totter. When one is up, the other is down and vice versa. He says, "Detoxification is part of your antioxidant system. Inflammation is part of a predominantly pro-oxidant system. Inflammation is where something comes in, eats you, and you respond to kill it with pro-oxidants: you're making bleach; you're making peroxide; you're making peroxyl radicals. When you're doing that, you're turning down detoxification."[cccxxxii]

Therefore, when there is a chronic situation involving inflammation, toxin overload develops – they can't get out; their exit door is blocked.

"Glutathione isn't there just to move mercury out of your system – or cadmium or other toxins. It's a big regulator. Glutathione controls Th1, Th2 responses to your immune system. When the glutathione goes down, you start hosting viruses. You've got herpes 1, 2, 3 just sort of wandering through your system; you begin rejecting a lot of food, becoming intolerant," Shade says.[cccxxxiii]

When the system begins to break down, it holds on to the garbage. As this garbage builds up, it stresses the body further. The liver becomes overloaded in the process. The situation further develops as the liver is overloaded, and the lungs become burdened.

Supporting the breakdown is the only effective long-term solution.

Shade says, "For the transport proteins to work, to actively transport nutrients in and actively transport toxins out, they need fluidity of the membrane. There can't be damage to the membrane."[cccxxxiv]

This membrane is what connects the processes in the tract.

"An adequate supply of essential phospholipids is going to allow fluidity of the membrane because all those transport proteins actually allow the movement in and out. They need that fluidity. You can't have oxidatively damaged proteins; you need to be rebuilding them all the time," he says. "Incidentally, the best way to get the highest source of phosphatidylcholine is raw egg yolks."[cccxxxv]

Phosphatidylcholine assists in proper liver function, maintains mental sharpness, including age-related decline, and promotes healthy skin elasticity.

Hepatobiliary Surgery and Nutrition says, "The intestinal microbiota produces TMA (trimethylamine) from dietary quaternary amines, like choline and L-carnitine, as well as from phosphatidylcholine."[cccxxxvi]

They go on to say, "Species of *Bacteroidetes* (particularly *B. thetaiotaomicron* and *B. fragilis*) may be involved in TMA formation, since they exhibit phospholipases hydrolyzing dietary phosphatidylcholine to choline. Moreover, it is reported that bacteria from the class of *Erysipelotrichia* (*phylum Firmicutes*) can produce TMA from choline. These evidences may be of great interest if we consider that *Bacteroidetes* and *Firmicutes* are the two main bacterial phyla among intestinal flora."[cccxxxvii]

Yolks should be eaten from pastured chickens that eat bugs, worms, and grass. As these chickens are outside, they soak up the sunshine, creating yolks rich in vitamins A and D. These nutrients are essential to repair.

Dr. McBride says, "Leaky gut and malabsorption are the typical results of vitamin A deficiency."cccxxxviii

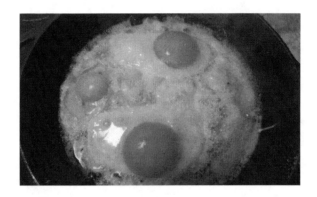

A science fair project was done in 2015 by an eighth grader in Chattanooga, Tennessee. The project included 20 chickens fed different types of feed: vegetarian feed, free-ranging vegetarian feed, free-ranging and foraging, free-ranging with non-GMO feed and raw organ meat feed.cccxxxix

His main objective was to show the obvious lack of nutrition in eggs fed vegetarian feed—because chickens aren't vegetarians.

The young man who did the project was a chicken lover if ever there was one. His school breaks didn't include getting a drink like normal people; he would go to visit the chickens. He talked to them; he named them; he even rode his bike with them on his handlebars. He is called the chicken whisperer. When he found out that store-bought chickens are fed vegetarian feed, he was baffled and said, "Chickens aren't vegetarians. Why would they feed chickens food they aren't meant to eat?"cccxl

In the desire to learn something, he went on an investigation mission. He studied the yolks and appearance, consistency, fluency, cooking response, and nutritional value. What he found was shady.

What should have happened was that the vegetarian-fed yolks would be pale in color, lacking vitamins A and D and other nutrients from the diet not designed for chickens. The vegetarian free-rangers should have had darker yolks, the free ranging non-GMO feed a bit darker, the free-ranging and foraging darker still, and the raw organ meat-fed chickens the darkest yolks.

The problem was that the vegetarian fed yolks were almost the same in color as the raw organ meat yolks – a deep vibrant orange. To find some answers, he picked up the phone and called the companies. After 3 companies were contacted, he found that they were all fed corn and soy, no matter if the eggs were labeled vegetarian or not. Since all their yolk colors were different, there was more to the story. Yes, the type of chicken house makes a difference – if they are in cages, or if they are roaming a dirt floor shoulder to shoulder, or if they are outside on pasture. But these yolks he tested, the yolks that competed with his raw organ meat-fed chickens, were from chickens in chicken houses. They were not basking in the sun. They were not eating ticks and worms along with grass and weeds.[cccxli]

He further researched the reason for the intensity of the yolk color and found that a lot of store-bought eggs have been manipulated to give them darker and more vibrant yolks.[cccxlii]

Apparently, back to 1966, people were doing experiments on this very same subject. *Poultry Science* published an article about adding carotenoids to chicken feed to change the color of their yolks to a darker yellow, "β-Cryptoxanthin biofortified maize increased β-Cryptoxanthin in the yolk and contributed to yolk color."[cccxliii]

Feeding the chickens dark colored carrots or tomato paste made the yolks darker and more vibrant, appealing in color.[cccxliv]

Feeding the chickens dark orange colored marigolds resulted in darker yolks, but the eggs were smaller for an unknown reason.[cccxlv]

Putting red pepper powder and pigment in the feed increased the weight and color intensity of the eggs.

Flax seed is a carotenoid (xanthophyll), but it lightened the color of the egg yolks. Since the companies were not looking for lighter yolks, as darker yolks are favored since they reflect more nutritious yolks in free-ranging chickens, flax was dropped from the feed, while the colored feed was emphasized to increase yolk color.[cccxlvi]

He found that the major chicken egg companies feed darker colored corn and soy to their chickens to get a darker and more vibrant yolk, in order to make it more appealing to the consumers.[cccxlvii]

Companies have been trying to manipulate the yolk color for years, using colored food methods as well as visible light spectrophotometer.[cccxlviii]

The *Journal of the Science of Food and Agriculture* reported that supplementing the feed of egg-laying hens with colored carrots efficiently increased yolk color parameters and carotenoid contents; this gives opportunities for improved nutritional value of eggs from forage material-supplemented hens.[cccxlix]

Journal of Lipids reported that the use of dark colored marigolds (*Tagetes erecta L.*) was reported to be a good source of xanthophylls and used for pigmentation of the egg yolks and poultry skin.

Xanthophylls are typical yellow pigments of leaves, oxygenated carotenoids.[cccl]

Asian-Australian Journal of Animal Science reported that the results of the present experiments indicate that dietary inclusion of both red pepper powder and pigment were successful in increasing the egg yolk score of laying hens, which would make these eggs more attractive to potential consumers. Neither product produced any negative effects on laying hen productivity, and both products tended to increase the weight of the eggs from treated hens.[cccli]

Poultry Science showed that adding flax to these diets seemed to depress yolk lutein content.[ccclii]

Journal of Agricultural and Food Chemistry showed that yolks from hens fed orange maize had scores indicating a darker, orange color.[cccliii]

Although he set out to show that proper nourishing feed would cause a darker yolk, reflecting a higher nutritional value, the child doing the science fair project found that manipulating the feed with tomato paste, colored marigolds, red pepper flakes, dark orange carrots and colored corn was by far cheaper. He thought it was sneaky, the work of a charlatan.

Lesson learned.

Chickens roaming free on pasture throughout the day do not have eggs of equal nutrition to store-bought eggs.

The deeper orange color shows higher vitamin D and A levels. The color variation doesn't often look different until you look at them side-by-side.

GAPS Shake

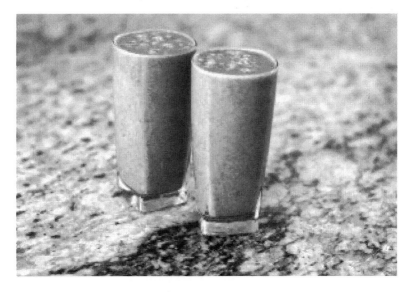

GAPS Shakes are also added on Stage Two. GAPS Shakes help to lubricate the bowel through increased bile flow. They are reported to gently massage the gallbladder while opening up the bile ducts. "Fat in stools means that not enough bile is being released from the gallbladder to emulsify fats. The most common reason in GAPS patients is gallstones. A gallstone is a clump of infection or a fragment of a worm, coated by bile: this is a defense reaction the liver has, when pathogens get into the bile ducts," Dr. Natasha says.[ccliv]

Fat in the stool is often recognized with stools that float. For most people, this is not a point of concern as it adjusts in time as the microbiome repairs. Dr. Natasha says that floating stools are not a concern and should not be used as a determining factor to lessen animal fat intake.[cclv]

Parasites can also cause a struggling gallbladder.

A struggling gallbladder can cause a person to feel nauseous or vomit when they eat more fat than the gallbladder can process. Feeling nauseous or vomiting after eating fats is just the body's way of telling you to support the gallbladder and work on gallstones.

McBride goes on to say, "[When] the liver does not get enough stimulation to empty the bile into the duodenum, the bile stones stay in the bile ducts too long and become calcified. As the stones accumulate calcium salts on their surface, they get larger and their surface becomes hard and rough, so they cannot be easily passed through the bile ducts."ccclvi

These stones grow in the liver and gallbladder. As they grow, they block the bile ducts and bile is not passed through into the intestines. This leads to inadequate digestion of fats.

A GAPS shake is fresh-pressed juice from a juicer with a large dollop or two of home-brewed sour cream and one or two yolks from pastured chicken eggs. The egg white can be used, as tolerated or desired. The juice should be comprised of 50% organic green apple as the malic acid in the apple assists in softening gallstones. The remainder of the juice should be organic greens and 5% organic beet, according to Dr. Natasha's recommendation.

Dr. Natasha says that the reason for a small portion of beet is "because beet is too powerful. It can make you nauseous if you put too much. It can make you vomit. It can really make you feel sick because it really cleanses – very powerful."ccclvii

If you don't have the nausea or the vomiting, Dr. Natasha says, "I would build it up gradually. You can have up to one beet root per one quart of juice."v

This author's favorite juice is 50% organic kale, one organic lemon, and two small organic green apples, with one or two dollops of home-brewed sour cream and one or two pastured yolks. If you cannot do GAPS shakes due to the sour cream, coconut oil is recommended as a substitute.

Drink the juice within 30 minutes of juicing as it loses its nutritional value quickly. The sooner you drink after juicing, the more nutrition is retained.

GAPS Shakes are best on an empty stomach, once or twice daily.

Russian Custard

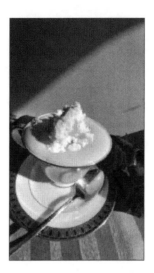

Russian Custard is a satisfying and satiating dish that will cause any cravings to be smothered. It is deeply nourishing, replenishing vitamin A deficiencies, vitamin D deficiencies, zinc deficiencies, and choline deficiencies, as well as many others. Russian Custard has been around for centuries. Martha Washington has a recipe for Orange Fool, which was orange flavored Russian Custard, in her cookbook. It can be made in a countless number of ways such as whipping it with a whisk, mixing it in a mixer, and blending it in a blender. The recipe is easy and leaves no hunger for hours.

For two to three servings, use:

　7 pastured egg yolks
　2 teaspoons local honey
　1 teaspoon vanilla

First, separate the yolks from the egg whites and place all the yolks in a blender or stand up mixer. The whites can be used later for meringue cookies.

With a blender, use the lowest speed or the next speed up until the yolks turn a soft, yellow-whitish color and become thick (emulsified). This usually takes roughly 20 minutes.

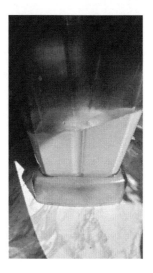

If using a mixer, set it to a medium speed for roughly 20 minutes. The result will be generally fluffier.

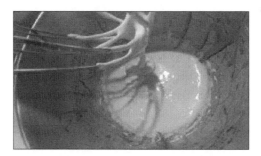

The custard can be flavored for variety. Add a bit of orange, lemon, or lime juice. Pour the ingredients into a beautiful cup and enjoy.

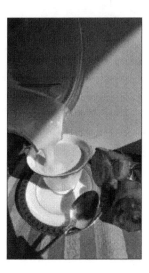

The color can vary due to several factors - number of yolks, color of yolks, time blended; all of these variations are fine.

Russian Custard can be eaten as is, or topped with whipped fermented cream or whipped cream, if tolerated. It can be served at room temperature or frozen – both are delicious.

Adrenal Support Stock

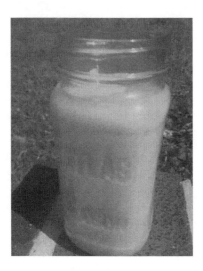

When the adrenals are blown, support is vital to function. Adrenal fatigue is growing more and more common. When someone suffers from advanced Adrenal Fatigue, that person spends the great portion of the day in bed, having no reserve of energy as well as no immediately available energy. The adrenals and thyroid gland work in a supportive fashion, meaning that when one is struggling, the other is pulled down, also.

For the adrenal-compromised person, all they can think is: *I'm so tired.*

Supporting the adrenals can be done through adrenal cortex, which, for most, only works for two months. It can also be done through adrenal supportive herbs. However, nothing works better than specific, cholesterol-rich foods, which support the adrenals on all levels. The Adrenal Shake, a shake made of yolks, home-brewed sour cream, and grass-fed butter, is a priority for supporting the adrenals; but the Adrenal Support Stock is an alternative that is warming and lighter in fare. Each can be a nourishing breakfast that will support sluggish adrenals to help the person function.

Pour one cup of Meat Stock over the amount of tolerated yolks, stir, and enjoy.

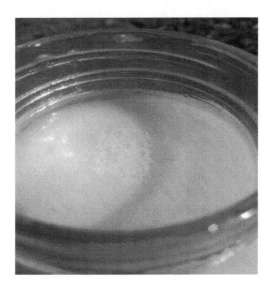

Adrenal Support Shake

This recipe is a Weston A. Price Foundation Recipe of the Month Winner, May 2018

To make the Adrenal Shake, crack open a dozen pastured yolks into a pint and a half Mason jar. This will make a cup of yolks. Yolks are highly nourishing, which will make the body stronger and cause it to kick out toxins or parasites. This can cause die-off, so yolks should be built slowly until tolerated.

Adrenal fatigue comes in four stages, each depicting the level of exhaustion for the person. Many things can cause adrenal fatigue, including an acute stressful event, pesticide consumption (which includes GMO foods), heavy metal toxicity, and an overloaded lifestyle without a supportive nutritional diet to compensate.

In an interview with Stephanie Seneff, Dr. Daniel Pompa asked how Glyphosate negatively impacts the adrenals. Dr. Seneff says, "Glyphosate is extremely damaging to the mitochondria (located inside our cells) where our body makes ATP energy. Mitochondria must be healthy and functioning in order to fix damaged cells, and if we don't have healthy, thriving mitochondria we experience exhaustion."[ccclviii]

Seneff is a senior research scientist at MIT and a leading expert on the damages of Glyphosate. She says, "The cell membrane of the mitochondria needs a good storehouse of cholesterol sulfate. But, if glyphosate has destroyed cholesterol sulfate stores, then our mitochondria will experience ion leaks (ATP is lost) and our energy flags. What's more, Glyphosate disrupts the production of DHEA sulfate, testosterone sulfate and cortisone sulfate in the adrenal glands, compromising proper hormone balance."[ccclix]

Stage one adrenal fatigue includes an overall state of alertness, but the sleep is not sound. Possible moments of depleted energy exist. They are often loaded with energy as they are pumping out adrenalin at a high rate. Most folks with stage one adrenal fatigue just push through, not even noticing there is an adrenal issue until they look back on the situation.

Stage two adrenal fatigue is a greater pronouncement of the wired but tired feeling; people in this category generally rely on coffee to make it through the day. They desire the flood of energy they had in stage one adrenal fatigue. They are tired. Their thoughts revolve around being tired. Their obligations in life are pared down so there is less drain. The desire to spend personal time with their spouse is depleted. Falling in bed at the end of the day is normal; exhaustion is normal.

Stage three adrenal fatigue is associated with the adrenals having burned out; depletion is the new normal. In this stage, people function throughout the day but are consumed with exhaustion and have no energy once they get home. They take naps to get through the day. Exercising doesn't energize them – it depletes them. They are just so tired all of the time. The desire to spend personal time with their spouse is nearly non-existent.

Stage four adrenal fatigue exists where there is a depletion of cortisol levels, no desire to spend personal time with your spouse, complete exhaustion, an inappropriate, emotionally downward spiral when encountering confrontation, shakiness with a greater demand on the adrenals, inability to fall asleep, and apathy for life events in general. There are no energy stores – just complete exhaustion. Usually the person cannot get out of bed, and if they do it's just to use the bathroom or possibly to throw together a bite to eat. They often tear up due to utter exhaustion.

Meanwhile, some professionals claim adrenal fatigue doesn't exist as stated by *BMC Endocrine Disorders*, published August 2016, displayed on the NIH.[ccclx]

However, the NIH also displays evidence to the contrary from *Alternative Medicine Reviews* regarding Adrenal Fatigue, saying, "Non-pharmaceutical approaches have much to offer such patients. This article focuses on the use of nutrients and botanicals to support the adrenals, balance neurotransmitters, treat acute anxiety, and support restful sleep."[ccclxi]

In early 2013, the *International Journal of Pharmaceutical Compounding* said that supporting adrenal fatigue can be done through several channels.[ccclxii]

The GAPS Protocol shows great success in supporting the adrenals so that the body can repair itself. However, support according to what the body requires is important.

The greater the fatigue is, the longer it takes to recover; however, supporting the adrenals properly can be done. Many people are spending the time it takes to allow the body to heal when it is supported correctly.

Rebuilding adrenals with the GAPS Protocol includes certain basics. Dr. Natasha says that adrenals love cholesterol, adrenals love salt, and adrenals need sleep.[ccclxiii]

This Adrenal Support Shake is an easy meal or snack to support the adrenals on two of these three needs.

12 pastured yolks
1/2 cup grass-fed butter
1 cup home-brewed sour cream
A handful of frozen berries (if you are Stage Five) or 2-3 tablespoons of
      lime juice
1 teaspoon of mineral salt

To make the Adrenal Support Shake, put 12 pastured yolks in a blender and blend on low to emulsify. This can take a few minutes or over twenty minutes, whichever you prefer. Add the grass-fed butter and continue to mix.

Next add the home-brewed sour cream and a handful of frozen berries or 2-3 tablespoons of lime juice, to taste. Sprinkle a teaspoon of mineral salt and enjoy.

For starting out, jumping into yolks can be too much due to die-off. For some, starting at half the yolks is best, building up from there. The butter can be omitted, depending on desire, taste, need, and stomach space. If a shake can't be added to your rhythm, making a deep effort to eat a dozen yolks a day can assist greatly.

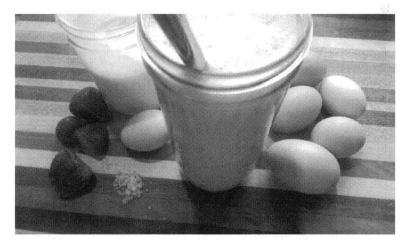

"Adrenals love fat and cholesterol. So, as far as the diet is concerned, eat lots of animal fats with every meal and cholesterol-rich foods, such as egg yolks, sour cream, butter. Another essential for the adrenals is sleep! Sleep is really not optional, so organize your life in such a way that you can have a nap every afternoon and a good long sleep at night," McBride says.[ccclxiv]

Instigating a mandatory 9 pm bedtime helps most of those with adrenal fatigue. Stopping the use of blue light screens[ccclxv] two hours prior to bedtime helps maintain sleep. The more sleep and the more cholesterol the person gets, the more the adrenals are supported.

Stage Two Soups

Soups on Stage Two are much the same as Stage One soups; however, yolks are added. Raw yolks stirred into a bowl of soup make it more of a cream soup. An egg dropped into the pot of soup for a minute or two make it more of an egg drop soup; adding the whites like this is Stage Three. Remember, yolks can cause the body to be stronger, making it able to kick the pathogens out all on its own, so they can cause die-off. Going slowly may be needed if the damage is deep. Raw pastured yolks are extremely nutrient-dense, while raw pastured egg whites are known as the champion for pulling out heavy metals. If eating the whites causes a yeast flare in any way, metals should be addressed.

Chowder

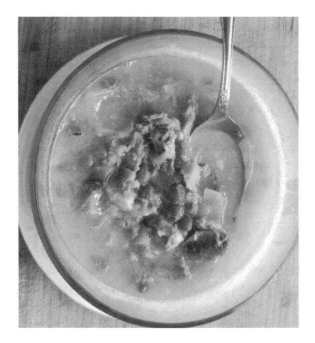

This recipe is best made with stock from the turkey, but can also be used with Meat Stock from beef, chicken, or fish. Each version creates a whole different meal.

To make the soup Stage Two:

2 quarts Meat Stock
3 tablespoons coconut oil
2 sticks grass-fed butter
11 green onion shoots, chopped into bite sizes
2 1/2 cups organic turkey
1-2 carrots, finely chopped
1 handful organic cauliflower
9 cloves garlic
8 pastured yolks

Combine all ingredients into a stock pot, except garlic and yolks, and cook on medium-low. Cook for 25-30 minutes, until vegetables are soft. Add chopped garlic for the last 5 minutes of cooking. Remove from heat and add all 8 yolks, stirring them into the soup. Warning: if the soup is too hot, the yolks will cook into soup, making clumps. If the soup is optimally warm, the yolks will give you a creamed soup effect, rich and irresistible.

Sweet Stock

Sweet Stock is a favorite recipe of Peter, a young GAPS husband who has seen major improvement with GAPS.

Peter says, "Since I was a boy, I would wake up with my eyes glued shut with so much eye gunk that I would have to hold a hot washcloth on my eyes for a few minutes until I could open them. I had also been taking allergy medications every day of my life and dealing with diarrhea. As an adult, avoiding all dairy and its derivatives cleared up these symptoms. After slowly implementing the Dairy Introduction while on GAPS Intro, I can now consume many forms of cultured, grass-fed dairy even though I still have symptoms if I eat conventional dairy."

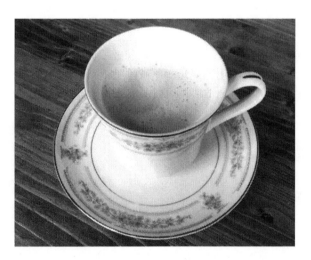

This recipe can be made with or without honey.

Step 1:

Make some beef stock with a few bay leaves and omit the salt, or use a very small amount of salt. Femur marrow bones work best for this recipe.

Step 2:

Steep 1 teaspoon chamomile, 1 teaspoon rooibos, and a bay leaf in 4 ounces of unsalted beef stock for 7 to 10 minutes. Chamomile gets bitter when crushed or when steeped too long. Strain.

Step 3:

When the infused stock has cooled, add 1 to 2 egg yolks, being careful not to cook them. Blend with an immersion blender until emulsified and creamy.

If this stock doesn't taste sweet enough on its own, stir in a little raw honey.

Honey Vanilla Ice Cream

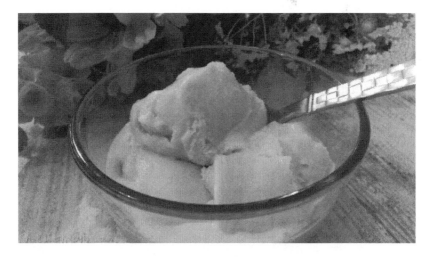

Enjoy this satiating ice cream any time of day because you just won't be able to resist! This healthy alternative is full of nutrition to heal your body while satisfying your mind.

These four simple ingredients are going to change your world forever!

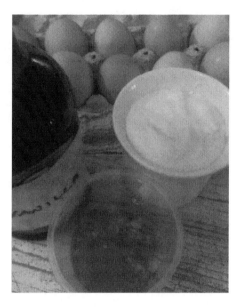

Add 8 pastured egg yolks to a Vitamix, and mix on low speed to emulsify for 10 minutes. If you do not have a Vitamix, a stand-up mixer, Cuisinart food processor or blender will work.

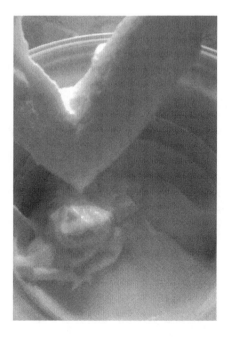

Add 1 cup of homemade kefir made from raw cream (making it kefir cream), 2 teaspoons of vanilla, and 2 tablespoons of local honey.

After the ingredients are combined, put them into an ice cream maker to chill while mixing and prepare to salivate. This recipe doubles well and freezes perfectly. Because of the high number of yolks, it scoops smoothly even directly from the freezer.

Eggnog

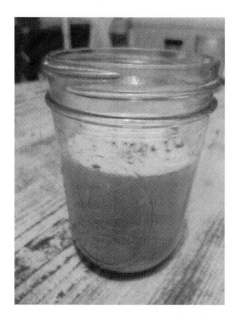

3 egg yolks
1 cup kefir cream (preferably made with raw cream)
Honey to taste
3 egg whites can be added in Stage Three

In a blender, on low, combine yolks and kefir for 10 minutes to emulsify. Add the remaining ingredients until combined. For a colder eggnog, serve chilled or blend in a few ice cubes. Nutmeg can be added in Stage Three.

Key Lime Pie Smoothie

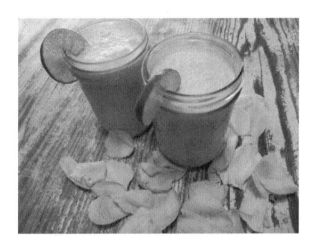

This spring treat will make your tongue so happy, it'll jump out of your mouth and slap your eyebrows!

    6-8 pastured yolks
    1 cup kefir (preferably made from cream)

    Blend the yolks and kefir together on low in the blender for ten minutes
        to emulsify. Then add:

    1 tablespoon local honey
    Add the juice from 3 limes.

Blend together briefly and enjoy. An ice cube or two can be added to make it colder and more enjoyable.

Fermented Fish, The Perfect Travel Food

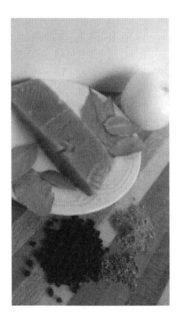

Fermented fish provides a plethora of probiotic strains.

Nutrients says, "Lactic acid bacteria (LAB) consist of homo and hetero-lactic acid organisms, and are a broad category of bacteria, including Lactobacillus, Streptococcus, Enterococcus, Lactococcus and Bifidobacterium, with the ability to produce lactate primarily from sugars. They are among the most commercially used bacteria today, contributing to yogurt, sauerkraut, kimchi and kefir production, the pickling of vegetables, curing of fish, and many other traditional dishes around the world."[ccclxvi]

The *Journal of Physiological Anthropology* says, "It is now obvious that household and artisanal fermentation of cereals, dairy, vegetables, fish, seafood and meats were a significant part of ancestral dietary practices."[ccclxvii]

Other findings are eye-opening. "A fish sauce product is also a fermented food made from different raw materials such as fish and shellfish. It was found that probiotic isolates such as *Lactobacillus plantarum*, *Saccharomyces cerevisiae* and *Staphylococcus arlettae* [...]possessed inhibitory effect against *S. aureus* and *Listeria monocytogenes*," says the *Journal of Animal Science and Technology*.ccclxviii

The *International Journal of Microbiology* says, "*Lactococcus lactis subsp. lactis* and *Leuconostoc citreum* were specifically associated with [fermented] fish fillet and [fermented] minced fish."ccclxix

The *Korean Journal for Food Sciences of Animal Resources* reported a study testing salted, fermented fish, specifically looking for large amounts of S-adenosyl-L-methionine (SAM). They found 169 different strains, most from the *Bacillus* genus. They reported, "The results of antibacterial activity for five indicators such as *Escherichia coli* O157:H7, *Enterococcus faecalis*, *Salmonella choleraesuis*, *Staphylococcus aureus*, and *Listeria monocytogenes* in the strains originating from the *jeotgal* showed that the antibacterial activity was not observed in the paper disc method and that 2 out of 10 strains did not show the inhibitory activity in the soft agar method, but the remaining 8 strains showed strong or excellent antibacterial effects."ccclxx

To make fermented fish, fill a pint-sized Mason jar with one serving of wild caught salmon, one small onion, a half of a tablespoon peppercorns, a half teaspoon of coriander (optimally seeds), two tablespoons mineral salt, a quarter cup of local honey (optional), five bay leaves, a half a teaspoon of dill seed, two tablespoons of whey, and filtered water to fill.

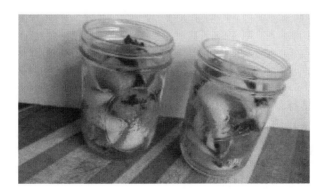

Cut up the onion and fish into bite-size pieces. Add all of the ingredients to a pint Mason jar.

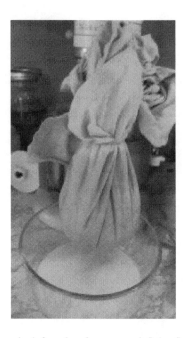

To make the whey needed for the fermented fish, first make milk kefir or yogurt. Be sure that the kefir or yogurt is fermented for 24 to 27 hours so that the lactose is digested and the casein is converted to paracasein, making it more digestible. To get more whey, ferment at a higher temperature, usually 110 degrees. Pour the kefir or yogurt into an old cotton t-shirt or cheese cloth, tie it up, and hang it from a cabinet knob over a bowl. The whey will drip out through the cloth. If there is any undigested lactose or casein, it will be more milk colored.

Whey is protein; when obtained in this manner, it is a live food, full of gentle probiotics. It is not to be confused with whey protein powders, sourced from the cheese industry after heating up the culture and dehydrating that whey into powder. Those are dead foods.

The whey assists in fermentation, pre-digesting the food. Salt does the same thing and is classified as wild fermentation. Using both in fish ferments is enough to ease anyone's preconceived concern with raw fish.

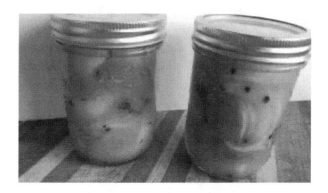

Put the lid on the jars, sealing out air, and let sit for three to five days on the countertop; then move them to the refrigerator. Take a pint jar for a complete, protein-rich lunch. If travel food is needed, it can be made, then fermented, while traveling.

Carrot Juice

Fresh-pressed juices are introduced on Stage Four, unless the person persistently suffers from chronic constipation. If this is the case, fresh-pressed organic carrot juice is introduced earlier, starting with one teaspoon. If one teaspoon is tolerated, the amount is increased until a full cup per day is tolerated. This is a long-time solution to assist with constipation.

Carrots are a sweet vegetable and must be watched for their yeast-feeding potential, which is not common but happens in those with excessive yeast. Yeast signs are commonly related to ethanol off-gassing, including things such as giggling or laughing inappropriately, bumping into walls, clingy behavior, slurring words, weepiness, fits, hitting, tantrums, as well as other signs. It is not common to experience yeast-feeding from carrots; is it common to experience healing.

Carrots and any other betacarotene-filled foods are imperative for supporting the body correctly. When betacarotene goes into the body, it goes to the liver where it is converted to vitamin A. Disease is a vitamin A deficiency. The more damaged the state of the body is, the more this detox channel is shut down and the conversion isn't made. When the betacarotene isn't converted to vitamin A, it's left floating around the body, loose, free, looking for a place to go; so, it comes out through the skin, turning the skin orange. Continuing with the betacarotene foods causes this conversion process to begin working again all on its own.

If constipation is an issue, carrot juice can help resolve it on earlier stages of GAPS. If constipation isn't an issue, fresh pressed-carrot juice should be introduced on Stage Four.

Extended Stage Two

Stage Two is the most detoxing stage. Some people who have a heavy toxic load stay at Stage Two for an extended period of time. Dr. Natasha classifies folks who stay at Stage Two for more than three months as practicing Extended Stage Two.

Foods on Extended Stage Two include all of Stage One and Stage Two foods, but can also step forward into some of the easier to digest foods that are part of the later stages, while avoiding those that are more advanced. This includes cooking meats and vegetables in different, more advanced stage methods, like sautéing, baking, broiling, and grilling, while holding off on fruits, nuts, and nightshades.

In addition to GAPS Shakes eaten on an empty stomach, Dr. Natasha says, "They build up to a cup of kefir. They're eating sour cream. They're eating lots of brine; by then they can have the sauerkraut. They can introduce juice, as well. So, basically, stay long-term on the Second Stage – it's modified, or extended – it's Extended Second Stage. So, they're eating all the soups; they're eating all the stews. They're cooking their vegetables; they're cooking their meats. But they can add the roasted vegetables; they can add the juices, the [GAPS] milkshakes, the fermented vegetables themselves – not just the fermented juice from them."[ccclxxi]

Cod liver oil, Fermented Cod Liver Oil, and fish oils can be added at Extended Stage Two.

One of the main reasons for Extended Stage Two, Dr. Natasha says, is that "people stumble when they try these pancakes – the nuts. Many people say, 'I can't.' They step back, and it's Stage Two. They modify."[ccclxxii]

She goes on to say, "For people who stay on Stage Two long-term: as they build up, gradually, to a certain level of fermented dairy, sour cream, kefir, and homemade cottage cheese, they can have large amounts. They can introduce fermented vegetables as well as their juices, sauerkraut, [and] vegetable medley. They can eat the vegetables. Introduce the vegetables themselves and they can introduce roasted meats and roasted vegetables at that stage."[ccclxxiii]

Extended Stage Two does not include nuts or fruits, but progresses through different types of cooking and more advanced foods.

On Extended Stage Two, parasites are often eliminated just though the protocol. Fermented foods are increased, and the body becomes stronger.

People with Crohn's, ulcerative colitis, diverticulitis, portions of their bowel removed, or other similar symptoms of a depleted microbiome, tend to thrive on Extended Stage Two.[ccclxxiv]

Dr. Natasha says, "If they've been on Stage Two for a year, after a year, it's a good idea to try and clean [parasites] out sometimes. And they may find out they may be able to move off the second stage."[ccclxxv]

She goes on to stay this if you find that you cannot get off Stage Two after a year: "Can't come off Stage Two[:] do the parasite cleanse; do the clay; do the Diatomaceous earth."[ccclxxvi] There are many parasite cleanses that work for GAPSters. An easy one to follow is to take Humaworm for two months, then take a two-month break, and then resume another two months to help with any newly hatched eggs. Dr. Natasha's recommendation for Humaworm is different from what Humaworm themselves recommend, which is less. Taking bentonite clay on GAPS starts with a quarter teaspoon a day, building up to three tablespoons a day. Taking Food Grade Diatomaceous Earth starts with a teaspoon and builds up to five tablespoons a day. Clay and Diatomaceous Earth can both be taken in water; however, clay needs to bloom or you will defecate clay in the same form in which it was taken. Putting it in a glass and letting it sit for 20 minutes before ingesting is enough.

Chapter 4:

Stage Three

GAPS Stage Three introduces more fiber.

• Ripe avocado is added to soups, one teaspoon at a time; then, when tolerated, it is eaten outside of soups.

• Egg whites from pastured eggs are added, if they have not already been introduced, as tolerated.[ccclxxvii] Raw egg whites are known to pull out heavy metals, which can cause a yeast flare. This should be monitored.

• The addition of nut butters allows the addition of pancakes. Nut butters include almond butter, pine nut butter, cashew butter, peanut butter, sunflower butter, or any other nut butter. [ccclxxviii] GAPS Pancakes are introduced, made from any nut butter (including peanut butter, even though it is a legume and not a nut), or seed butter, any allowed summer squash, and eggs. Any squash allowed on GAPS up until this point can be used, including zucchini, yellow crookneck squash, patty pan, white scallop squash, or pumpkin, as well as winter squashes if they are tolerated. For those who are most sensitive, it is recommended to first ferment the nut butter before introducing homemade nut butter, then store-bought nut butter can be introduced. Fermenting nut butter is done by adding whey to the ground nuts and allowing it to sit for a day or two. The general ratio is one to two tablespoons of whey per quart of ground nuts.

• Scrambled eggs and gently fried eggs (such as over easy eggs, also known as over medium eggs, depending on where you live) are introduced.

• Sautéed onions are added made by cooking them in 4 to 5 tablespoons of fat and covering them with a lid and cooking for 20 to 30 minutes until they are soft and translucent.

- All other Stage One, Two, and Three vegetables are cooked in the same way – 4 to 5 tablespoons of fat and covering them with a lid while cooking for 20 to 30 minutes, as tolerated.[ccclxxix] Vegetables cooked this way are not firm in any way; they are softer and easier to digest.

- The vegetable portions of vegetable ferments are added.

- Celery root can be added if not already tolerated in Stage Two.[ccclxxx]

- Olives can be introduced. Dr. Natasha says, "Organic fermented olives done only with salt and no chemicals can be tolerated when sauerkraut cabbage is being introduced, but this may be individual. So, introduce with care."[ccclxxxi]

- All fresh, powdered, or dried herbs and spices are added including rosemary, thyme, coriander, fennel, or any other herb.[ccclxxxii] These can be used as seasonings or actual food ingredients. Hot spices, such as red pepper, are introduced later, since they are more difficult to digest.

- Shellfish is added cooked in Stage Three.[ccclxxxiii]

- Fish oils, cod liver oil, and fermented cod liver oils are added into the protocol at Stage Three.

Avocado is a flag telling you the status of healing. If avocado is not passed, it is best to stay back on earlier stages instead of pushing through. It's a signal telling you more healing needs to happen.

Once getting to Stage Three, with the addition of nut butters and moving forward to baked goods using nut flours in the later stages, sometimes people revert to the Standard American Diet method of eating. This includes things like pancakes or muffins for breakfast, bread sandwiches, cookies, rolls, sliced bread with butter, and so forth with meals. When these foods become the staple, symptoms often creep back to the surface. The GAPS Protocol relies heavily on nourishing foods, not baked goods which provide much less nutrition. GAPSters have compromised microbiomes, which means that they do not readily get the nutrition from their food – this is known as a Secondary Nutritional Deficiency. Most people need to use the stomach space on deeply nourishing foods such as egg yolks, organ meats, and animal fats so that the food that is absorbed is highly nutritious.

When adding nuts, the method of introduction depends on the person. Some people who are healthier can just add nuts. Others who have more damage in the microbiome need to begin by first fermenting the nuts. GAPS Chef Monica Corrado, MA, CNC, CGP, is a specialist on the matter. Corrado is an author and a Teaching Chef for GAPS and The Weston A. Price Foundation and is a Holistic Nutritionist at Simply Being Well. She says that making your own nut butter is optimal; "Because so many of them are rancid in the jar, you get your nuts, you ferment your nuts, and then you make your own nut butter from there. Sometimes people add coconut oil or ghee or tallow to make it smoother."[ccclxxxiv] Corrado can be reached at simplybeingwell.com.

Many people go to the SCD (Specific Carbohydrate Diet) way of eating or blur the lines of GAPS and SCD, since the basis is similar. This can include lots of baking with nuts. Many GAPSters have yeast overgrowth. Nuts often feed the yeast, which makes the fussy eater desire only products made with nut bases.

Dr. Natasha says, "Naturally these families did not see the expected improvements, because no child or adult can live on ground almonds and honey most of the time. Nuts are very fibrous and hard work for the digestive system, that is why they are introduced in later stages of the GAPS Diet, and only when the severe digestive symptoms are gone. I recommend to many patients to ferment nuts in the initial stages, as it makes them more digestible. If the GAPS Introduction Diet is followed correctly and nuts are introduced at the right time, majority of patients find no trouble with eating sensible amounts of nuts."[ccclxxxv] Fermenting nuts is done by adding whey to the water when the nuts are soaking – one teaspoon of whey to one quart of water.

• Olive oil, sesame seed oil, and avocado oil can be added in Stage Three. Dr. Natasha says, "Sesame seed oil and other vegetable oils like olive oil – Stage Three. I would have it raw. All of these vegetable oils can be used on Full GAPS or started from Stage Three when we introduce olive oil."[ccclxxxvi]

She is not a fan of heating these oils since it changes the molecular structure of the oil, making it less recognizable to the body than in its natural cold-pressed state.

• At Stage Three, we can start having crunchier bits on our cooked food. Bacon is a quality food on GAPS, especially when it is sourced from pastured animals. Regarding bacon cooked in the oven with crunchy bits, Dr. Natasha says, "Crunchy bits? Oh, it's lovely! Stage Three."[ccclxxxvii]

• Dried herbs and spices are added at Stage Three. Dr. Natasha says, "They are fine to add to the water when we make Meat Stock or tea, but after the infusion is over, we strain them out. If they are finely shredded (or powdered), we can use it in stew or other dishes from the 3rd stage onwards."[ccclxxxviii]

Fermented Nut Butter

Regarding fermented nut butter, Dr. Natasha says "That's a new thing we should add there – Stage Three. Nut butter pancakes should be homemade and fermented prior to blending into nut butter. Just add a little bit of whey."[ccclxxxix]

Fermented nut butter is designed for those who are most sensitive and must take each step slowly. To make fermented nut butter, we make nut butter at home and add a teaspoon of whey to every two to three cups of nut butter.

Put a lid on and let is sit for 24 hours before using. The addition of whey assists in predigesting the nut butter, making it gentler on the digestive tract.

After the nut butter is fermented, it can be used anywhere and in any method that nut butter is used at this stage. It can be used as nut butter or as an ingredient in cooking pancakes.

Once the fermented nut butter is tolerated, gradually increasing the amount as needed, nut butter that has not been fermented can be used.

This method of introduction is particularly useful for those who suffer from issues with nuts.

Pancakes

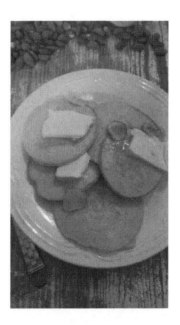

For those who are not on GAPS, these pancakes, made with real food ingredients, will satiate and not cause sugar swings.

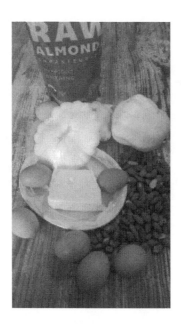

3/4 to 1 cup nut butter (or seed butter)
1 cup cooked squash (zucchini, yellow crook neck, patty pan, white
    scallop, pumpkin)
5 eggs
1 teaspoon vanilla (or any other extract)
Butter
Local honey

Add the nut butter, squash, and eggs to a mixer, Cuisinart, or blender. Blend until smooth.

Now add the vanilla extract and blend just a bit more.

Pour it onto a hot skillet or griddle greased with lard, butter, ghee, duck fat, or goose fat.

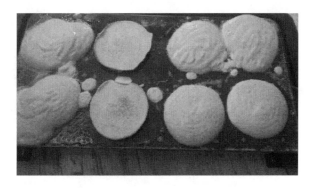

Cook as you would Standard American Diet (SAD) pancakes; in other words, when the surface of the pancakes is no longer shiny, there are bubbles in the pancake, and the outer edges look more solid and dull in color, flip them to cook the other side.

Serve with lots of butter and a small taste of local honey.

Using pumpkin as the squash and adding a tablespoon of cinnamon, 2 teaspoons of nutmeg, and 1 teaspoon of ginger powder makes an amazing pumpkin Thanksgiving pancake all year long. A favorite of mine is to use cashew butter and white scallop squash or zucchini.

Vanilla extract, or any other extract, can be introduced at Stage Three and added to the pancakes.

Maple syrup is best added when Coming Off GAPS, but butter and honey are great additions at Stage Three.

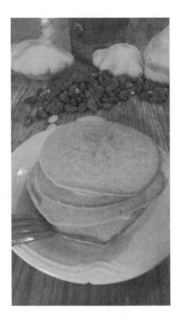

Using less nut butter or adding butter, milk kefir, or water thins the batter, allowing you to create crepes. Of course, you would use a small skillet or crepe pan for this.

Peanut Butter Marshmallow Mousse

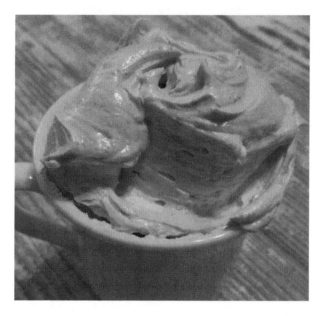

"This reminds me of having marshmallow fluff and peanut butter sandwiches when I was a kid. I'll stop eating it whenever you're ready for me to," my husband said when I gave him my latest experiment to hold while I climbed into bed. Needless to say, he ate it all.

This version of Peanut Butter & Marshmallow Mousse contains no marshmallow but has the flavor of the two.

    1 cup pastured butter
    2 tablespoons local honey
    2 tablespoons organic peanut butter
    1 teaspoon vanilla (preferably homemade)

Put all ingredients into a mixer and beat until fluffy – ten minutes or more. Just before it is finished, you can optionally add 1 teaspoon Celtic sea salt, course ground. This adds a delightful salty crunch which amplifies the sweet. If this is mixed in too early, the salt dissolves into the mixture and it's just too salty overall.

Instead of measuring out two tablespoons of peanut butter, some folks stick a butter knife deep into the peanut butter tub, which comes out thick with peanut butter on both sides. This is roughly two tablespoons and it's not as messy as measuring the peanut butter with a measuring spoon.

Fermented Nut Flour

Dr. Natasha says, "I think this recipe (Monica's fermented almond flour recipe of cake or bread), fermented, even nut butter can be fermented. Just add a little bit of whey. That's stage three. The nut butter pancakes."[cccxc] This recipe is found in the Full GAPS section.

Vanilla Extract

Dr. Natasha says, "You can do your own extract as soon as you introduce your own pancakes."[cccxci] Making an extract is as simple as adding the ingredient to gin or vodka to soak for six weeks. The products are true, meaning vanilla beans make vanilla extract, lemon peels make lemon extract and the like, except for almond. Almond extract isn't made from almonds, it's made from peach pits, cherry pits, or apricot pits in the alcohol.

Vanilla extract can be used in specialty baking or given as Christmas gifts.

Be sure to use grade B beans; they are less oily and produce a superior product.

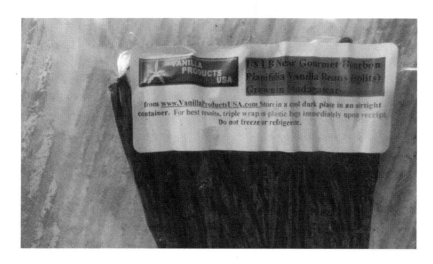

1-pound vanilla beans, cut into half inch-long strips
1-gallon vodka, 70-90 proof

To make a quart of vanilla, use 1/4 pound of beans cut into half inch strips. Then fill the rest of the quart jar with vodka. Once you make homemade vanilla, ice cream will never taste the same. The flavor is far superior. Double-strength vanilla extract can be made by just covering the vanilla beans instead of adding more vodka to fill the vessel. Once you try double strength, you'll never go back. Over the past eight years, the vanilla crop has been struggling. It has gotten worse and worse every year. Speculations over the vanilla bean decline have abounded, ranging from Glyphosate and pesticide poisoning to cyclical changes. Regardless, making a batch of vanilla has often been reduced to using one or two beans in a small glass bottle, which is still more flavorful and less expensive than store-bought.

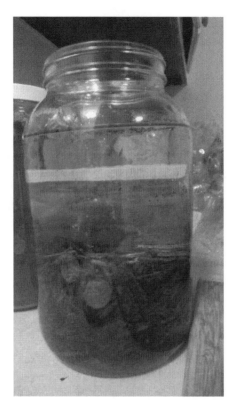

Put the cut beans into a gallon jar, add the vodka, and screw on the lid. Place the jar in a dark spot. Different recipes call for different directions, and here's where the recipes differ: some say leave for one month and shake contents daily, others say leave for six months and shake contents every few days. Vanilla that has been brewing for a year has a deeper flavor. After you brew your beans, you can brew the same ones again a second time and a third time.

Lemon Extract

Making lemon extract at home is more flavorful and less expensive than store-bought. The recipe is simple. First take organic lemons. Wash them twice, being sure to rinse them well. Pat dry.

Peel the skins off the lemons with a potato peeler. Be sure not to dig deep. You do not want the white portion of the lemon, just the skin. Pour vodka or gin over your lemon peels. Vodka is usually used; rum can also be used. Lemon extract can be made in a quart Mason jar. It's easiest to peel your lemons as you use them and keep filling the jar as time passes. Top with a lid and store the jar in a dark cabinet. Every once in a while, shake the jar or turn it over and back. It's best to do this every day, but, in reality, some jars are never shaken and they end up fine. The longer you let it brew, the better the flavor will be. Some folks like it after a month; others let it go at least 6 months.

The cost of homemade lemon extract is roughly $7 a quart.

Lemon extract is often paired with yellow food coloring in recipes. Yellow food coloring is a product associated with behavioral problems in children. In fact, the Center for Science in the Public Interest is trying to get the FDA to ban Yellow No. 5.[cccxcii]

Europe revisited their stipulations on food colors, reevaluating their dangers. They found, "Exposure to synthetic colors or a sodium benzoate preservative (or both) in the diet result in increased hyperactivity."[cccxciii]

Lemon Drops

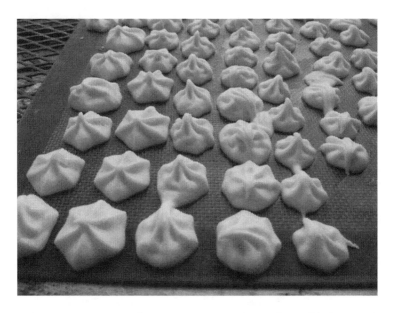

Lemon drops are sweet and sour, a pure goodness that will change the way you dessert forever!

Memories of a buttercream candy will swim through your head as you nourish your insides with the powerful benefits of coconut oil. They make a great after dinner dessert or a refreshing snack.

Lemon zest makes this recipe a Stage Three recipe. If omitted, it can be introduced earlier. Rebuilding starts small and builds.

> 1 cup coconut oil
> 1/4 cup fresh-squeezed lemon juice
> 2-3 tablespoons local honey
> Zest from 1 1/2 lemons

Blend up all ingredients in Vitamix, food processor, or other appliance until smooth. Place contents into a frosting bag with the flower tip. Squeeze out flowers onto a parchment paper covered cookie sheet. Freeze. Enjoy!

Butter Cream Mints

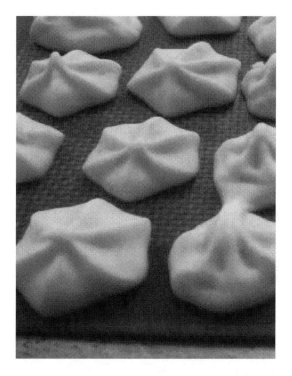

Adding animal fats can be done by adding the fats to stock or by making animal fat treats like Butter Cream Mints. Any animal fat can be used, according to each person's individual taste and tolerance.

Buttercream mints are a favorite and can be duplicated for a delicate creamy treat that is healthy and indeed beneficial.

Mix together:

    1 cup grass fed butter
    1 cup home-brewed sour cream
    1 tablespoon mint extract
    1/4 cup local honey

Blend all ingredients until smooth. Add contents to a zip top bag or frosting bag. Immediate use depends on how long the mixture was blended and its liquid consistency. Some blenders or food processors heat up the mixture while blending, causing it to be too liquified to use immediately. If the mixture is too runny, put it in the refrigerator until ready to use. It may need to be kneaded when taken from cold storage in the refrigerator.

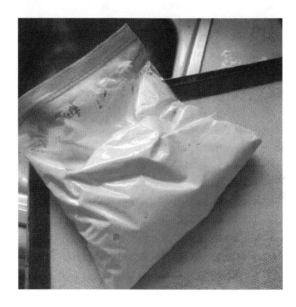

Cut a corner out of the bag. The bigger the cut is, the bigger the Meltaways will be. A small cut will make them bite-sized; a larger cut will make them big enough for two bites each, causing the person to hold a melting treat in their fingers. The choice is yours.

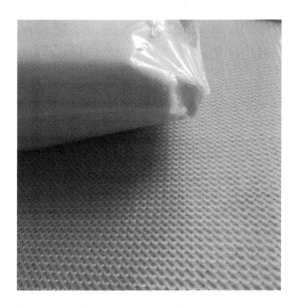

Drop small dollops onto parchment paper lined cookie sheets. Freeze for 30 minutes. Store in an airtight container or zip top bag in the freezer.

Liver Pâté

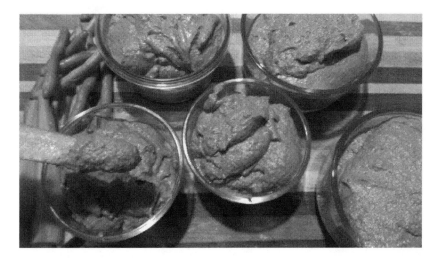

Organ meats are the powerhouse of nutrition. They've held a long-standing position on the dinner table until recent years. Traditional societies offered them to the most highly honored member of their community first. When tribal men hunted, the first thing removed from the animal was the heart or the liver, and the first bite was given to the elder or shaman on the hunt. Fried liver and onions were a weekly tradition in most homes in the '50s. Our current society is depleted in nutrition, while it's sitting right at our fingertips.

The B vitamin load in liver dwarfs any supplement. B9 is folate; B12 is methylcobalamin; B6 is pyridoxine. The B12 content is so high, some consider it to be the B12 jackpot! The iron levels in liver can stop anemia dead in its tracks. Liver contains copper, zinc, chromium, phosphorous and selenium, essential fatty acids EPA, DHA, vitamins A, D, E, and K, and CoQ10. When there is damage in the intestinal tract, nutritional deficiencies are present, and few things rank as highly as liver.

Dr. Natasha recommends liver on a regular basis; "An anemic person should eat liver and other organ meats once a week, at least. A child needs a small amount: one to two tablespoons of cooked liver every other day... or a full liver meal once a week."[cccxciv]

She recommends liver, daily. In a health crisis, it is measured with proportions the size of your hand – not the palm, the hand.[cccxcv]

It is recommended that liver be soaked in lemon water, whey, kefir, yogurt, or raw milk for a roughly four hours to remove the bitter taste. This is called washing the liver.

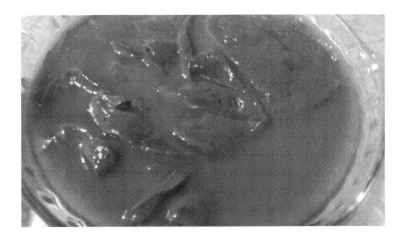

One of the easiest ways to tell if liver is a benefit to you is to eat liver and exercise. One teenage boy said, "Mom, when I eat liver, I can do seven pull-ups and it's not hard. When I don't eat liver, I have a hard time doing one!"

Making liver taste good is important to consumption. One of the most important steps in this process is washing the liver. As described above, in order to wash the liver, lay the pieces in a shallow pan (this recipe calls for a pound of liver) and cover it with lemon juice, real milk, home-brewed kefir, or home-brewed yogurt. After it has been on the counter for 4 hours, remove the liver from the washing and pat dry.

Put a cup of grass-fed butter in a properly seasoned, cast iron skillet on medium. Add four onions, chopped. It is very important to use organic onions as they soak up pesticides like a sponge.

On top of the cooking onions, add:

    1 pound of washed liver
    1 8-ounce package portabella mushrooms
    5 cloves garlic
    1 teaspoon dry mustard
    1/2 teaspoon dill
    1 teaspoon dried rosemary
    1 1/2 tablespoons lemon juice
    A sprinkle of salt and pepper.

Cook this mixture on medium low until the liquid is cooked down. The more you cook down the liquid, the firmer the pâté will be. The more liquid you leave the liquid, not cooked down dry, the easier it is to scoop.

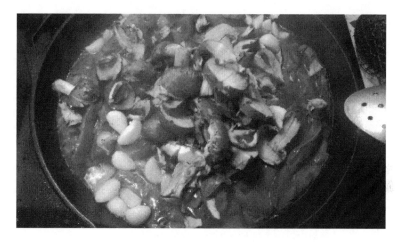

Place all the ingredients into the Vitamix and blend until smooth.

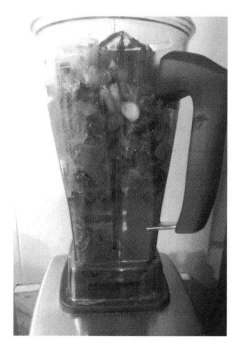

Pour into Pyrex containers and serve or freeze. This makes an easy travel food for lunch or a classy dip for a party.

Mint Meltaways

This wholesome, healthy snack is a refreshing treat without the guilt.

>   1 cup coconut oil
>   1/2 teaspoon mint extract
>   1 tablespoon local organic honey
>   2 tablespoons avocado

Put all ingredients into your blender or Vitamix and blend until thoroughly blended. Put contents into a frosting bag and drop onto baking sheets. Put in the freezer. After 30 minutes, scrape into zip bags and store in the freezer.

If you blend too much and it becomes too runny or thin, put the frosting bag in the refrigerator for 10 minutes. Knead with hands to break up any hard coconut oil clumps. Continue to make flowers.

Pumpkin Spice Latte

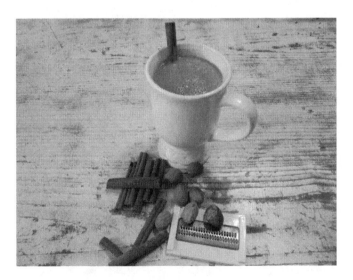

The spin of this treat is taken from the pumpkin spice latte at Starbucks which contains ingredients (taken straight from the bottle) such as sugar, condensed nonfat milk, sweetened condensed nonfat milk, annatto (E160b, colour), natural and artificial flavours, caramel colour (E 150d), salt, and potassium sorbate (E202, a preservative).

Their pumpkin spice latte contains no pumpkin.

It doesn't take much research to find that these ingredients aren't real food.

While following the GAPS diet, treats should be limited as honey should be used sparingly and coffee should be brewed weak. Coffee can be used if you are on Full GAPS; it should be weak, where you can read the paper through it. On intro, dandelion root granule tea, which tastes like coffee, should be used. You can adapt yours to use less honey and weaken the 'coffee' to your liking.

To get the biggest punch out of your treat, use freshly ground nutmeg.

This version is 130 calories, compared to 510 calories from the Starbucks pumpkin spice latte, but the important thing is eliminating the chemicals.

    1 cup cooked pumpkin
    1 cup home brewed kefir from real milk
    2 tablespoons local honey
    1/2 teaspoon cinnamon
    1/2 teaspoon nutmeg
    1/2 cup dandelion root granule tea (coffee if you are Full GAPS, weak
        in strength)

Blend together all ingredients until smooth.

Sauerkraut

With billions of probiotics in each bite, sauerkraut is being ranked as one of the highest forms of probiotics you can eat, including out-ranking over-the-counter probiotic pills. It's also one the easiest things to make in your kitchen where, literally, the chopping of the cabbage is what takes the most time.

First, take a medium to large organic head of cabbage (about five pounds) and chop it up as fine as you like it. The finer the chop is, the faster it ferments. Some prefer to make kraut by chopping it in the Vitamix, floating the cabbage in water. It takes 4 minutes to chop the whole head this way.

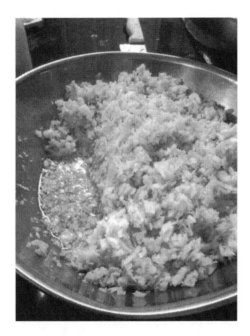

Add 2 tablespoons of mineral salt and stir. You want to have all of the salt equally distributed throughout the cabbage pieces. Some people go on to pound their cabbage with a cabbage pounder or a meat tenderizer; some even use a clean baseball bat. Other people massage and squeeze it with their hands, while others just let it sit and allow the salt to break open the cell walls. Either way, let it sit or pound it until the cabbage is limp and liquid has come out of the cabbage. This is called salting.

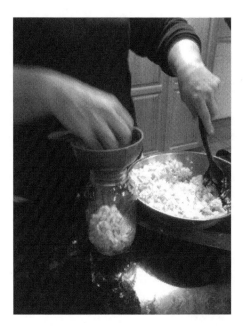

Place the cabbage into Mason jars, packing it tightly so that there are no air pockets. Be sure that the top of the cabbage is covered by the liquid; this protects it from rising above the brine and going moldy. Leave one inch of head space between the top of the cabbage and the lid. Brewing in a Mason jar is an anaerobic ferment, meaning without oxygen. This only takes four to seven days to brew. The warmer the temperature is, the faster it brews. If you need it to brew faster, use one tablespoon of mineral salt and one tablespoon of whey. The warmer your climate or home is, the faster it brews. Most GAPSters brew the sauerkraut for 12 days. Once it is brewed to your taste preference, put it in the refrigerator to slow fermentation.

Take note, if any cabbage rises over the top of the water brine, it is fine. If it is left long enough, white mold will form. Traditionally, instructions have been to scrape it off and eat what is beneath. It sounds disgusting, but that mold is not a damaging mold to your body, according to Sandor Katz, the Godfather of Fermentation and author of *Wild Fermentation*. He says (if the mold does form) to scrape off the white top before the layer gets too thick and reaches deep down into the jar; then put it in the refrigerator to slow down the fermentation process.[cccxcvi]

Since this is an anaerobic recipe, it is important to leave the jar with the lid on; do not open it to see how it's doing. Go by the look of how limp the cabbage is; the lighter the color is, the more it has been brewed. If you just can't stand waiting, then open it and taste it. Be aware that when you do this, you are letting oxygen in and halting the anaerobic environment; so it'll take longer to brew once you put the lid back on, and you risk bacteria growth. People do this; you haven't ruined it if you open it – it's just not optimal.

RECIPE RECAP:

1 medium to large head of organic cabbage, roughly 5 pounds

2 tablespoons mineral salt

Chop, salt, pack in jar, put the lid on, leave on the counter for four to twelve days (preferably under a towel, as it likes a dark spot).

The FDA has never found any incidence of someone getting ill or dying from sauerkraut.

Probiotic count of sauerkraut ranks in the high billions.[cccxcvii]

To reduce the bad microbes, you need to feed the good microbes through probiotics and cultured foods.

McBride says that most probiotics on the market today are prophylactic and GAPSters should find one made out of as many species of bacteria as possible.[cccxcviii]

Cultured foods are foods that have been fermented, like sauerkraut, kimchi, kefir, yogurt, and the like. Fermentation preserves the food for years.

McBride say, "With every mouthful of sauerkraut, you're consuming billions of beneficial microbes, which will be killing the pathogens in your gut, driving them out and replenishing the beneficial flora in your digestive tract."[cccxcix]

Fermented Garlic

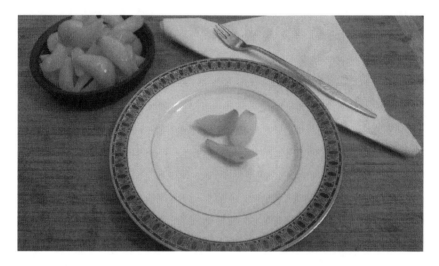

Garlic is well known as a natural antibiotic, shows antifungal properties, and is a natural testosterone boosting food.

Fermenting garlic can be done with the skins on or with the cloves peeled. Cloves can change color during fermentation, representing a few potential factors.

In an Epicurious article, Dr. Luke LaBorde of Penn State University's Department of Food Science says 'It's definitely enzymatic and nonenzymatic reactions occurring in the garlic, but we really don't know entirely why."[cd] Some say this is connected to variations of different nutrients in each clove.

"The bioactivity of some natural products is increased by fermentation," says *Nutrition Research*. They reported that fermented garlic protected diabetic, obese mice through the antioxidant activity of the fermented garlic versus the unfermented garlic. The study showed remarkable liver support and anti-obesity effects.[cdi]

Plant Foods for Human Nutrition, a publication of the Netherlands, reported a study on fermented garlic which showed "superoxide dismutase (SOD)-like activity, scavenging activity against hydrogen peroxide and the polyphenol content of the garlic extract were increased 13-folds, more than 10-folds, and 7-folds, respectively, as compared with those of the control garlic extract."[cdii]

They go on to say, "The fermented-garlic is suggested to possess desirable anti-oxidative properties."

What's specifically interesting is, as they say, "Hydrogen peroxide is generated from the scavenging reaction by SOD."[cdiii]

Fermented garlic powder was used in a study with 144 pigs that had just been weaned. The 5-week trial showed an increase of total tract digestibility after use of the fermented garlic powder.

The *Journal of Animal Physiology and Animal Nutrition* reported the study concluding, "Dietary fermented garlic powder decreased the blood total cholesterol. The triglyceride concentration was decreased. Dietary fermented garlic powder can also increase the nutrient digestibility, lymphocytes and RBC concentrations, but decrease the fecal E. coli concentration in weaning pigs."[cdiv]

Peeled and blanched garlic and garlic that had not been blanched were compared during fermentation. The findings were reported by the *International Journal of Food Microbiology*. The blanched garlic was prepared by pouring boiling water over the peeled garlic for 15 minutes prior to fermentation. They reported, "The starter grew abundantly in the case of blanched garlic, producing mainly lactic acid and reaching a pH of 3.8 after 7 days, but its growth was inhibited in unblanched garlic. Ethanol and fructose, coming from enzymatic activities of the garlic, and a green pigment were formed during the fermentation of unblanched garlic, but not of blanched garlic."[cdv]

Sometimes, when fermenting garlic, the cloves change colors to green, blue, and, sometimes, variations of orange.

Epicurious says, "As far as they can tell, garlic enzymes—which give it that distinct flavor—break down over time. Naturally occurring sulfur in the garlic interacts with those enzymes, occasionally turning it slightly green or blue. Sometimes the color change happens; sometimes it doesn't. Shifts in temperature, pH, and the age of the garlic can also come into play."[cdvi] Older garlic turns blue or green more frequently than fresh garlic.

Trends in Food Science in Technology reported a study where they tested all 22 amino acids with garlic fermentation. They said, "Blue–green pigments are easily generated by mixing juice from heated white onions, a good source of 1-PeCSO (1-propenyl-L-cysteine sulfoxide) [, which causes the] formation of thiosulfinates, 'color developers'."[cdvii]

They further concluded, "Green discoloration" in crushed garlic represents a mixture of yellow and blue pigments, and the blue color results from at least 8 pigments, depending on amino acid composition, rather than a single blue pigment. Results indicated that amino acids other than glycine have the potential to form blue pigments."[cdviii]

The *Journal of Agriculture and Food Industry* posted another study testing the pigmented fermented garlic, saying, "Alliinase and acetic acid were required for the color formation. UV-vis spectral measurements and pH results suggest that the color formation occurs by two kinds of processes: one enzymatic and the other nonenzymatic."[cdix]

Some traditional cultures make Black Garlic, a totally different product from fermented garlic. Black Garlic is made by putting dried, unpeeled garlic in the slow cooker on the warm setting for 12 to 20 days without opening the lid. This is not a probiotic food; it's still good for you – just not a probiotic.

Probably the most telling aspect of fermented garlic is its incredible strength against Staph and the bacteria MRSA (Methicillin-resistant Staphylococcus aureus). MRSA that is specifically resistant to antibiotic use consistently is no match for fermented garlic.

Microbiologist and Pharmaceutical Scientist Michelle Moore says, "Unlike antibiotic drugs, garlic is very complex, containing 27 known active ingredients and dozens more that work in unknown ways. Many of these ingredients can work together synergistically inside the body in intricate ways to fight infections. The herb is highly effective against resistant MRSA bacteria because it is too complex chemically for the bacteria to become resistant to. In contrast, the antibiotic drug Zyvox, which is prescribed for many MRSA cases, has only one active ingredient: Linezolid."[cdx]

The *British Journal of Biomedical Sciences* says, "Resistance to mupirocin in MRSAs is increasing. Allicin is the main antibacterial agent isolated from garlic." They tested garlic isolates and found, "88% of clinical isolates had MBCs of 128 microg/mL, and all were killed at 256 microg/mL. Of these strains, 82% showed intermediate or full resistance to mupirocin; however, this study showed that a concentration of 500 microg/mL in an aqueous cream base was required to produce an activity equivalent to 256 microg/mL allicin liquid."[cdxi]

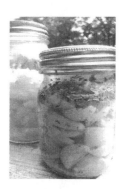

Fermenting garlic is one of the easiest and most potent things people can do for their health.

Fill a quart Mason jar full of garlic cloves (peeled or unpeeled, your choice); add a tablespoon of mineral salt. Fill the jar with filtered water, leaving an inch of headroom. Let the jar sit for a few weeks or longer.

Any additional herb or spice can be added, according to your desires.

Eggnog Ice Cream

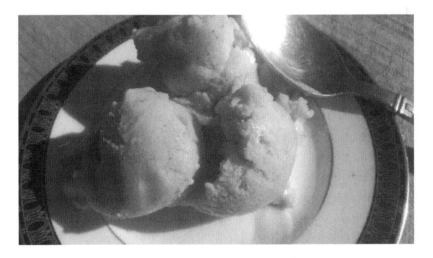

There's nothing more delicious at Christmas time than Eggnog Ice Cream. This nutritious and delicious treat is a crowd pleaser, but it's so good, it'll make you hide somewhere just to get it to yourself. With a dish like this, no one needs to share!

Eggnog is delicious but also healing. Rebuilding the microbiome includes specific steps, one of which is copious amounts of yolks and sour cream. Add a sprinkle of honey and a chilling process—boom, eggnog ice cream.

A quality ice cream maker needs to be easy to operate; otherwise, you won't use it.

3 to 12 egg yolks
(more yolks make the ice cream more scoopable straight from the
freezer)
1 cup kefir (preferably kefir cream, kefir made with raw cream)
2-3 tablespoons Honey (to taste)
1 teaspoon vanilla
3 egg whites
1 teaspoon nutmeg

In blender, on low, combine yolks until they change color to a soft yellow or white. This is emulsifying the yolks. Add the remaining ingredients until combined. Do not blend kefir long as it changes the structure.

Add mixture to an ice cream maker. When the mixture is firm, enjoy or freeze.

Probiotic Pickle Relish

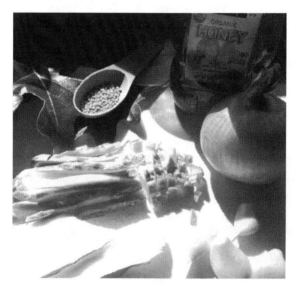

Chop up two pickling cucumbers – the finer, the better.

In a pint Mason jar, add an oak leaf (a grape leaf can also be used) to the bottom or the jar.

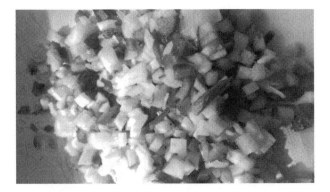

Mix together cucumbers, one diced garlic clove, one onion, one teaspoon mustard seed, one tablespoon local honey, half of one red pepper, and two teaspoons mineral salt. All ingredients should be organic.

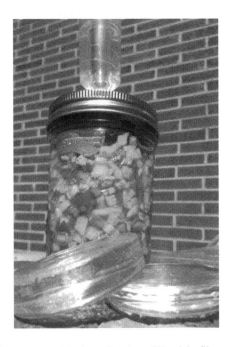

Once the ingredients are added to the jar, fill with filtered or spring water up until one inch from the top. Add another oak leaf to the top for crispier relish. Press the ingredients down below the water line with the oak leaf.

For best results, use an air lock or crock rocks. Leave on the countertop for 3 days; then refrigerate.

Probiotic Pickles

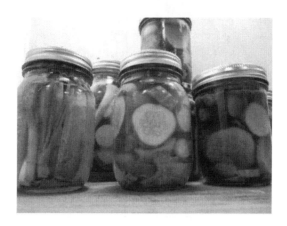

These GAPS-approved pickles are a fermented vegetable high in beneficial digestive aspects.

The base recipe for a quart-sized jar is:

2 oak leaves or grape leaves
Cucumbers (be sure to cut off the flower end as it contains enzymes that make wimpy pickles).
Chopped green onions or white onions, quartered
1 tablespoon mustard seed
1 teaspoon dill (use fresh if you can find some)
Organic garlic, chopped or sliced to your liking
1 tablespoon mineral salt

Chop the pickles, onions, and garlic to the sizes you desire. Make sure the pickles are short enough to stay covered with juice when in the jar.

Next pack all the ingredients into the quart jar. Start with an oak leaf. Then add the pickles, onions, garlic, and spices—leaving about an inch of room at the top. Top the pickles with the second leaf. Add filtered water to just cover the contents.

Put the lid on and leave it on the counter for 3 days; then refrigerate.

This recipe is also delicious with some ginger added.

* 1 tablespoon local honey can be added but is optional—honey is antimicrobial and will create a different variety of probiotics. It will, however, add other beneficial microbes.

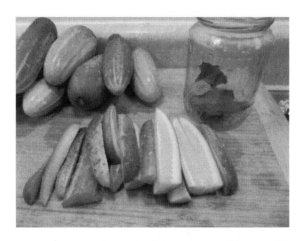

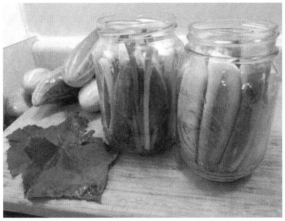

The oak leaf, or grape leaf, on the bottom and top produces crispier pickles.

Fish Oils

Fish oils on GAPS come in three forms, including Fermented Cod Liver Oil, Cod Liver Oil, and Fish Oil. The oils taken are determined by the person's individual needs.

Vitamin supplementation is not generally recommended on GAPS. The supplement industry is not regulated; often included in the supplements are extra ingredients that feed the very pathogens we are trying to starve and drown out with beneficial flora.

The *American Journal of Clinical Nutrition* says that, as it was traditionally, we should be eating a blend of omega-3 and omega-6 fatty acids; however, the deficiency we see in today's food is causing chronic disease. They say, "There has been an enormous increase in the consumption of n−6 fatty acids due to the increased intake of vegetable oils from corn, sunflower seeds, safflower seeds, cottonseed, and soybeans,"[cdxii] which adds to the imbalance.

Beneficial essential fatty acids fitting for a GAPS protocol can be found from several sources.

Physical signs that the body is deficient of essential fatty acids are hangnails and dry flaky skin, rash on the skin, lack of growth in a child, slow wound healing, weakened immune system, and dry patches of skin, including dry patches in the ears and nose.

Wound Repair and Regeneration reported a study showing, "Polyunsaturated fatty acids (PUFA) alter proinflammatory cytokine production."[cdxiii]

They reported research that "found improved reconstitution of epithelial integrity with both ω-3 and ω-6 PUFA-treated intestinal cells in rats following mucosal injury."[cdxiv]

In 1929, George and Mildred Burr studied the effects of Essential Fatty Acids in the body. They fed rats a diet devoid of fats and found that fat-deprived rats developed visible skin abnormalities, increased water loss across their skin (also referred to as transepidermal water loss (TEWL)), stunted growth, and impaired reproduction.[cdxv]

The *Journal of American Science and Biotechnology* studied pigs and the effect of EFAs saying, "Short chain fatty acids are essential for maintaining the normal metabolism of colon mucosa, regulating colonocyte growth and proliferation. The beneficial effect of SCFA is not restricted to the colon, and SCFA also stimulates cell proliferation and growth of small intestine. This effect on distant mucosa is likely mediated by a systemic mediatory mechanism."[cdxvi]

Fish oil, olive oil, evening primrose oil, hemp seed oil, flax seed oil, and egg yolks from pastured chickens are all wise choices. Dr. Natasha recommends that when taking hemp oil and flax seed oil, they should be combined with olive oil to balance the omega-3 and omega-6 ratio. Oils such as these should be cold-pressed and stored in a dark green or amber bottle that is not exposed to sunlight, and preferably refrigerated.

These oils are officially Stage Three; however, GAPS can be very bio-individual. Seeking a qualified Certified GAPS Practitioner can guide you with this process. For cases such as those on Extended Stage Two, supplemental oils are added earlier.

Dr. Natasha says, "In the first two stages of the Introduction Diet, I recommend not to introduce any supplements, just introduce fermented foods. In a small number of patients, no fermented food can be tolerated, so for these patients I recommend introducing a probiotic gradually starting from a tiny dose. From the third stage, if fermented foods have been successfully introduced, you can start introducing the probiotic and the cod liver oil in tiny amounts, gradually increasing the daily dose."[cdxvii]

Regarding cod liver oil, she says, "When cod liver oil has been introduced (the full dose is taken daily), introduce fish oils. When olive oil is being introduced, you can introduce cold pressed nut/seed oils gradually with meals. For those who started from the Full GAPS Diet, probiotics and cod liver oil can be introduced from the beginning, starting from a tiny amount and gradually increasing the dose. When cod liver oil has been successfully introduced, start the fish oils and the nut/seed oils."[cdxviii]

Finding a clean and beneficial cod liver oil takes some research and can be costly. The benefits far outweigh the cost. Some people consider it their insurance policy for health. Cod liver oil should be sourced from wild-caught fish, processed without heat, and stored in an amber-colored bottle to prevent oxidation.

"In order for the body to give birth to healthy, well-functioning enterocytes, it needs two factors. It needs building blocks because they're made out of certain nutrients. They're made out of proteins and out of certain fats, out of certain vitamins and enzymes. All these building blocks need to be provided for these enterocytes to give birth," McBride says.[cdxix]

She goes on to say, "We need to drive out pathogens, we need to replace them with beneficial flora, and we need to provide all the building blocks for the gut lining to give birth to those enterocytes."[cdxx]

Many fish oils have added tocopherols, which are most often sourced from soy, an endocrine disruptor.

Dr. Natasha does recommend Norwegian cod liver oils as favorable. One the most popular among Norwegians being Carlson Norwegian Cod Liver Oil. Many Norwegians consider this oil a religious part of their day. Some say this is a weaker therapeutic oil, more suited for those who are hypersensitive.

It's important to use only unflavored oils unless the company has been contacted to ensure the ingredients hidden under the labels "lemon flavor" or similar titles are clean. Unspecified ingredients, such as flavorings, are often the source of upset in a damaged gut.

Most people see optimum results by taking FCLO along with another cod liver oil at night before they go to bed.

After Codlivergate [the storm of accusations by Kaayla Daniel, PhD., against Fermented Cod Liver Oil (FCLO), made by Green Pastures], many practitioners were inundated with questions on whether or not FCLO was still part of the GAPS protocol. For some practitioners, this question is encountered multiple times a day.

Dr. McBride spoke on this topic of Fermented Cod Liver Oil, post-Codlivergate, in her presentation Gut and Psychology Syndrome (Part 1) at Wise Traditions 2015, the 16th Annual International conference of The Weston A. Price Foundation. She said that for "vitamin A & D, the good supplement is cod liver oil. The recent controversy about Fermented Cod Liver Oil has confused a lot of people. I use both the Fermented Cod Liver Oil and the Rosita oil. I have many people who take them. They have taken them for many years with good results. I use both. I don't take any sides because neither side has any solid science or any solid testing. I wouldn't be afraid of either of these," McBride said.[cdxxi]

One of the easiest ways to determine if a product is tolerated well by the body is to see how parents see success with the product when their child has an extremely damaged microbiome, in cases such as severe autism, Crohn's, celiac disease, lupus, MS, and the like.

Having imbalanced yeasts in the stomach can sometimes cause the Fermented Cod Liver Oil to shoot up the esophagus. In these cases, the yeast in the stomach should be addressed.

"They're very useful, but again, it is a supplement. Be careful with the supplements. We want foods," McBride says.[cdxxii]

One of the main things seen with GAPS is that there are many different paths to the end goal. It is very bio-individual. This specifically addressed in McBride's article "One Man's Meat is Another Man's Poison," specifically saying to listen to the body and what it needs nutritionally. This means that no one can tell you what your body needs in its course of healing. Only the body can tell you.[cdxxiii]

This includes Fermented Cod Liver Oil.

Not all Fermented Cod Liver Oils are GAPS-compliant, and some may be the cause of some digestive upset. Cinnamon Tingle contains cassia oil and processed stevia, which are best for when a person is Coming Off GAPS. It often causes upset in the stomach when bacteria and yeasts are in abundance.

Many times, when a person is healing and supporting his or her system, people tend to get very scientific, saying we need this balance of this vitamin and that balance of another vitamin. However, the body doesn't necessarily work the way a lab deciphers or breaks down vitamins. "Too scientific," is how Dr. Natasha responds.

"We get a lot of vitamin A from GAPS. It's very rich in vitamin A. The recent testing that I became aware of has demonstrated that the values of vitamin D in foods, that [have] been put into all of our nutritional textbooks, and dietician textbooks, are incorrect. That two quality egg yolks a day can provide your daily amount of vitamin D. A good helping of butter can provide a daily amount of D, particularly pastured butter," she says. "That certainly makes far more sense from the logical point of view because so many people in our western world spend the whole winter without sunbathing. Yet we all don't drop off and we all don't have osteoporosis and tooth decay."[cdxxiv]

Her stance has not changed. Her protocol of repair comes from supporting the body correctly. Foods provide us the nutrients to support the body to heal.

McBride doesn't lean on supplements, saying, "I only use the supplements at the beginning of the program until the diet is fully introduced, fully going, and the person starts healing. Then we can discontinue supplements because the diet provides everything necessary."[cdxxv]

It is not necessary to continue taking supplements for life. Our bodies are perfectly and wonderfully made. We are not designed to be reliant on popping supplements.

"So again, cod liver oil is not something you will have to take forever. The diet will provide you with everything," McBride said.[cdxxvi]

The more damage a person has, the longer they need the support until their system is absorbing nutrition from their food. "Children with dyslexia, hyperactive children, schizophrenic people, autistic people and people with other mental and behavioral issues benefit dramatically from supplementing fish oils. Studies were done without changing the diet, without changing anything else in the lives of these groups of patients apart from supplementing them with a particular brand of fish oil," she adds.[cdxxvii]

The goal is food, not supplements.

"Based on that, I used these supplements particularly at the beginning, particularly with those groups of children and adults. Then after two, three months of supplementation, we usually discontinue that as well – because there is no need anymore. Once we are up to having good amounts of animal fats every day, and we build animal fats consistently – the more animal fat a person consumes, particularly with mental illness, the quicker they recover. That is an observation that is very solid – many years of observation."[cdxxviii]

McBride's clinical practice has been extensively working with canaries-in-the-coal-mine. This is the basis for her statements.

Fish oil, cod liver oil, and Fermented Cod Liver oil are three different products, each used for different situations.

"Dr. Natasha says, "Fish oils will work as an anti-coagulant and anti-inflammatory agent better than aspirin."[cdxxix]

Dr. Natasha say, "In the first two stages of the Introduction Diet, I recommend not to introduce any supplements, just introduce fermented foods. In a small number of patients, no fermented food can be tolerated, so for these patients I recommend introducing a probiotic gradually starting from a tiny dose. From the third stage, if fermented foods have been successfully introduced, you can start introducing the probiotic and the cod liver oil in tiny amounts, gradually increasing the daily dose. When cod liver oil has been introduced (the full dose is taken daily), introduce fish oils. For those who started from the Full GAPS Diet, probiotics and cod liver oil can be introduced from the beginning, starting from a tiny amount and gradually increasing the dose. When cod liver oil has been successfully introduced, start the fish oils and the nut/seed oils."[cdxxx]

In some folks with seizures, involuntary movements, and tics, fish oils and cod liver oil should not be used until enough healing has happened that the movements have stopped. Those with diarrhea should also wait longer, until the loose stools have passed.

Most folks need more fish oils during the winter months.

Navigating which fish oils are beneficial is not easy. Many are simply a waste of money, only good for the garbage can. Again, the supplement industry is self-regulated, which means that they themselves determine what is safe and beneficial for the supplement. Many supplemental oils are cut with canola oil or corn oil, making the manufacturing process less expensive and the profits higher. Moreover, many fish oils, including cod liver oils, are sourced from farm-raised fish.

Many studies have been done on people with cancer and the use of essential fatty acids EPA and DHA, omega-3 fatty acids. The results are remarkable. *JAMA Internal Medicine* reported a study on non-Mediterranean people with cancer using the Mediterranean Diet (high in omega-3 oil). Their cancers showed such great reduction that omega-3 oils were labeled anticancer.[cdxxxi]

Another study done by the University of Michigan showed that omega-3 fatty acids had anticancer effects on prostate cancer.[cdxxxii]

The Cochrane Collaboration reported a study showing that omega-3 fatty acids preserved cognitive function.[cdxxxiii]

The Marine Stewardship Council evaluates fisheries for sustainable practices, awarding those who have a low impact on the environment and comply with applicable laws for the "blue label," a 5-Star rating.

Fish oils can oxidize and go rancid; therefore, they are stored in colored bottles. If there is ever a time where you won't be using your fish oil, keep it fresh by putting it in the refrigerator.

These fish oils show good results and rank high in testing. GAPSters should be aware of added ingredients that can feed the pathogens, such as natural lemon flavor, rosemary extract, ascorbyl palmitate, and tocopherols, which are usually sourced from soy. They are listed in no specific order.

Viva Naturals has an extremely high omega-3 content, showing 2200 mg omega-3 every two capsules, tested by a third party. The manufacturer says that their fish are cold water, wild-caught, and never farm-raised.

Nordic Naturals Omega-3 comes from wild-caught, deep sea fish, such as anchovies and sardines. Two capsules contain 1280 mg of omega-3. This supplement ranks very high in independent laboratory testing; however, the natural lemon flavor and rosemary extract can be troublesome for some GAPS folks.

Nutrigold Omega-3 Gold Triple Strength ranked highest by the Marine Stewardship Council, showing one of the highest per serving doses. It is free of corn and soy.

Sardines are an easy food that can be grabbed on the go. A sardine is enormously high in omega-3 fatty acids – 1300 mg, depending on the size. Overall, small, wild-caught fish is the safest source of seafood. Bigger fish, which eat little fish, which eat smaller fish, which eat tiny fish, which eat itty bitty fish, build their accumulation of heavy metals with each passing size. For this reason, bigger fish should be used in rotation with other foods, not as a daily delight.

Fish Stock, as described in Stage One, is another fantastic source for nutrition, especially omegas.

Most folks on GAPS just supplement with Fermented Cod Liver Oil – unflavored, orange, or mint.

Chapter 5:

Stage Four

Stage Four keeps all previous foods but adds:

• Cooked meats and vegetables, cooked in the oven without the lid. The meat and vegetables are exposed directly to the heating element, giving them a harder outside, making them even crunchier than earlier stages.

• Roasting meats and vegetables and cooking in the oven in an open dish, on whatever temperature, is introduced. Frying and cooking meats and vegetables on the grill comes later, on Full GAPS. It is important that there are no charred pieces as these is harder to digest.

• Pork cracklings, the crunchy bits that float to the surface while rendering lard, are introduced at Stage Four. This delicious treat is best served scooped right out of the oil, salted with mineral salt, and eaten.

• Broiled foods are added in Stage Four. In the UK, where Dr. Natasha lives, grilling is the term used when food is set in the oven, exposed to heat from the top, the same term used for broiling in America. Dr. Natasha says, "You can just set it on the rack or a tray and then, after a few minutes, flip it – if you're doing lamb chops for example, leaving them medium rare in the middle. Rare meat is great."[cdxxxiv]

• Cold-pressed olive oils, flax seed oil, hemp oil, and the like, can be added to meals if they have not been added already. Oils that are cold-pressed, unrefined, and organic are added here, such as sunflower oil and avocado oil.[cdxxxv]

• Sautéed vegetables can be cooked without the lid, giving a less soft vegetable.

• Roasted vegetables are added at Stage Four. Dr. Natasha says Stage Four adds "baking vegetables, I quite often put vegetables in cubes, in a tray, in a mixture, you can have onions, you can have zucchini, you can have turnips and radishes and daikon – handful, literally a handful of fat. What I do is I take it with my hand and go over all those pieces (of vegetable) with my hand, with the fat. Every piece is covered, and in it goes. The juice, the jelly from the bottom of the (Meat Stock) jar goes in there. That's the flavor. It goes in the oven for about 40 minutes, 50 minutes. Until the vegetables are soft, they've absorbed all the fat, they're translucent. And a handful of garlic in there, too."[cdxxxvi]

In America these are called roasted vegetables. Dr. Natasha says, "Roasted vegetables can be done at Stage Four. Very satisfying, particularly for people who are losing weight."[cdxxxvii]

Grilling is a separate matter and should be monitored closely. Dr. Natasha says, "When the fire gets in direct contact with food it burns it and turns its outer layers into toxic chemicals. We need a heat source without direct fire. Grilling is done with the heat source above the food; there is no contact between the food and the fire. Barbecue has the heat source under the food, so the fire from burning gas comes in direct contact with the meat. As a result, the barbecued meat burns on the outside. The exception are the old Mediterranean grills where they burn wood for a long time to create glowing embers (there is no fire anymore), then the meat is placed above this heat source on a grill. This does not apply to the modern barbecues which use wood or charcoal, but then a very toxic chemical is poured on top of it to light it up."[cdxxxviii]

• Seed flours are generally easier to digest than nut flours and can be introduced first. Fermenting these flours with a bit of whey, salt, or apple cider vinegar is the optimal place to start. Dr. Natasha says, "Seeds should always be soaked for 12 hours at least and better sprouted a little. If there is still a reaction, then grind soaked and sprouted sunflower seeds into paste and ferment for 24 hours; then bake with it." Once digestion has healed, down the road, seeds no longer need to be soaked or sprouted.[cdxxxix]

• Nut flours and seed flours are introduced, including almond flour, cashew flour, sesame seed flour, as well as others. Nut flours or seed flours can be used to create baked breads made from nut or seed flours, eggs, and animal fat; however, these are not a staple to the diet eaten with every meal, just an occasional treat. Baked sweets come later in Stage Six. Again, these flours should be first introduced as fermented flours, adding whey, salt, or apple cider vinegar to the water covering the flour.

• Baking soda can be added to baked goods.[cdxl]

• Coconut cream and coconut milk can be added in Stage Four if they are homemade or bought in the store in glass jars with no pathogen feeding ingredients.[cdxli]

• Cured meats such as salami can be added in at Stage Four if they are, "Not too spicy, too many chilies," says Dr. Natasha.[cdxlii] Cured meats should not contain any chemicals or added nitrates or nitrites, and absolutely no MSG.

• Miso, a traditionally fermented dish from Japan, can be added at Stage Four.[cdxliii] Usually, it is made from fermented soybeans and barley but can also be made with soybeans and rice malt.

• Fruit kvass is added. Here are the directions to make this: put fruit in a jar a third of the way full; add a teaspoon of whey and fill with water; put on the lid and let it sit for 3 days or until fizzy.[cdxliv]

• Juicing is added in Stage Four, starting with carrot juice. Once carrot is tolerated, other vegetable juices are added. Juicing fruit is not introduced yet due to the high sugar content, unless they are made as a GAPS Shake. Juices should be made and consumed within 20 minutes of juicing. Carrot juice is the only juice that has a refrigerator shelf life, lasting 2 days, according to the Gerson Protocol.

Juicing Vegetables

Purchasing a juicer can cost anywhere from $30 to $1,500. Finding something that works for you and produces healthy juice is important. Dr. Natasha says, "I use a centrifugal juicer myself because it's quicker and easier. You want something that is practical, affordable, and doesn't take hours to clean."[cdxlv]

The Juice Man Juicer and Jack LaLanne Juicer both produce economical versions. Unused Jack LaLanne Juicers are often available on Craigslist or in resale shops for a quarter of the original price.

Juicing vegetables starts with carrot juice. The goal is at least one cup a day. Some have to start slowly with a teaspoon or even with watered-down juice; only your body can tell you what your body tolerates. Once carrot juice is tolerated, other vegetables can be used.

Dr. Natasha says, "Introduce freshly pressed juices, starting from a few spoonfuls of carrot juice. Make sure that the juice is clear, filter it well. Let your patient drink it slowly or diluted with warm water or mixed with some homemade yoghurt. If well tolerated gradually increase to a full cup a day. When a full cup of carrot juice is well tolerated try to add to it juice from celery, lettuce and fresh mint leaves. Your patient should drink the juice on an empty stomach, so first thing in the morning and middle of afternoon are good times."[cdxlvi]

Some practitioners say that juicing cruciferous vegetables is dangerous to your health, damaging your thyroid. Adverse side effects like malaise, weight gain, and exhaustion are being blamed on specific raw vegetables.

The GAPS Protocol uses these juiced vegetables in appropriate amounts.

The *New England Journal of Medicine* reported a case where an 88-year-old Chinese woman was trying to control her diabetes through eating bok choy, a Chinese cabbage. This goitrogenic vegetable is healthy but for her it became deadly.[cdxlvii]

When she ate 3 to 4 heads a day, a ghastly amount, it damaged her thyroid to the point of crisis. After several months of her "healthy habit," she was so lethargic that she could not walk. Her throat began to close on her, and soon, she could not swallow. After three days of extreme lethargy and an inability to swallow, she was taken to the emergency room.[cdxlviii]

Her thyroid was not palpable, which means it could not be felt to the touch, was not engorged, and was not filled with life.[cdxlix]

She was suffering because vegetables from the brassica family were not being well tolerated by her body.[cdl]

The journal reported that she experienced "respiratory failure and [was] admitted to the intensive care unit with a diagnosis of severe hypothyroidism with myxedema coma. She was treated with intravenous methylprednisolone and levothyroxine [thyroid medicines] and was eventually discharged."[cdli]

Some practitioners consider brassica family vegetables to contain compounds that are termed goitrogens because they inhibit the thyroid uptake of iodine. GAPSters are not to be eating three to four juiced heads of cabbage a day, as the lady discussed did for many months. The quantity consumed while on GAPS is not a concern.

In 1920, *The New Zealand Medical Journal* reported the deaths of two teenage girls and one teenage boy as the result of exophthalmic goiter, a result of thyroid deficiency.[cdlii]

The *NZMJ* reported, "In 1928, Chesney and colleagues at Johns Hopkins found they could produce goiters in rabbits by feeding them a cabbage diet.

This was the forerunner of medical treatment for thyrotoxicosis. Cabbage contained a positive goitrogenic substance, as opposed to the negative goitrogenic effect of iodine deficiency."[cdliii]

Dr. Barbara A. Hummel says, "There are no food [sic] that reverse hyperthyroidism or make it worse." Dr. Hummel is a Family Medicine Doctor and contributor on *HealthTap*. Dr. Ed Friedlander, a pathologist agrees with her statement, as does another unrecognized MD on the site.[cdliv]

The term goitrogen means goiter producer. A goiter is a growth on the thyroid gland.

Goitrogenic foods are known as being very beneficial for breast health, yet large amounts of uncooked goitrogens suppress the thyroid by causing inflammation.

Cooking or fermenting goitrogens removes the problematic oxalic acid but some people receive this information too late.[cdlv]

Goitrogenic foods are: kale, cabbage, collard greens, mustard greens, canola, kohlrabi, broccoli, Brussels sprouts, bok choy, rutabaga, turnip, cauliflower, kohlrabi, radishes, millet, cassava, soy flour, soybean oil, soy lecithin, soy, strawberries, pears, peaches, rapeseed, and turnips. These vegetables are not the heavy content of juicing for a GAPSter, but rather, just a complement.

However, avocado, coconut, caffeine, and saturated fat have shown that they stimulate the thyroid.

Juicing goitrogens is a major cause of negative goitrogenic side effects. A better source for juicing would be cucumber, carrots, or celery, which contain high quantities of potassium with a low sugar hit unlike apples, carrots, and pineapple. To keep your health at an optimum level, eat all vegetables in an organic form.

Meat Pie

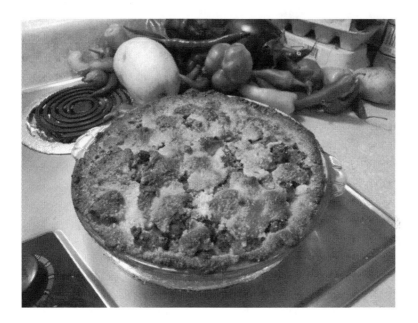

Pie Crust

    3 cups almond flour
    2 tablespoons local honey
    5 tablespoons grass-fed butter

In a mixer, blend together the almond flour and local honey.

Continue by adding the butter, one tablespoon at a time, until the butter is fully incorporated.

Press the "dough" into a pie pan.

Meat Pie Filling

    1 pound ground beef
    1 pound ground pork
    1 pound pork sausage
    2 large onions

2 carrots
1 cup of peas (frozen is fine)
Broccoli bits and pieces
2 tablespoons almond flour
1/4 cup dry red wine (Full GAPS)
1 cup block shredded cheddar cheese (preferably raw)

In a pan, sauté the onions until they're caramelized. Set them aside.

Next sauté the ground beef, the ground pork, and the pork sausage (all free-ranging, grass-fed, grass-finished). When mostly done, add the caramelized onions.

To this mix add the carrots, peas, and broccoli and salt and pepper to your liking.

The next ingredient, almond flour, helps give the mix a little body, holding some of the juices in the mix instead of leaching into the shell. Sprinkle the almond flour over the mixture.

For those on Full GAPS, you may add a 1/4 cup of dry red wine—poured over the mix. NOTE: any wine you drink from a measuring cup is not considered drinking – it's considered cooking!

Add the meat pie filling into the pie shell and top with the remaining crust, leaving spaces for steam to escape.

For those on Full GAPS or for those working their way through intro for a second or third time—top with the shredded cheese (preferably raw).

Cook at 350 degrees for 25-35 minutes or until the top is lightly browned (crust or cheese).

Bacon-wrapped Asparagus

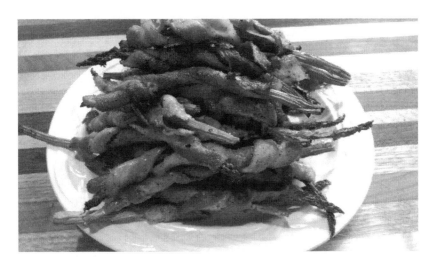

Bacon-wrapped asparagus is quite possibly the simplest recipe there is.

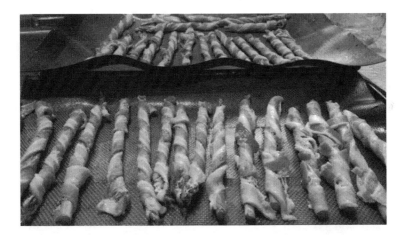

Wrap each piece of asparagus with a slice of sugar-free bacon, optimally pastured. Lay them side-by-side on a baking sheet. Cook at 400 degrees for 25 minutes, or until desired crispiness is achieved.

Don't tell anyone you've made this—or they disappear.

Roasted Pig's Head

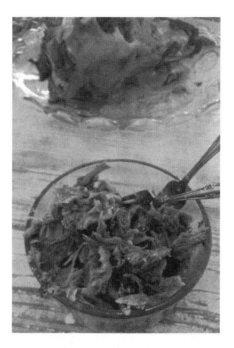

Cooking a pig's head is daunting, but honestly, it is one of the easiest things to cook. The local processor or pastured meat sales business can provide you with a head. Some are sold without the cheeks, jowls, as they are used as a form of bacon. The price of a head ranges from free to $40. Pastured meat is best.

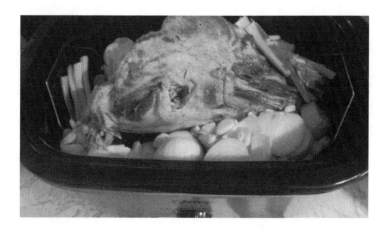

In a roaster pan, add the head, onions, garlic, and whatever other vegetable you desire and can tolerate. Salt and pepper the head for seasoning. Cover the bottom of the pan with water.

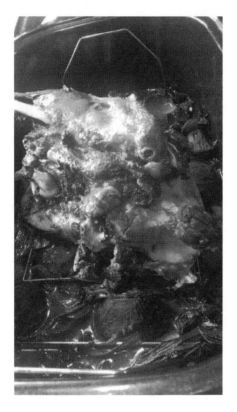

Put the lid on and cook at 225 for 6 to 8 hours.

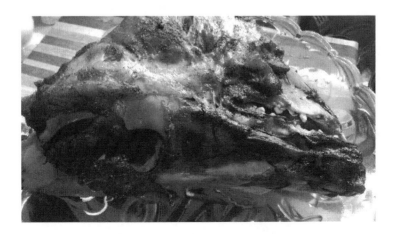

With two forks, remove and shred the meat, including the tongue, which is, frankly, the best part. The delicacy is the meat between the upper jaw and lower jaw, where the jaws connect.

Place all the shredded meat and some (or all) of the fat on a serving dish with the vegetables.

Bacon-wrapped Hearts

*This recipe is a Weston A. Price Foundation Recipe of the Month Winner, January 2018 *

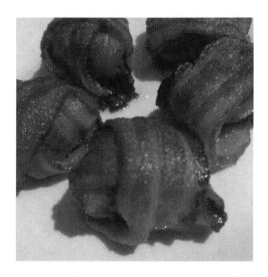

It's no secret that organ meats are a champion in nutrient-density. Their nutrient content is easily absorbed, especially for those with a damaged intestinal tract. Many nutritional deficiencies can be satisfied through organ meats. The problem is... they're organ meats.

This delectable dish goes against all understanding, defies reality, and will even leave teenage boys begging for more. In fact, that's happened on more than one occasion here.

THIS dish is a food you will not have to hide in meals—it shines right out in the open, proud to display its nutritional value!

Bacon wrapped hearts are delicious, mouthwatering, and make the whole-body tingle as it's flooded with nourishment. It's a true treat! More importantly, this dish is about the easiest dish a girl can make! Then, when you consider the fact that three bacon wrapped hearts will satisfy your hunger for over 3 hours, it's a must-have food.

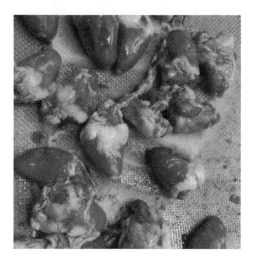

A whole tray can be made as an appetizer dish with, literally, a few minutes of prep time.

Finding chicken hearts from pastured chickens that have not been treated with antibiotics or other medicine is important. Chickens raised on pasture contain more vitamins and minerals, satisfying the body with the nutritional support it needs. It is important to eat organ meats for regaining health, rotating different organs throughout the week.

Any heart will do; just cut it up into bite-sized pieces.

The hardest part is finding clean bacon where the pork has not been fed soy or other starchy grains. Pigs are very difficult to contain in a paddock, making secure fencing expensive for acres of paddock space. Electric fencing is most praised by farmers. If the fence is not secure, where the pigs cannot root under the barrier, the fence is really more of a suggestion than a secure perimeter. They are much like dogs and often come back for their food, but for safety reasons, keeping them penned up tightly causes most pig farmers to raise pigs in small paddocks or on a concrete floor inside a building. This is not optimal.

It is important to note that a pig that is kept on plush green grass where he can forage for grubs and turn over the soil is so happy, he won't stop wagging his tail with delight.

For optimal results, find a local farmer who raises pastured pigs in the sunshine and supplements with fermented organic feed only. Using the pork belly, sliced thin and seasoned with mineral salt, pepper, and local honey (optional), is best and the least amount of work. If that is not available, bacon can be sourced from your local health food store but be careful of the sugar content. Finding prepackaged bacon without sugar is nearly impossible. Sugar feeds pathogens in the gut, even in the tiniest amounts if you have great gut damage. Health food store bacon is costly and often very thick, which causes for a longer cooking time for this bacon-wrapped hearts dish.

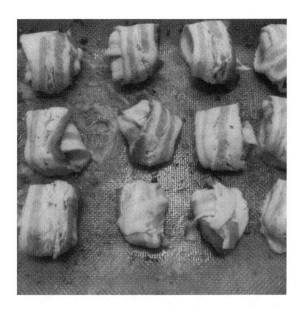

The recipe is simple: wrap each heart with a slice of bacon. Cook in the oven at 350 degrees for 30 minutes until done. Again, thicker bacon takes much longer. Some people like crisp bacon and well-done hearts, others like chewy bacon and less-done hearts. Adjust your cook time accordingly.

Breaded and Baked Liver

Liver makes some folks curl up their noses, but this treat is one that even the picky eater will enjoy.

Organ meats are highly nutritive. Some people think that, since liver is a filter organ, it contains toxins; however, studies show that it does not retain the toxins.[cdlvi] This is similar to how people used a bladder or stomach as a wine skin.

Liver sourced from a grass-fed, grass-finished, free-ranging animal is optimal. Be aware of grass-fed beef that isn't grass-fed. Many folks favor lamb, sheep, or chicken livers.

> 1 pound liver
> 3 eggs, beaten until smooth
> Almond flour (or other nut or seed flour)
> Rendered tallow, rendered lard or unrefined coconut oil
> Salt and pepper to taste

First, remove any connective tissue from the liver and slice the liver, or cut it with scissors, into edible-sized strips.

To wash the liver, place it in a mixture of lemon juice and water, or apple cider vinegar and water, or whey and water, or salt and water. Leave it to soak for about four hours.

After washing, liver has a less dry, more delicate taste. Some people even do their "washing" in kefir, yogurt, or raw milk as well.

Place the liver strips in an egg wash. A glass pie pan makes a great dipping station.

After the strips are bathed in the egg wash, place in a shallow dish of almond flour, or other nut or seed flour. Push the pieces of liver into the flour to help the flour stick. Be sure both sides are coated.

Place the strips into a baking dish (9×13 pan or cast iron skillet), the bottom covered with your tallow, lard, or coconut oil.

Bake at 350 degrees for 15 to 20 minutes, or until done and browned to your liking. Season and serve with a heap of sautéed onions and garlic or other tolerated side.

Believe it or not, this dinner causes this family to throw elbows. There are never leftovers.

Homestyle Chicken Casserole

Homestyle Chicken Casserole is the creation of Autumn, a young mother who changed her family's health with GAPS. Autumn started GAPS for their 2-year-old son, Gunnar, with the diagnosis of Failure to Thrive three separate times. He ranked in the 10th percentile. He only had one food intolerance, but it was a severe dairy issue. After an accidental exposure to a large quantity of dairy, he became nonverbal with only 5 words and developed new food intolerances. He began to tolerate less and less until he was on a small number of foods. Autumn says "Many people call the GAPS Diet restrictive, but for our family, it added foods in right from the start. He had profuse diarrhea, was pale with red rims and very dark circles under his eyes." He was painfully thin with a remarkably hard, bloated belly.

At age 4, and being on the GAPS Diet for 2 years, his doctor said he was in the 60th percentile for his weight. Today, he is fully verbal and spends his days as a responsible older brother, playing in the woods and thriving in school. You would never know that he ever had an issue. It is clear that on the GAPS Diet, he thrives. "We are so grateful for all the foods his body has learned how to digest thanks to the GAPS Diet."

This is Autumn's recipe:

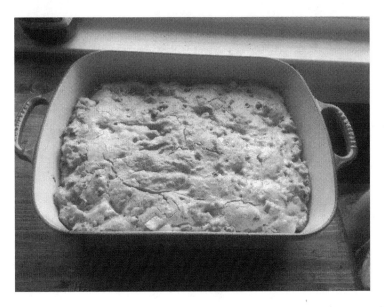

This is a very forgiving recipe that can be tailored to your GAPS family; it may even be made nut and egg free by adding more soft tissues or using fewer vegetables. Nut free would make this recipe Stage Two compliant.

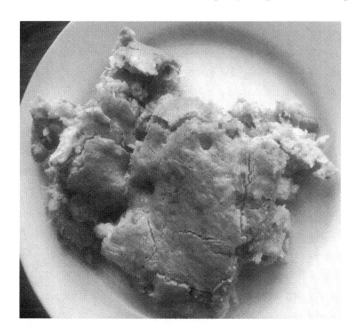

The most important part of this recipe is the soft tissues from Meat Stock. These tissues help create a 'cream of chicken' batter for your casserole. I used the minimum amount of tissues necessary for the recipe to work, but there is no maximum!

Sautéed Onions:

4 diced onions
6 cloves minced garlic
2 tbsp fresh herbs of choice, optional (like parsley, thyme, rosemary, marjoram, or tarragon)
1/2 cup fat of choice (pork lard, beef tallow, duck fat, goose fat, chicken schmaltz, ghee, or butter)

Cream of Chicken Batter:

1/2 cup soft tissues, however, more is even better
1/4 cup Meat Stock in warm, liquid form, not cold gelatin form
1/2 cup chicken
4 eggs
1 cup soaked and still wet cashews or 1/2 cup of nut butter of choice
2 teaspoon mineral salt

Meat and Vegetables:

2 cups chicken cut into small chunks
6 cups chopped leftover vegetables that were cooked in Meat Stock (like
     leafy greens, carrots, peas, turnips, rutabaga, green beans, zucchini,
     yellow squash, etc.)
1 cup melted fat of choice
Salt and pepper to taste
Extra herbs of choice, optional

Step 1- Sautéed Onions:

Melt fat onto skillet and add diced onion and 1/2 teaspoon salt or salt to taste. Cover and simmer until sweet and translucent (about 20 minutes); add 1 tablespoon of Meat Stock before covering for faster cook time. Once translucent and sweet, scrape onion to the sides of the pan like a ring and add minced garlic and herbs in the center; sauté for 5 more minutes. Remove from heat to cool.

Preheat oven to 375F and grease a 9×13 baking pan or bakeware of choice.

Step 2- Cream of Chicken:

If your soft tissues and stock have been cooled in the fridge, gently warm them on low heat in a saucepan. Set a timer for about 2 minutes so that it doesn't get so hot it cooks the eggs in the process.

Add 1/2 of the sautéed onions mixture, soft tissues, stock, chicken, soaked and still wet cashews (or nut butter), salt, and eggs to a food processor and blend until smooth. If the stock got too hot, blend all ingredients until smooth except the eggs; then blend the eggs in after the mixture has cooled.

Set aside approximately 1/2 cup of your batter for the top of the casserole.

Step 3- Meat and Vegetables:

In a large mixing bowl, combine meat, vegetables, melted fat, and the other half of your sautéed onions. The chicken will absorb the melted fat well. Then fold in the remainder of your cream of chicken batter and pour it into your greased pan. Spread the mixture out and then top it with the batter you set aside.

Cook Time: 1 hour for 9×13 baking pan or 30 minutes for ramekins.

Zucchini Bread

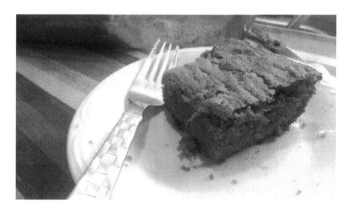

Zucchini bread is summer comfort food. This recipe makes it healthy.

This mix does well as muffins, baked in a 9×13, or made as a bread in a loaf pan.

    1 cup grass-fed butter
    3 tablespoons local honey
    1 tablespoon cinnamon
    1 teaspoon baking soda

2 teaspoons vanilla
1 teaspoon almond extract
2 cups grated zucchini—packed tight
4 eggs
4 cups almond flour
1 cup chopped walnuts optional

First, put the butter and honey in a mixer and beat until frothy – about 20 minutes.

Add the cinnamon, baking soda, vanilla, almond extract, and grated zucchini to the mix. Lightly blend them in.

Add the eggs and almond flour, alternating them (i.e., one egg, mix thoroughly, one cup flour, mix thoroughly, one egg, mix thoroughly, one cup flour, etc.), until blended. Add the chopped walnuts, if desired.

Pour the mix into either a lined muffin pan, a buttered 9×13, or a buttered loaf pan. Bake at 350 degrees for 50 minutes (less for the muffins) or until cooked thoroughly so the top has browned and cracked and doesn't jiggle.

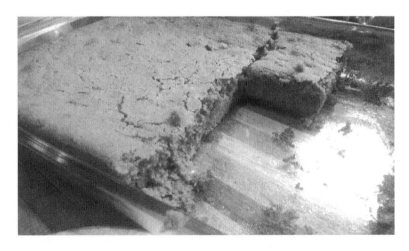

Pumpkin Pie

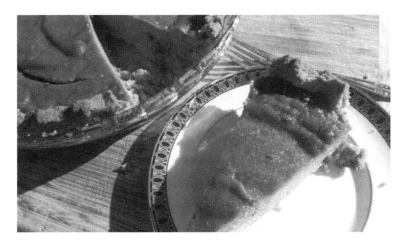

There are few things better at Thanksgiving time than pumpkin pie; however, once you begin making pumpkin pie out of real ingredients, you'll soon see how much of a difference sugar and binder ingredients make. This recipe is a pleaser with both GAPS folks and Standard American Diet lovers.

It's so good, you may never return to another pie.

Crust

>   2 cups cashews in the Vitamix (blend until finely ground)
>   or 2 cups cashew butter
>   1 egg
>   3 tablespoons organic grass-fed butter
>   1 teaspoon vanilla
>   1/4 cup coconut flour

Add all ingredients to a Vitamix or food processor and blend until smooth. Turn the mixture out into the pie pan. Press it into the pie pan until it covers the pan. Decorative topping can be made with your fingertips at the top of the pie pan. Press into the pie pan with your fingers. This recipe fills one pie pan with thick crust or can be made thin and cover two pie pans.

After the pie crust is ready, prepare the pumpkin mixture.

Pumpkin Pie Filling

15 ounces pumpkin
4 ounces kefir made from cream
4 tablespoons pastured butter
2 pastured eggs
4 pastured yolks
3/4 cup honey
2 teaspoons vanilla
3 teaspoons cinnamon
1 teaspoon ground ginger
1/4 teaspoon ground cloves
2 teaspoons nutmeg

In the Vitamix, blend until smooth. Pour ingredients into a pie shell and cook at 350 degrees and for one hour or until the topped is cracked, showing it is cooked.

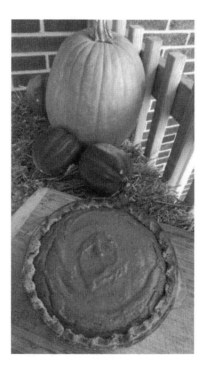

Pumpkin Pie Pumpkin VS Jack-O-Lantern Pumpkin

Pie pumpkins are small, often darker in color and cost roughly $2.86. They yield roughly 4 cups of pumpkin.

Jack-O-Lantern pumpkins are four times the size of pie pumpkins, nearly the same color and cost $4.00. They produce roughly 18 cups of pumpkin.

Canned pumpkin isn't really pumpkin, but instead a relative of butternut squash, and costs $2-$5 a can. It contains just under 1.9 cups of pumpkin.

The two pumpkins were compared. Pumpkin was cooked, baked, eaten alone, and made into pies, cookies, and breads. It was not a job for the faint stomach. The task was a large one, but the results were favorable.

Thirteen samplings were used. Two separate tests were done, each one month apart, showing the same results each time. Tasters did not know which samples were from which pumpkin.

Pumpkins were cut in half, deseeded and cooked in the oven face down on a cookie sheet at 350 degrees for an hour or until done. The skin was removed, and the pumpkin was utilized.

Samples of fresh, hot, cooked pumpkin were tested; cooled pumpkin, pumpkin pie, and pumpkin cookies were all tested, using identical recipes with different pumpkin types. Of the nine samples, the testers could not determine which tasted more like pumpkin.

No identifying colors, textures, or sizes were noticeable.

The only remarkable difference between the pie pumpkin and the Jack-O-Lantern pumpkin is that the Jack-O-Lantern pumpkin contains much more water. The pie pumpkin had the consistency of a meaty squash. The total liquid expressed measured roughly two tablespoons per cup. The Jack-O-

Lantern pumpkin was poured into a piece of cotton fabric and squeezed, expelling roughly eight cups of liquid total. After the liquid was extracted, the pie pumpkin yielded four cups of squash. The Jack-O-Lantern yielded 18 cups after the water was expressed.

The test results showed no identifiable favorite. Of the three samples chosen as favorable in taste, all three testers changed their minds after a second sample, saying the choices were no different. Samplings of the cooked hot pumpkin, cooked, cooled pumpkin, and sliced pie showed the results were inconclusive.

Pumpkin Bread

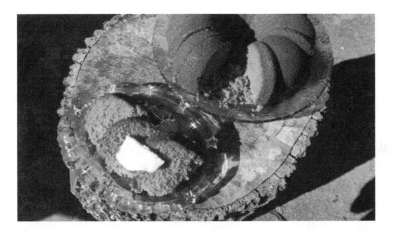

Few things fill the house with the smell of love like pumpkin bread! This gluten-free, sugar-free recipe quickly disappears. It freezes well and transports for camping like a charm.

1 cup grass-fed butter
1/3 cup local honey
2 cups pumpkin
4 eggs, bug eating chickens free-ranging in the yard preferred
3 1/2 teaspoons baking soda
3 1/2 cups almond flour
2-3 teaspoons cinnamon

2 teaspoons ground nutmeg
1/2 teaspoon ground ginger
1 1/2 cups Greek yogurt (home brewed)
1 teaspoons vanilla (preferably home brewed)

Cream pastured butter and honey for 10 minutes until frothy. Add the eggs, yogurt, and vanilla, alternating with almond flour. Add the cooked pumpkin until combined.

Your mixture will be smooth. If you still have chunks of pumpkin it's, OK; you'll just get bites of pure pumpkin in a slice. A pumpkin from Halloween or a baking pumpkin are both fine to use. Halloween pumpkins have a higher water content and may need to be strained of water first. To cook the pumpkin, cut it in half, scoop out the seeds, lay it face down on a cookie sheet, and cook at 350 degrees for 45 minutes to an hour, depending on the size. The skin can be peeled or cut off and pumpkin meat used for cooking.

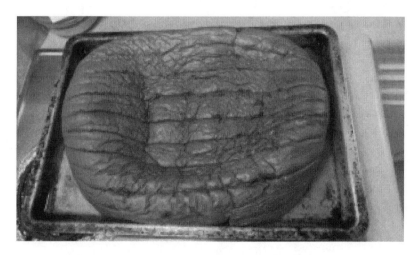

Add each egg one at a time until each is incorporated.

Mix in the remaining ingredients. Fresh nutmeg nuts, grated into the mixture, will make the product taste divine! It'll make your cooking compete on a whole different level!

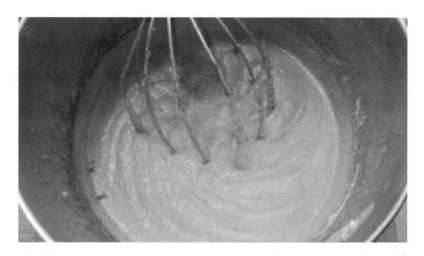

Butter the Bundt pan heavily.

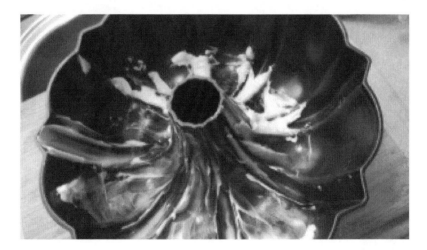

Bake at 350 degrees for 40 min. Stick a butter knife into the cake, and if it comes out clean, it's done. Other visuals to show a finished bread are a cracking top, a light browning color, and the edges pulling away from the sides.

Serve with lots of grass-fed butter and enjoy!

Shepherd's Pie

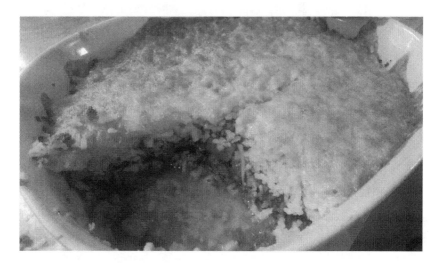

Shepherd's pie is a comfort food that is easier to bake in large batches and freeze for easy meals in the future. This is a great meal to take to a GAPS family as a gift when baby comes, or to someone who just needs a little encouragement.

The only problem we've ever had with this dish is that it disappears!

  2 lbs pastured ground beef
  3 medium onions
  4 chopped carrots
  1 chopped rutabaga
  2 cups chopped green beans
  6 diced garlic cloves
  2 cups peas
  6 cups Riced cauliflower
  Raw cheese to cover
  Salt and pepper to taste

Cook the ground beef until just done.. Remove it from the pan and cook the onions, carrots, rutabaga, chopped green beans, garlic, and peas.

Add the cooked ground beef and stir to combine.

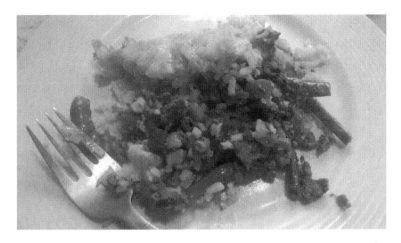

Place the cooked mixture in the bottom of a casserole pan and/or 9×13. This recipe fills both for us. Top with riced cauliflower and raw cheese. Cook at 500 degrees for 25 minutes or until the cheese is golden brown.

Thanksgiving Turkey with Gravy

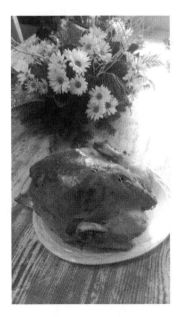

The Thanksgiving turkey isn't just the centerpiece of the table; it's a nourishing dish that can satisfy and satiate. The meal can be made Stage

Two on the GAPS Protocol, made just like the Italian Casserole described in the yellow GAPS book.

Turkey

First, choose an organic bird, optimally a pastured turkey, so that glyphosate isn't involved in your nourishing meal. Soaking the turkey in a brine adds flavor but also breaks up the muscle tissues, making the meat easier to digest. Soaking the turkey in brine can be done in a large, stainless steel pot; some even use a food-grade, five-gallon bucket, if you're comfortable with that.

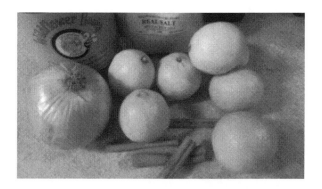

The brine base is
    1 cup mineral salt
    1 cup local honey
    4 oranges
    4 lemons
    3 onions
    6 garlic cloves
    4 cinnamon sticks
    Filtered water

The brine base is the mineral salt and local honey. From there, any flavor group can be used. One blend liked here is listed above. You can experiment but make sure the ingredients are the appropriate stage and tolerated.

If the turkey is too big to be fully submerged in the brine, half can be submerged one day, then flipped, and then the other half marinated the next day. The container with the turkey should be covered and kept in the refrigerator.

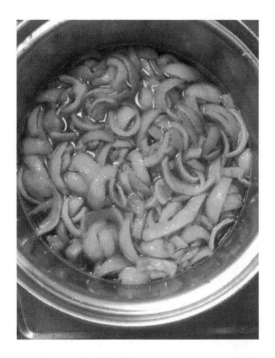

When it comes time to cook the turkey, remove the bird from the brine and drain the liquid trapped in the turkey's internal cavity. The brine ingredients have been soaking in raw turkey juice—so please discard the brine.

Place the turkey in a roaster on the support rack to keep the bird lifted out of the drippings as it cooks, giving you crispier skin. Using a roaster instead of an oven allows the drippings and steam to keep the turkey moist without having to baste the turkey every fifteen minutes, prolonging the cooking time. Cooking the bird in the roaster is like cooking it in a turkey bag, but without the toxicity from plastics.

Gravy making vegetables:

2-3 onions
4 garlic cloves
1 sliced rutabaga
1-2+ carrots
2-3 stalks of celery

Add gravy making vegetables to the bottom of the roaster.

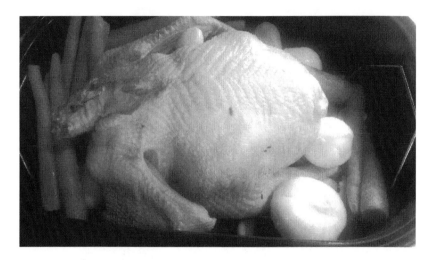

Cook time is calculated according to the size of the bird, 20 minutes per pound. When using a roaster, the time is greatly reduced.

This 25-pound turkey would be cooked for roughly 3 hours.

A 16-pound turkey would cook for roughly 2 1/4 hours.

A 12-pound bird would take roughly 1 1/2 hours.

If this bird were cooked in the oven, it would take roughly 8.3 hours. The roaster keeps the space, steam, and heat quarantined, which greatly reduces cook time—just like a turkey bag.

The internal temperature of the bird must be 165 degrees when a meat thermometer is inserted into the breast of the bird. When the turkey is cooked, lift it out of the roaster and let it sit on a large platter for 15 minutes before carving so that the juices saturate the muscle tissues. While the turkey is resting—make the gravy!

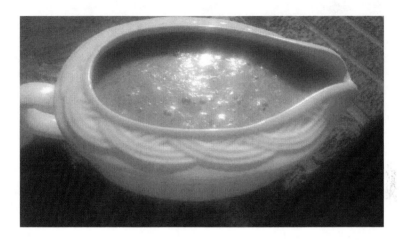

Gravy

Put the vegetables from in the roasting pan in the Vitamix along with enough of the turkey drippings in the roasting pan to make the gravy the desired thickness. More drippings mean thinner gravy.

The selection of vegetables is purely up to you. Again, the more carrots you use, the more yellow or orange your gravy will appear. For a traditional white gravy, use half of a carrot and organic onions, garlic, and rutabaga.

Your great-great-grandmother may have had a blend that you just love. So experiment and go with it when you can.

Quiche

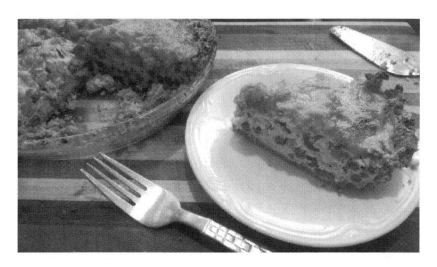

Breakfast quiche is a delicious all in-one-meal that can be made ahead of time and served warm or cold. This meal can save time and satisfy many.

Start with a GAPS-approved pie crust that is a savory, gluten-free, and sugar-free recipe; this works in dessert pies like pumpkin pie as well as quiche.

In a Vitamix or food processor, blend a full two cups of cashews with three tablespoons of grass-fed butter. Add one egg and one teaspoon of home-brewed vanilla. Blend until smooth.

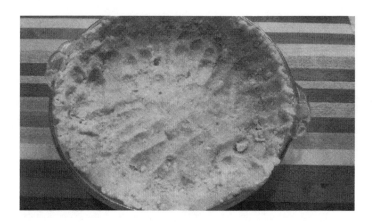

Press the pie crust mixture into a pie pan.

Put 9 pastured eggs in a bowl and whisk until combined. Add one teaspoon of mineral salt and half of a teaspoon of ground pepper. Pour mixture into the prepared pie crust. Add two cups of peas and one cup of chopped approved vegetable of choice. Fermented sour cream or butter can be added if you choose – it'll make the quiche smoother and fluffier.

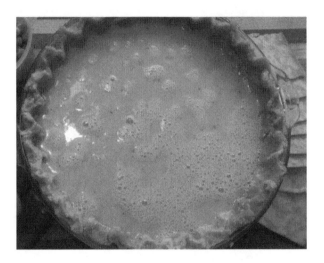

Top with cheese. Here, Monterey Jack is used.

Cook at 350 degrees for one hour or until done.

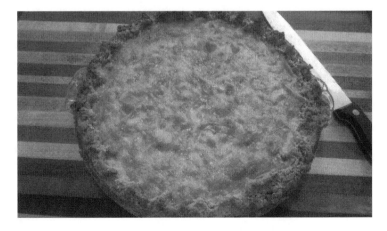

Cut and enjoy. This recipe can be served warm or cold.

Tom Kha Gai (Thai coconut soup)

Serves 4, Adult Portions

By Autumn for her son Sebastian.

From birth, Sebastian was not an obvious candidate for the GAPS Diet because he was thriving and happy; but because he was starting solids when his older brother started the diet for diarrhea, GAPS Intro offered wonderful first meals. When we introduced egg, he would immediately projectile vomit. We very slowly followed Dr. Natasha's Egg Introduction Protocol, and once he was successfully eating as many eggs as he pleased, we were surprised his mild eczema and constipation disappeared. If it hadn't been for his brother's obvious GAPS symptoms, we would have never addressed the underlying problem causing his subtle symptoms.

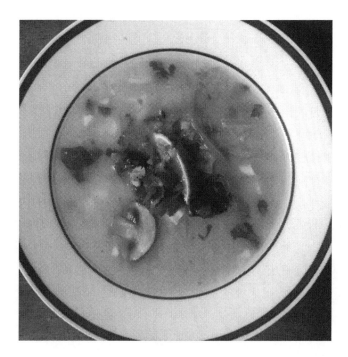

Base:

1/2 gallon chicken stock
1 teaspoon fresh, minced ginger
1 lemongrass shoot (if cut and sifted, use tea infuser)
2 cups sliced mushrooms
4 cloves garlic
Salt to taste

At least one or more of the following ingredients:

1/2 cup sour cream, optional
1 cup homemade nut milk (Stage 4), optional
2 tablespoons coconut oil, optional
1 cup coconut milk (Full GAPS), optional

Optional Ingredients by Stages:

Stage 1:
    onion, leeks, shallots, green onion, garlic scapes, seaweed
Stage 2:
    fresh cilantro
Full GAPS:
    fresh turmeric, lemon-zest, lime-zest, jalapeno, chili oil, chili flakes

Optional Proteins:

Calamari or Squid cut into rings (our favorite)
Chopped Chicken
Salmon
Scallops
Shrimp
Whisked Eggs (Stage 3)
Caviar

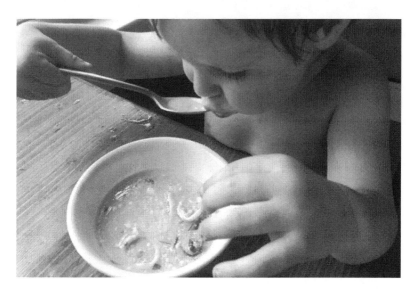

Step 1:
Have all ingredients chopped and prepared because this soup cooks
quickly.

Step 2:
Bring chicken stock, coconut oil, coconut, or nut milk to a boil.

Step 3:
Add all your prepped ingredients except the garlic and calamari. Bring
back to a boil, and then simmer for 10 minutes.

Step 4:
Add garlic and simmer for 3 more minutes. Calamari, salmon, scallops,
shrimp, and whisked eggs may be added at this time as well.

Step 5:
Serve over optional leftover chicken.

When cooled off, add optional probiotic ingredients: sour cream, kimchi, or (our personal favorite) a drizzle of fermented cod liver oil. Caviar may also be added when cooled.

Serve with a side of chili oil, coconut oil, sour cream, or lemon or lime wedges for more personalization.

Olive Oil

Cooking with olive oil is a common practice. Restaurants do it, personal chefs do it, and even housewives do it. The topic has been debated for years. Many "experts" say that cooking with olive oil is beneficial; however, doing so may be more than harmful.

The way we treat olive oil on GAPS holds it as a sacred food, as it has been traditionally.

"NEVER cook with olive oil. Never heat, never cook with it. Nut and seed oils are extracted in cold conditions and in the dark. They can be easily damaged. Never cook with cold-pressed olive oil. The value of olive oil is in its micronutrients—salicylates, phytonutrients. The aspects that make it green and spicy – this is the healthy aspect of olive oil," Dr. Natasha Campbell-McBride tells her Practitioners in Certified GAPS Practitioner Training.[cdlvii]

Olive oil is best pressed cold when it contains higher nutrition from ripe olives. The olives are pressed to extract their oil. Some olives are so ripe that when you lay them on the tray, they drip oil without any pressure from the machine. This oil is optimal.

The *Olive Oil Times* reported, "A three-year study by Australian scientists confirms that oxygen, light and heat are indeed among extra virgin olive oil's worst enemies."[cdlviii]

Jamie Ayton, Rodney J. Mailer, and Kerrie Graham were researchers in the study establishing stability in processing, packaging, shipping, and shelf life. They found that olive oil should be stored at cool temperatures, away from light and without exposure to oxygen. Otherwise, "the olive oil can deteriorate so much that it can no longer be classified as extra virgin olive oil."[cdlix]

They found that high temperatures and oxygen negatively impact the olive oil on many levels. The sensory profile declined, free fatty acid levels rose, antioxidants were lost, and rancidity developed.

Tocopherols were lost, meaning the vitamin E content of the nutritious oil was greatly depleted, if not diminished altogether.

The *Journal of Agricultural and Food Chemistry* reported a study saying, "Two monovarietal extra virgin olive oils were subjected to heating at 180 degrees C for 36 h. Oxidation progress was monitored by measuring oil quality changes (peroxide value and conjugated dienes and trienes), fatty acid composition, and minor compound content. Tocopherols and polyphenols were the most affected by the thermal treatment and showed the highest degradation rate."[cdlx]

The publication said, "We conclude that despite the heating conditions, [virgin olive oil] maintained most of its minor compounds and, therefore, most of its nutritional properties."[cdlxi]

This statement ranks in the same category of *everything in moderation*. Eating food, if it's not food, is not healthy. Drinking lighter fluid in moderation is not acceptable; eating antifreeze in moderation is not healthy– yet these are the ingredients are in processed foods today. The preservative tertiary butylhydroquinone, or TBHQ, is lighter fluid, used in chicken nuggets. Propylene glycol, antifreeze, is used in ice cream and frozen yogurt to prevent them from turning into a block of ice.

If food is not in its real-food form, the body cannot recognize it for digestion. This is true for olive oil in its original, unadulterated state.

Some "experts" say that olive oil has been heated for centuries by the ancient Greeks, Romans, and Italians. Others say that they never heated olive oil, unless it was being used as lamp oil – it's only the later generations that have heated the oil.

Atherosclerosis, a journal which analyzes disturbances of lipid and lipoprotein metabolism, says that olive oil is altered and suffers oxidative stress when heated.[cdlxii]

The *World Journal of Gastroenterology* says, "Virgin (unrefined) olive oil contains a significant amount of antioxidants and α-tocopherol and phytochemicals. However, when refined or heated, olive oil loses these natural compounds. The exact composition of olive oil depends not only on the growth conditions in the year preceding the harvest, but also on the degree of ripeness of the fruit and the technical processing (cold pressing, refining)."[cdlxiii]

If heat in the extraction damages the oil, we would be naive to believe that heating the oil in cooking doesn't damage the oil.

Quality olive oil should be green in color and taste spicy. It should be stored in a colored glass container to deter sunlight from damaging the oil. Cooking is best done with grass-fed tallow, pastured lard, or unrefined coconut oil if high heat is used. Pastured butter can be used if the heat isn't too high, as it has a low smoke point.

As a Stage Four food, olive oil is most often used by drizzling it over a cooked meal prior to serving.

Mushroom Caps

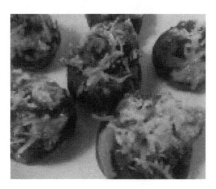

Many people mistakenly believe that mushrooms feed the pathogens that feed yeast, giving a person a yeast infection, when in fact, the opposite is true. These mushroom caps taste just like traditional mushroom caps; however, with these clean ingredients, they don't feed pathogens. The only problem will be that there are never enough of them!

The mushroom itself has anti-yeast properties to it – spores that reside on the mushroom protecting it from other mushrooms or fungi. This keeps the mushroom intact and stable. It's what protects the mushroom, keeping it as its own species and subgroup.

If you take mushrooms and put them out in the sunshine for 20 minutes, they will absorb vitamin D from the sun. Mushrooms are incredible for holding vitamin D, and they become a free vitamin source, a great way to increase your natural vitamin D levels. When vitamin D levels are high, it is more difficult for the body to get ill.

MedlinePlus says, "Vitamin D helps the body absorb calcium. Calcium and phosphate are two minerals that are essential for normal bone formation. If you do not get enough calcium, or if your body does not absorb enough calcium from your diet, bone production and bone tissues may suffer."[cdlxiv]

Fungi Perfecti, a site dedicated to mushrooms and the education thereof, says, "Even sliced and dried mushrooms—including wild ones picked the year before—will soar in vitamin D when placed outdoors under the sun. Now, the summertime, from June until September, is the best seasonal window for people in northern latitudes to make vitamin D enriched mushrooms!"[cdlxv]

They go on to say, "Mushrooms and animal skins create vitamin D when exposed to sunlight. Mushrooms are rich in the vitamin D precursor ergosterol, which ultraviolet B (between wavelengths of 290 nm to 315 nm) converts to ergocalciferols, also called provitamin D2. Mammal epidermis has cholecalciferol, which ultraviolet light converts to D3."[cdlxvi]

An experiment was done by placing organically grown mushrooms divided into three testing groups. The first group was dried inside, away from the sun. The second was dried outside in the sun, gills down. The third was dried gills up outdoors. Before sun exposure, vitamin D levels tested at 100 IU/100 grams. "The most vitamin D was found in shiitake dried with gills up exposed to sunlight for two days, six hours per day. The vitamin D levels in these mushrooms soared to nearly 46,000 IU/100 grams. Their stems, though, produced very little vitamin D, only about 900 IU. Notably, vitamin D levels dropped on the third day, probably due to over-exposure to UV."[cdlxvii]

With this trick, these mushroom caps become vitamin D supplements!

For this recipe, fresh mushrooms, not dried, are used, but both are fine. Exposing the mushrooms gills up outside to the sunshine for any length of time will increase the vitamin D content. Placing the mushrooms outside should be done with common sense regarding flies or other pests to avoid contamination.

Remove the stems from the mushrooms and place the caps gills up in a shallow cardboard box or on a cookie sheet.

   24 oz baby portabella mushrooms
   1 pound pastured, ground sausage
   2 small onions
   3 tablespoons almond flour
   1/3-2/3 cup grated Parmesan cheese
   1/2 teaspoon ground thyme
   1/2 teaspoon ground sage
   2 cloves garlic
   Salt and pepper

In a cast-iron skillet, or other pan, place a pound ground sausage, preferably pasture-raised, with two small, chopped organic onions and sauté until cooked. Add 3 tablespoons almond flour, 1/3-2/3 cup grated Parmesan cheese (depending on tolerance and taste), salt and pepper to taste, the mushroom stems, 1/2 teaspoon ground thyme, 1/2 teaspoon ground sage, and 2 garlic cloves, chopped fine. Continue cooking for just a couple more minutes.

Spoon the cooked ingredients into the mushroom caps, pressing firmly to fill. Sprinkle with more Parmesan cheese to garnish and cook.

Snickerdoodle Cookies

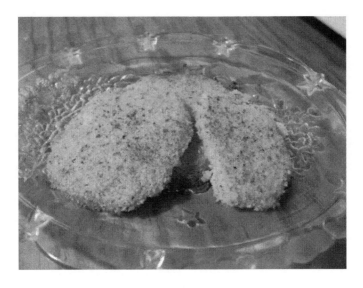

6 tablespoons grass-fed, grass-finished butter
2 tablespoons local honey
1 teaspoon vanilla
3 cups almond flour
Cinnamon
Nutmeg

Cream 6 tablespoons grass-fed, grass-fed butter with honey for 10 minutes until frothy, scraping down the sides as you go. Add vanilla and continue to mix. Add almond flour and stir until incorporated. Drop onto buttered cookie sheet, press flat to about 1/4-inch-thick, sprinkle tops with cinnamon and fresh grated nutmeg. Cook at 350 for 10-14 minutes until lightly browned.

Snickerdoodles are a delightful marriage of butter, cinnamon and nutmeg. These cookies will make you feel like you're not missing a thing as you heal and seal your gut lining.

Key Lime Pie

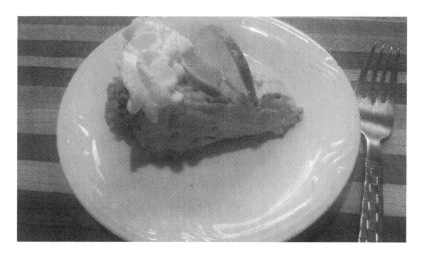

Key Lime Pie is a seasonal favorite that is refreshing and smooth. Making
Key Lime Pie in a healthy manner will satisfy even the most sensitive palate.

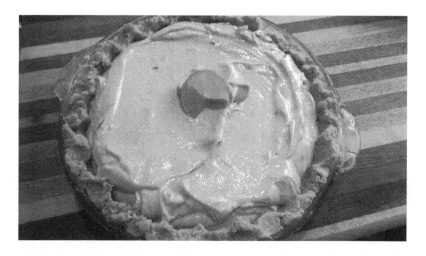

Crust

2 heaping cups of cashews (or two cups cashew butter)
1 egg
1 teaspoon of vanilla
1/4 cup of coconut flour

Add ingredients to your Vitamix or food processor. Blend until smooth. Press the mixture into a pie pan, covering the bottom and sides evenly. Cook for 12 minutes at 350 degrees. Let cool; then add the filling.

Filling

3 ripe avocados
1 cup of organic, grass-fed butter
1/2 cup of local honey
1 teaspoon of vanilla extract
1/2 cup of home-fermented sour cream
the juice of 4 limes (about a 1/2 cup)

Blend all of the ingredients in your Vitamix or food processor. Pour the filling mixture into the cooled pie shell and refrigerate. Serve chilled, with whipped fermented cream, as tolerated.

Pumpkin Donuts

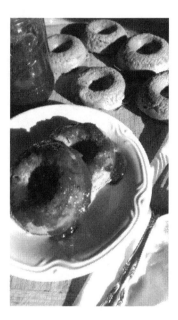

Donuts are unrivaled comfort food. Donuts that are healthy are not easy but are certainly doable. This recipe is a tweaked form of Stage Two GAPS Pancakes. The pan used to make the reminiscent shape is hard to find without a Teflon coating, but finding one makes it that much more valuable.

To make Pumpkin Donuts, combine:

  2 cups cashew butter or any other nut or seed butter
  2 cups pumpkin, squeezed dry of liquid
  5 pastured eggs
  4 yolks
  1 stick grass-fed butter
  3 tablespoons local honey
  2 teaspoons home-brewed vanilla
  5 teaspoons cinnamon
  4 teaspoons nutmeg
  3 teaspoons ground ginger
  1/2 teaspoon allspice

Blend all above ingredients in the Vitamix or food processor and pour into a ceramic doughnut pan.

Tap the pan on the counter to release air bubbles and spread throughout the pan evenly.

Cook at 350 degrees for roughly 25 minutes.

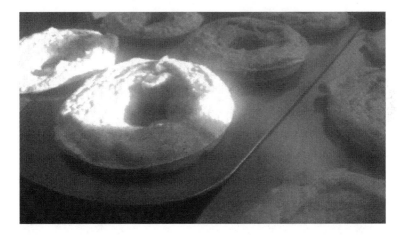

Allow to cool for a few minutes; then turn out onto a cooling surface.

These are best served warm. They are delicious with an additional drizzling of melted pastured butter, poured on just as you would a glaze. Pumpkin Donuts are fantastic topped with Green Tomato Raspberry Jam, cinnamon, or drizzled local honey.

Chapter 6:

Stage Five

Stage Five adds:

• Cooked, peeled and cored apple, made into a puree after cooking, starting slowly and building as tolerated. Butter can be added to the puree, along with cinnamon and nutmeg, if desired. If butter or ghee are not tolerated yet, any animal fat will do. It is very important to watch yeast flares with apples, especially if heavy metals are present.

• Cooked cabbage and cooked celery are added in Stage Five due to the higher fiber content.

• The stem from kale, collards, chard, and others of a similar type can be added in Stage Five, cooked.

• Raw vegetables are added. Good vegetables to start with that are often favored are lettuce and the soft parts of cucumbers. Once they are tolerated, the next to add are carrot, tomato, onion, cabbage, celery, and others. Vegetables are added according to what is ripe and fresh, in season from your local farmer or garden.[cdlxviii] Undigested vegetable may appear in the stool. If this is the case, encourage more chewing and wait until the body processes it better. It is not a sign to go back – just a sign that more healing needs to occur before progressing off GAPS.

• Eating lemons is introduced on Stage Five. Dr. Natasha says, "When you introduce raw vegetables, that's when you introduce actually eating the lemon."[cdlxix] Other citrus fruits are added at the same time, such as eating grapefruits, oranges, or limes.[cdlxx]

• Dr. Natasha says, "In Stage Five we can leave tomato here when we introduce raw vegetables, just tomato."[cdlxxi] When introducing nightshades, tomato is added first. She says, "What I would do at this stage is use raw tomato, spit out the skins. You don't have to remove the skins specifically but spit them out. The seeds can go in, but the skins should be spit out."[cdlxxii]

• Regarding hot peppers, Dr. Natasha says, "Stage Five, because they can be quite irritating. Bell peppers and jalapeños and chili peppers, all varieties of those and eggplant as well."[cdlxxiii]

• Horseradish is added.[cdlxxiv]

• Capers can be added.[cdlxxv]

• Juices that are fresh-pressed can include fruit, as tolerated, again, watching for yeast flares. Green apple, pineapple, and mango are good places to start because they are sour. From there, other apples and fruits can be added. Fresh-squeezed lemon juice, of any quantity, is Stage Two, as tolerated.

• Nightshades are added. It is important to remember when adding certain foods, like nightshades, that we observe closely for adverse responses. This group of foods is added in Stage Five in a marinade or cooked (Full for raw); however, some folks have to wait for more healing to happen. [cdlxxvi] Marinating eggplant, as in many Middle Eastern dishes, makes the eggplant slimy, not to be confused with mucilaginous foods.

• Vinegar, Apple Cider Vinegar with The Mother, or other vinegar without pathogen feeding ingredients are fully introduced in Stage Five. This includes recipes such as pickled beets or other vegetables.

• Juicing is done with more variety. Dr. Natasha says, "If the juice made from carrot, celery, lettuce and mint is well tolerated, start adding fruit to it: apple, pineapple and mango. Avoid [juicing] citrus fruit at this stage."[cdlxxvii]

Probiotic Ranch Dressing

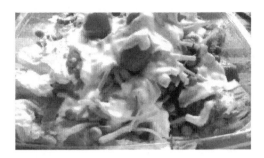

Ranch dressing is a refreshing salad topper, and quite possibly one of the easiest things to make at home. Ranch dressing on the store shelf is filled with chemicals and genetically modified ingredients. For example, Hidden Valley Ranch Dressing, owned by the Clorox company, contains soybean or canola oil (genetically modified foods), sugar, natural flavors (hidden, unlisted ingredients), phosphoric acid, xanthan gum, modified food starch, monosodium glutamate, artificial flavors (hidden, unlisted ingredients), disodium phosphate, sorbic acid, calcium disodium, EDTAS, preservatives, disodium inosinate, and disodium guanylate. Making your own dressing at home takes less than five minutes.

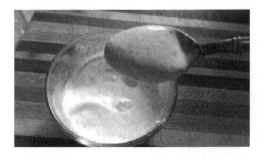

To make homemade ranch dressing, combine these ingredients in a bowl and stir:

   1 cup kefir cream (cream fermented with kefir grains)
   1 teaspoon apple cider vinegar
   1 teaspoon dill weed
   1 teaspoon parsley

1 teaspoon chives
1 tablespoon finely chopped onions
1 teaspoon finely chopped garlic
1/4 teaspoon ground mustard
Salt and pepper to taste

Store in a Mason jar in the refrigerator. Homemade ranch dressing can be served cold or used warm directly after combining the ingredients. It is thicker after being refrigerated. This is not just a refreshing dressing; it's a probiotic food.

Pizza

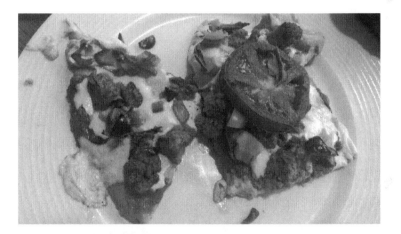

Pizza is a comfort food that is both easy to make and good to take as a lunch on the go. This recipe holds together well and is an unrivaled favorite.

First mix together 4 cups of quality cheese (gouda is easy to shred and adds depth of flavor), 6 eggs, 1 cup of almond flour, and salt and pepper to taste.

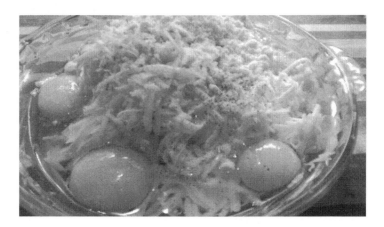

Spread the mixture with a spoon onto a baking sheet; placing it on top of parchment paper makes for easy clean up and serving. Spread it as thin as you can without there being holes.

Cook at 350 for 25 minutes, until the edges and top are slightly browned.

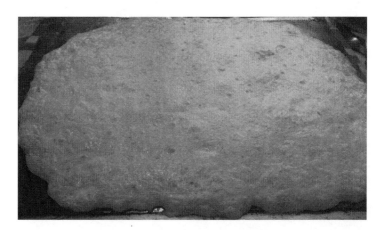

Top the pizza with your desired toppings. Make a note, this crust doesn't absorb any liquid, so the tomato sauce should be thicker, not runny or watery. If the sauce is filled with too much liquid, the liquid will run off the tray and drip onto your stove and cause smoke.

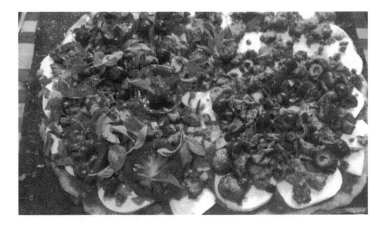

Cook at 500 degrees for 12-15 minutes, or until the cheese is melted and browned.

Mozzarella cheese has too much lactose for the GAPS tract and is best for those who are Coming Off GAPS. Cheeses that are GAPS-approved and easier to digest are asiago cheese, blue cheese, camembert cheese, cheddar cheese, Colby cheese, gorgonzola cheese, gouda cheese, Havarti cheese, limburger cheese, muenster cheese, Romano cheese, Roquefort cheese, stilton cheese, swiss cheese, and any other hard block, quality cheese.

Meatloaf

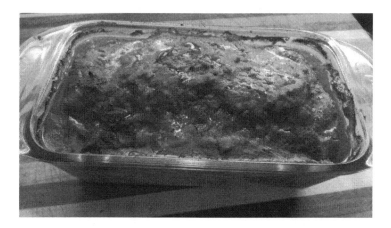

Meatloaf is probably the easiest thing to make when in a pinch. Everyone loves it, it's highly nutritious, and, if the batch is doubled, is easy to reheat for another meal.

In a large bowl, mix whatever meat is available. This recipe uses three pounds of ground venison and three pounds of ground, pastured beef. Any ground meat can be used.

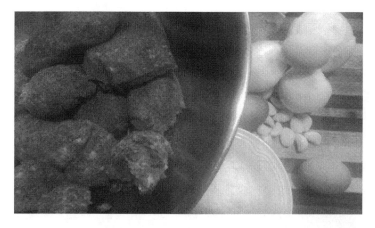

Add four small chopped onions, 5 large garlic cloves, three pastured eggs, 1/3 of a cup of finely ground almond flour (or seed flour is there is a nut allergy), and salt and pepper to taste.

*This recipe is an easy way to hide ground organ meats like liver, heart, kidneys, tongue or anything else you can source. Ounce for ounce, organ meats are the most nutrient-dense food. It also makes great meatballs and hamburgers.

Meatballs made with ground beef can be added to Stage One soups and cooked from there. Organ meats and salt can be added to the meatballs, along with chopped onion and garlic.

Mix together all the ingredients.

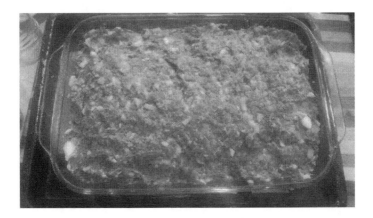

Tightly pack the mixture into a glass 9×13 pan and/or bread loaf pan, depending on how much mixture you have. This recipe fills both pans.

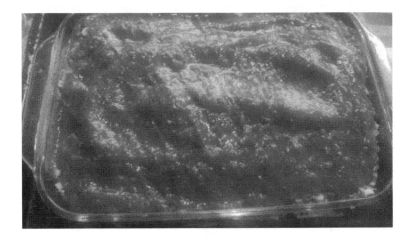

Spread tomato sauce on top of the meat.

Cook at 375 degrees for one hour or until cooked through.

Almond Veggie Wrap

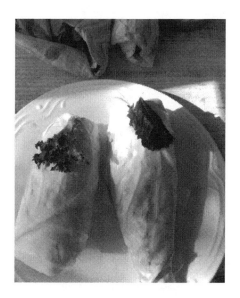

The almond veggie wrap is a raw treat that is filling, crunchy, sweet and satiating. One roll gives you energy and removes hunger, two of these rolls and you are set, three rolls and you don't think about food for at least 4 hours.

Rolls are easily kept in the refrigerator for a quick snack or quick meal.

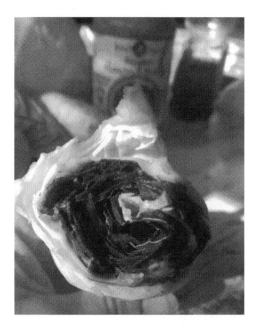

Take a cabbage leaf or collard leaf and cut out the thickest part of the spine as it makes the wrap harder to chew. Cabbage leaves are sweeter (unless the collards have been through a frost); collards have a deeper taste but are easier to achieve in one piece with no rips or holes. Removing the cabbage leaf from the head is the hardest part of the process. This is done most easily by picking a large head that is loosely bound. It's easier to remove the leaf in one piece by cutting the leaf close to the stem with a knife and pushing it gently away from the head.

Peeling the leaf from the outer edge often ends in split leaves. If the leaf is difficult to remove, it often helps to put a spoon gently under the leaf and lift.

Smear organic almond butter down the center area or the long area of the leaf. Drizzle some raw, unfiltered or local honey on top.

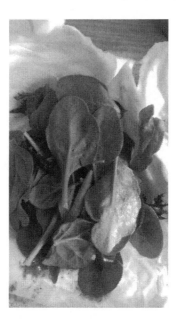

Add organic baby spinach. Add organic spring mix.

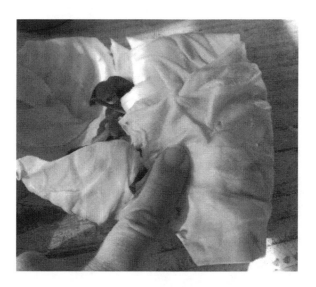

Fold in the sides. Roll up long end to long end. Each roll transports and holds in the refrigerator nicely.

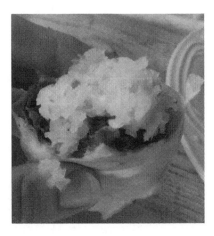

For variety, adding some home-brewed sauerkraut is fantastic!

Pickled Beets

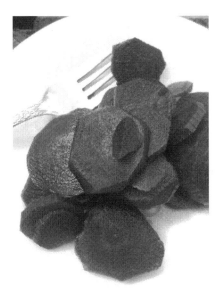

Pickled beets are a different dish than probiotic fermented beets, such as kvass.

Pickled beets use apple cider vinegar. Apple cider vinegar, with the mother, replicates hydrochloric acid in the stomach. GAPS folks generally have low stomach acid and need a regular dose of HCl stimulation.

Harvesting beets fresh from the garden can happen twice a year, so pickled beets often happens at the same time.

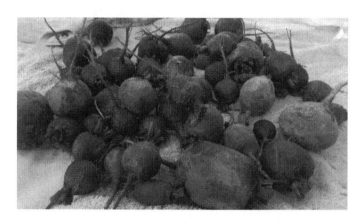

Peel beets and slice roughly 1/4 inch thick.

This picture count was used in this recipe. Peel and slice the beets to desired thickness.

Toss cut up beets into the 3-quart saucepan and cover with filtered water. Bring to a boil and cook until soft. This process only takes a few minutes.

Drain the pot until there's roughly a half-cup of water remaining. This will be less than it looks. Add a half cup of local honey and one cup apple cider vinegar. Stir until combined.

Stuffing

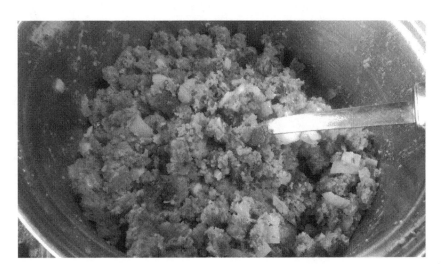

This stuffing recipe is the perfect complement to a holiday meal. It's always the first thing to go with barely enough leftovers to make a second meal.

Prepare a loaf of bread two days before this dish is to be eaten. The bread needs to dry in order to make it into breadcrumbs.

Bread

> 1 loaf of bread cut and dried into cubes, recipe for bread is first.
> 1/2 cup filtered water
> 1/2 cup cold yogurt, kefir, or sour cream (preferably home-brewed)
> 1/4 cup pastured butter (4-5 tablespoons)
> 1/2 cup local honey (optional)
> 2 pastured eggs
> 1 teaspoon baking soda
> 3 1/2 cups almond flour
> Dash of salt

Mix the ingredients in a mixer and cook in a greased bread pan at 350 degrees for 40 minutes, or until done. After cooked and cooled, cut the bread into breadcrumb sized pieces and put in the dehydrator to dry thoroughly.

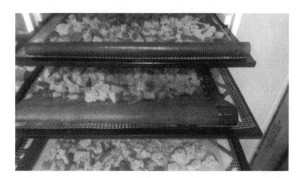

Be sure the pieces are small enough. If you do not have a dehydrator, spread crumbs on a cookie sheet in the oven on 200 degrees or simply fill cookie sheets in thin layers and let them sit on the table for three days to dry.

Stuffing:

> 1/4 cup pastured butter (4-5 tablespoons)
> 1/2 quart Meat Stock
> 4 stalks celery chopped
> 2 medium organic onions, chopped
> 1 cup peas (chopped celery can be used in Stage Five)
> Salt and pepper to taste

Add butter, Meat Stock, onions, and celery to a large Dutch oven pot with a lid. Heat on medium, just until the onions and celery are cooked but not mushy. Optimally, there should be some crunch left in the vegetables. Add the breadcrumbs and gently stir so breadcrumbs are coated with butter, onions, and celery. Be quick yet gentle. Cover with a tight-fitting lid and turn off the heat to the pan. Let sit for 15 minutes. Gently stir again and serve while hot.

This is a traditional stuffing recipe.

Fermented Cranberry Sauce

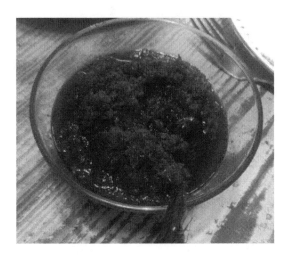

Fermented cranberry sauce is an easy dish for Thanksgiving prep, especially since it gets made 12 days before eating. Another dish can get checked off the list early, leaving you with less to do for a big holiday celebration. It keeps in the refrigerator for months.

Fermenting this recipe has a lot of flexibility. When you take the rinds off the oranges and lemons, it's best to remove the seeds before chopping both up for the ferment. You can use the sliced-up oranges and lemons or just the juice – it's your choice.

The product will not be salty – the salt helps to ferment the food as well as add flavor. The cranberry sauce will be more of a sour-tart flavor; adding more honey will make it a sweet, sour, and tart dish.

Fermenting this dish is best done by putting the ingredients into a Mason jar with a lid fingertip tight and setting it on the counter under a towel or in a cabinet for 7-12 days. Then refrigerate.

To make the sauce, use:

   1 package cranberries, 12 ounces
   1/2 cup local honey
   3 oranges, no seeds, rinds removed
   Rind from two oranges, pith removed, cut into thin strips about an inch
       long.
   2 lemons, no seeds, rinds removed
   2 teaspoons ground cinnamon
   1/4 teaspoon ground clove
   1 tablespoon mineral salt

Coarse chop cranberries to desired size. Combine all ingredients into a large bowl – everything, including lemons – and let sit for 20 minutes. Pack into Mason jars, pressing down ingredients until liquid covers the top. If there is not enough liquid to cover the top, add a small amount of filtered water. Cover with the lid, fingertip tight, and let sit in a cabinet or under a towel on the countertop for 7-12 days. Refrigerate and enjoy.

Sweet, Salty, Spicy, Fermented Pineapple and Peppers

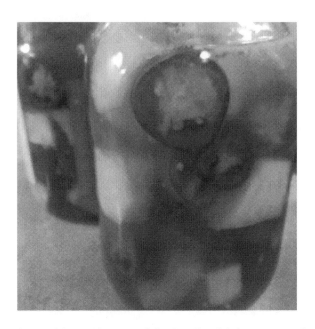

Pack Mason jars with a mixture of fresh, sliced jalapeños and pineapple. When the jars are packed tightly, fill each with the desired mineral salt according to the size of jar (1 quart = 1 to 2 tbsp mineral salt, less for smaller jars). Then fill the jar halfway with filtered water, halfway with local honey, leaving one inch of head space at the top. Screw tops on fingertip tight.

The heat from peppers is amplified when made into a probiotic food—beware.

Choose your ratio according to your desires. If you like hot and spicy, add more hot peppers. If you like sweeter, lean more heavily toward the pineapple and add more honey.

Leave jars to brew on the counter for 3-7 days, depending on your taste.

The honey will sink to the bottom. It is important to flip the jars daily to keep the honey flowing instead of settling. This makes an even sweetness throughout.

Refrigerate and enjoy.

Chapter 7:

Stage Six

In Stage Six, we add:

● Peeled, ripe, raw apples are added. If this is tolerated, other fruits are added as well. Fruits are added according to what is in season, fresh from farmers. Store-bought fruit is not GAPS recommended.

● Dried fruit can be added in Stage Six, including using dried dates for baking.

● Baked cakes and other sweet pastries can be added. Using dried fruit as a sweetener is recommended and preferred.

● Raw cabbage and raw celery can be introduced if they have not already been added.

● Fried foods can be added. This includes french fries using rutabaga fried in tallow or lard, beet fries, carrot fries, or celery root fries. Butternut squash fries, buttercup squash fries, and other winter squash fries are Full GAPS when winter squashes are added. Pumpkin is the only winter squash added early (Stage One). Vegetables or meats can be put through an egg wash and then battered in almond flour and fried in tallow or lard.

● In Stage Six we also add cooked nightshades, if they have not yet been introduced in Stage Five, (except tomato which was introduced previously, on Stage Five, and peppers which will be introduced at Full GAPS). Dr. Natasha says, "In the first stage, I would remove the nightshades (the peppers and the eggplant and the tomatoes – nightshades). So many people react, they don't realize. I would add it in on Stage Six cooked, and raw on the full diet (Full GAPS)."cdlxxviii

● Dehydrated foods can be added.

She goes on to say, "I think we need to make a note about all of these nightshades. Many people react without knowing it. So, when you introduce it, watch for it. Be aware. Many people react to the nightshades, so watch for it. If there is no reaction, great. Celebrate it. Great, you can tolerate it – fantastic."[cdlxxix]

She amplifies this by confirming, "Aubergine we can add cooked in Stage 6."[cdlxxx]

• Homemade mustard can also be added in Stage Six.[cdlxxxi]

Skillet Meals

A skillet meal is a meal made in one skillet. It's easy cooking and easy cleanup. The basic premise is first to add oil (tallow, lard, or butter) to a heated skillet. Next, add the longer cooking foods, such as chopped onion or meat. When they are nearly done cooking, add whatever vegetable or vegetables are in season and cook until desired tenderness.

This is one example, but the options are endless:

Remove bits of ground beef from the package with a spoon and shape into balls. This doesn't have to be laborious rolling and pressing; it can simply be scoop, press the edge twice, and drop in the pan. Drop balls one by one into a pan heated on medium heat, filled with butter or another animal fat. When the edges brown, turn them over.

On top of the turned meatballs, add cut vegetables such as the cabbage, carrots, and peppers shown here.

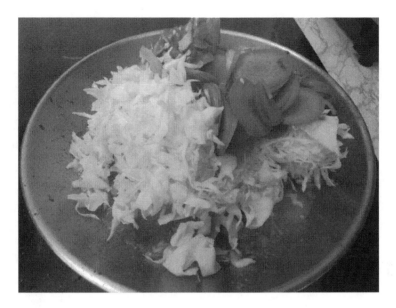

After the vegetables have steamed for a few minutes, gently turn the contents with a spoon.

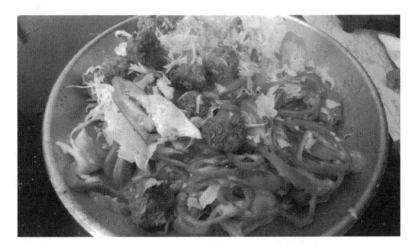

Top with more butter, if desired, salt, and pepper to taste and enjoy.

Fried Salmon Patties

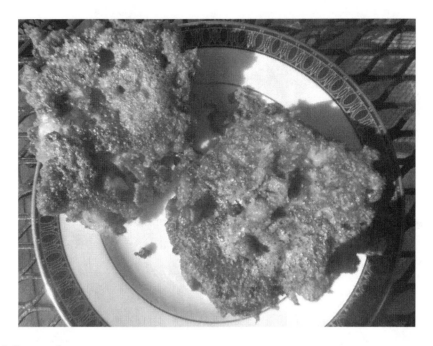

Mix together:

    24 ounces cooked salmon, shredded with a fork
    1 chopped onion
    1/2 cup almond flour
    2 pastured eggs
    1/4 of a diced red pepper
    3 sprigs chopped green onions, chopped
    4 tablespoons homemade mayonnaise

Mix together the ingredients and form into patties. Drop into skillet on medium heat and cook until the edges turn brown. Turn and cook on the other side.

Serve as they are or dip in mayonnaise or mustard, or the two mixed. They disappear quickly.

Fried Zucchini

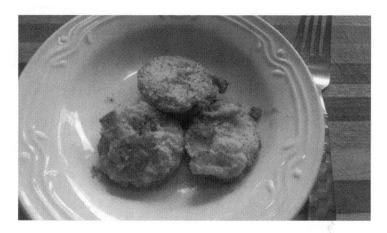

When zucchini flows from the garden, the kitchen heats up with delicious treats. Fried zucchini is just one option that pleases even the most critical palate. To make fried zucchini, slice zucchini circles about a quarter of an inch thick or slightly thicker. Too thick is difficult to eat. Place each slice into an egg wash. An egg wash is simply pastured eggs beaten with a fork. Some use a small bowl; a pie pan makes an easy vessel to do the egg and flour wash. Salt and pepper sprinkled in the egg wash adds flavor. Flip the zucchini circles so that both sides are bathed in egg. Put each ring from the egg into the almond flour.

Place each circle in hot lard or tallow.

Cook until the sides start to brown; then flip to cook the other side.

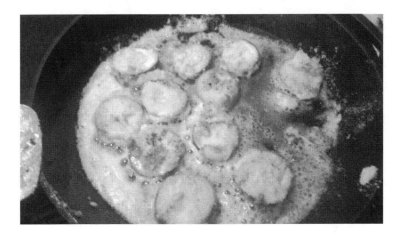

Sprinkle salt and pepper to taste and enjoy. The only problem with this dish is that they disappear as fast as you make them.

Mustard

Mustard is a delicious condiment that is extremely easy to make. These two variations on mustard are standard recipes. Mustard is hot – the longer it sits the more the heat mellows.

Two-ingredient Mustard

Pour mustard seeds into a glass jar and cover with Kombucha a half-inch over the seeds. Put a lid on top of the jar and let it sit on the counter for three days. Blend to desired smoothness and refrigerate.

Traditional Mustard

Fill a glass jar with a quarter of a cup of mustard seeds, two cloves of sliced garlic, and half of a teaspoon of whey and fill with water until covered. Let it sit on the countertop for three days with a lid on top. Blend to the desired smoothness.

Bacon Mayonnaise

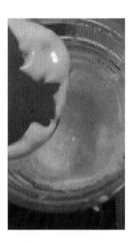

Bacon mayonnaise may be the best food accessory of the modern world. It's an easy condiment to make and whips up in literally eight minutes.

This recipe is a modified version of Sally Fallon's mayonnaise recipe in *Nourishing Traditions*.

The hardest part of this whole recipe is reserving the bacon grease. If you cook bacon on a cookie sheet (with sides to contain the grease) you will get more fat. After you cook your bacon on the cookie sheet, pour the grease into a heat-tolerant standby container until you're ready to make bacon mayonnaise.

This will be your biggest challenge.

When you make eggs, you'll see the bacon grease waiting for use—and you'll want to use it! The same goes for when you're frying vegetables—there it is again, just sitting there, smiling at you! For this purpose, I have found it is best to cover the dish of bacon grease with a paper towel. This way, it's out of sight and doesn't scream at you, "Oh, I'm so yummy – use me NOW!"

The ingredient list is simple:

> 1 egg from a free-ranging, bug-eating, sun-soaking chicken, room
>   temperature
> 1 egg yolk, room temperature
> 2 teaspoons Dijon mustard
> 1 1/2 tablespoons lemon juice
> 1/2 cup bacon grease
> 1/2 cup organic avocado oil
> 1/4 teaspoon mineral salt

Mayonnaise is easily made with a stick blender, but it can be made with other types of mixers, also. A lot of blending on low speed is the secret to good mayonnaise, so a tall vessel is important as it will splash over the top of a low vessel.

Add all of the ingredients except the oils to a container and mix on low to emulsify the eggs properly. This will take a couple of minutes.

On low, heat the bacon grease until warm enough that it is liquefied. If it is too hot, you will cook the eggs and ruin the mayonnaise. Add organic avocado oil to the bacon grease so that both oils are in one container.

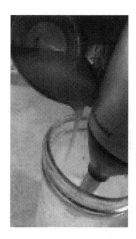

Pour both oils into the emulsified egg mixture in a slow, steady stream, mixing on low the whole time. The secret is to pour the grease slowly – patience will make the best mayonnaise as the slow, steady pour is vital.

Some cooks put their mayonnaise vessel in a bowl filled with ice so that it has a constant chill from below, causing a thick and rich mayonnaise. After all of the oil is incorporated, blend for a few minutes longer.

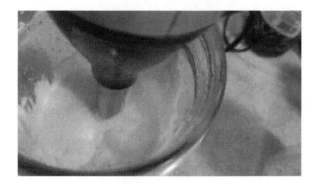

Transfer the mayonnaise to a smaller jar for the refrigerator. Be sure to label it "dog saliva" – otherwise it will disappear before you get the chance to use it. It is necessary to not tell anyone in the family that you have made bacon mayonnaise for the same reason.

Bacon Mayonnaise Deviled Eggs

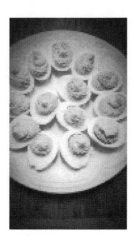

This is one of those *step away from the plate* kind of meals. If you don't step away, the plate will be empty – quickly.

Take a dozen eggs from a pastured chicken and place them in a pot. Fill with filtered water to cover the eggs. Add one teaspoon of baking soda and one teaspoon of apple cider vinegar to assist in peeling the eggshells.

Bring the pot to a rolling boil. Turn off the heat, cover, and let it sit for 10 minutes. Pour the eggs into a clean kitchen sink filled with ice, allowing them to break as they hit the sink. Immediately rinse with cold water and return the eggs to the pot or large bowl filled with cold water and a good portion of ice. Let them sit for 20 minutes. This will make the eggs easy to peel.

Peel all of the eggs under a slow, thin stream of water. Cut all eggs in half lengthwise and pop out the yolks into a separate bowl. Add one cup of bacon mayonnaise, a handful of fresh chopped cilantro, and a dash of salt. Mix the ingredients together until smooth. Add this filling to a zip top bag or frosting bag and fill the egg white halves.

For variety, but qualifying as a Stage Five food, mix chopped cilantro into the filling and top each egg with a slice of jalapeno.

Breaded Fried Liver

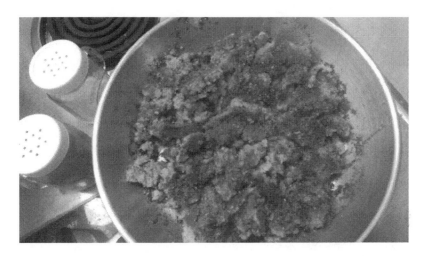

Fried liver makes some folks curl up their noses, but this treat is one even the picky eater will enjoy.

First, remove any connective tissue from the liver.

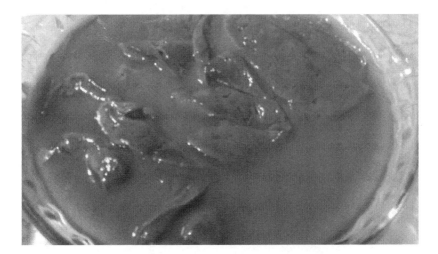

Slice liver, or cut with scissors, into edible-sized strips and soak one pound of liver in enough water to cover; add one tablespoon organic lemon juice and lightly stir to mix. Allow 4 hours to soak, fully submerged. This will remove any "dry sandy taste."

Place liver strips in 3 bug-eating-free-ranging eggs, stirred until smooth.

After the strips are bathed in the egg wash, place in a shallow dish of almond flour. Push the liver into the almond flour and flip to be sure both sides are coated. Place strips into a cast iron skillet with heated, home-rendered tallow, lard, or unrefined coconut oil. Medium to medium-high heat is perfect – the strips of liver should cause the oil to bubble slightly when you put them in the oil.

Fry until sides have changed to a light tan color, roughly 5 minutes depending on your range-top. Flip. Repeat. Enjoy.

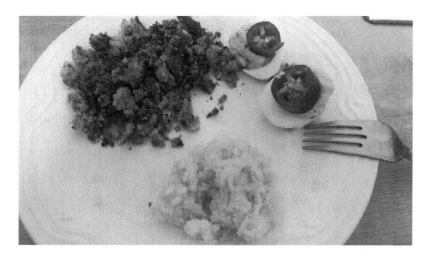

Enjoy while warm!

Bacon and Kale

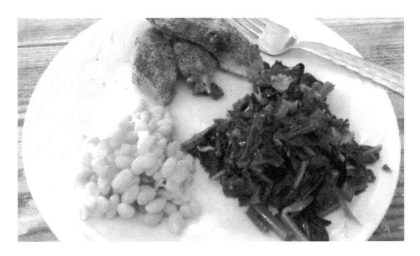

This is probably one of our most favorite meals and is absolutely easy-peasy. It's two steps.

1. Cut approved bacon and fry in a Dutch oven.
2. When it's almost done cooking, add chopped kale to fill to the top of the pot. Stir as it cooks. Top with salt.

There is an optional third step.

3. Hide in the closet and eat (so you don't have to share).

Kale from your own garden, grown organically, is always best. It makes a beautiful ornamental plant.

Smiley Sour Cream and Apple Sauce

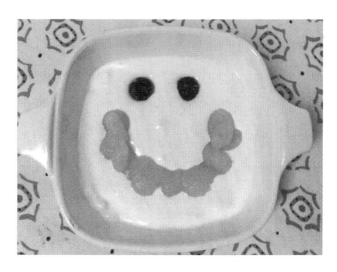

By Emili Hashimoto Litster NTP, CGP

Emili says:

The GAPS diet has been a wonderful journey in my life. Without it and without the guide from GAPS practitioners and my mom, I wouldn't have been able to fight Lyme disease, start a family of my own, and feel real joy that comes from eating nourishing food. I am now a happy and strong wife, a mother to a beautiful 12-month-old girl, Avery, and expecting another child soon. When I had Avery, my husband and I had made a mission to not let her suffer with poor health like her mother, and since day one we decided that we would follow the GAPS diet to nourish her gut. She's smarter and happier every day, which fills us with joy in seeing that we had made the right decision.

Add the amount of your homemade sour cream (recipe in Stage One section) that you and your child tolerate into bowls. Be creative with your apple sauce! Cinnamon and vanilla, local honey, or any other tolerated ingredient can be added. I like to do a smiley face: the apple sauce as the smile and two little frozen blueberries as the eyes. Avery loves that! I started giving her my apple sauce in a small amount—1 tablespoon. I gradually increased it to 2 tablespoons as I saw her doing very well with the homemade, organic apple sauce. Enjoy it!

Meals don't have to be complicated.

Carrot Cake

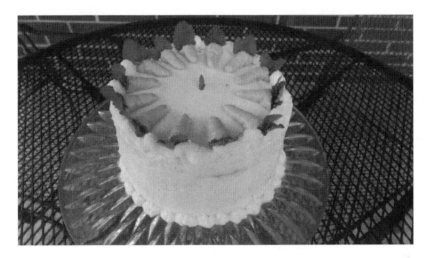

One Easter tradition that never gets old is carrot cake. This delicious GAPS recipe is a favorite, even with those who eat the Standard American Diet.

Cake

   1 cup grass fed butter
   3/4 cup local honey
   1 tablespoon vanilla
   1/2 cup home-brewed kefir (preferably made from cream)
   1 teaspoon baking soda
   3 teaspoons cinnamon
   3 cups almond flour
   4 pastured eggs
   2 cups shredded carrots
   1 cup chopped walnuts

In a mixer, whip together one cup butter and 3/4 cup local honey. Mix until fluffy, about 20 minutes.

Add 1 tablespoon vanilla and a 1/2 cup kefir cream. Mix to combine.

Add in 1 teaspoon baking soda and 3 tablespoons cinnamon.

Alternating ingredients, add in 4 eggs and 3 cups almond flour (i.e., add one egg and mix, one cup almond flour and mix, one egg and mix, etc.).

Once combined, add in 2 cups carrots, shredded on a cheese grater; then add 1 cup chopped walnuts (soaked and sprouted if needed). Pecans can also be used. Soaked and sprouted pecans taste more like maple syrup and add a whole different flavor to the cake.

Cook at 350 degrees for 40 minutes, or until done, when the top of the cake pulls away from the sides of the pan and begins to slightly crack.

Frosting

> 16 ounces homemade, properly fermented cream cheese
> 1 cup grass-fed butter
> 3/4 cup local honey

Mix together all the ingredients on high until fluffy, about 20 minutes.

To color decorative carrots on the top of the cake, take a portion of the frosting in a bowl and add 1/4 teaspoon turmeric, or the amount that is a pleasing yellow, and then set one slice of beet in the frosting bowl and let sit. It doesn't take long, but once the desired amount of red has been added to make a glorious orange, remove the beet and mix. We use lemon balm leaves for decorative carrot leaves because they pass as complementary and are ready for picking at Easter. The cake can also be topped with chopped almonds or pecans, soaked and sprouted if needed.

Serve and enjoy. This cake is better the next day. Lemon balm leaves are best added just before serving or presenting.

If a stronger cream cheese flavor is desired for the frosting, add a third of a tub, or 8 ounces, of cream cheese. If using store-bought cream cheese, be sure there are no non-GAPS ingredients, most especially no gums.

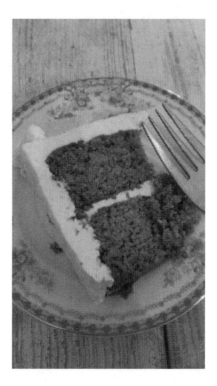

Dr. Natasha say sweet treats such as this "should be rare treats and not a staple."[cdlxxxii]

Meringue Cookies

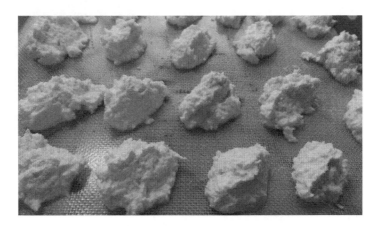

Using up extra egg whites can be done by making meringue cookies. Take the whites, beat them until they are stiff peaks, and add some local honey and vanilla extract. Cooked in the dehydrator is Stage Six.[cdlxxxiii]Save the whites in a separate Mason jar in the refrigerator until you have 3/4 of a quart full. If you don't eat them yourself, this is an inexpensive treat to leave a plate with a friend, the music teacher, or anyone stuck on sugar and flour looking for proof that real food can make a delicious treat.

These meringue cookies dissolve in your mouth like cotton candy with a slight exterior crunch.

Making these treats in bite-sized cookies is optimal since they dissolve easily. If they are too big, taking a bite leaves a lot of messy crumbs. As they dehydrate, they shrink, so dropping the cookies larger than bite-sized works well.

Using parchment paper is difficult as the cookies do not peel off easily; coating the parchment with butter prior to dropping the cookies is helpful.

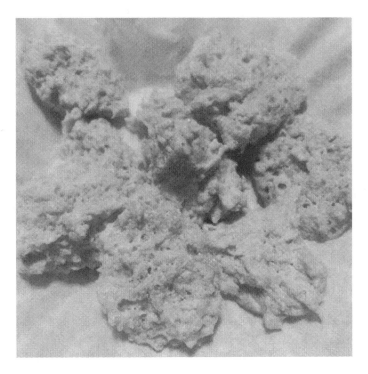

The finished cookies are irresistible!

Bacon Jerky

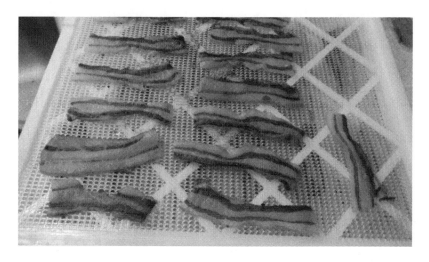

There are numerous meals we can pack for on-the-go-food, but let's be serious here: nothing tops bacon jerky. It's easy. It's tasty. It's an energy-giving food being that it's a healthy fat. Plus, it holds you over forever with consistent fuel.

Parasites and worms can be acquired from pork. Be careful with your meat; be sure it has been deeply frozen for 4 weeks prior to using to kill any potential pathogens. Watch your temperature and cook thoroughly.

First, start with a good source of bacon. Pastured pork is best.

Cut the slices of bacon in half so they're easier to eat. Marinate them for four hours if you choose. A delicious marinade is tomato sauce, honey, garlic, salt, and pepper to taste.

Lay the bacon slices out onto dehydrator trays.

Leave space for plenty of air movement. Dehydrate on 145-200 degrees for 8-12 hours, being sure the meaty part of the bacon is cooked through when it's done. Let it dehydrate to your preferred crispness. The longer it dehydrates, the more fat will cook off the bacon, making the whole slice crisper. Bacon jerky stores perfectly in snack zip-top bags.

Prosciutto Jerky

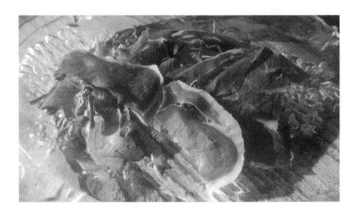

It doesn't get much easier than cutting and laying slices of prosciutto on dehydrator trays and letting them turn to jerky. However, the flavor and texture will make you run for more. This treat has a crispy, salty satisfaction that makes chips desirable.

To make prosciutto jerky, simply cut prosciutto into strips with scissors and lay them directly on the dehydrator trays. Choosing the proper prosciutto means selecting ingredients that do not contain inferior ingredients such as preservatives, chemicals, and sugars. Dehydrate at 120 degrees for 8 hours.

Prosciutto is made from select ham shanks that have soaked in a brine, usually around 10 days, and then dried for roughly a year. Different companies choose different variations to the process, giving each a flavor all their own.

Yogurt Taffy, Sour Cream Taffy, Kefir Taffy

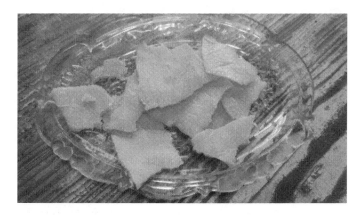

Yogurt taffy can be flavored with any fruit or sweetener. This one is flavored with local honey as, in small amounts, it does not feed pathogens and is easily transportable.

Spread yogurt on a non-stick sheet, preferably using home-brewed yogurt from real milk.

Flavoring yogurt taffy with strawberries or drizzling with local honey as shown are both delicious.

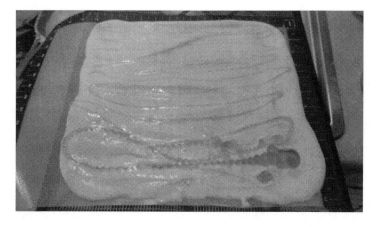

Dehydrate on trays until desired firmness at 115 degrees. Cut with kitchen scissors and store in snack pack bags. This works well as kefir cream taffy also. The thicker the cream is prior to fermenting, the thicker the taffy will be, making it more delicious.

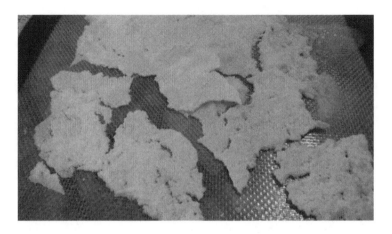

The thinner you spread the yogurt or kefir, the thinner and more cracked your taffy will be.

Using higher fat dairy, like organic heavy whipping cream, makes the best taffy.

Kombucha Taffy

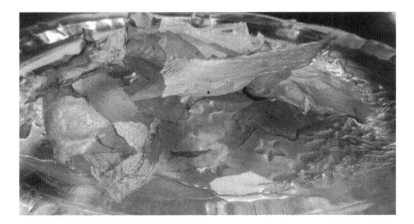

Taffy is a healthful probiotic treat that travels well and provides a tasty alternative to candy.

When your kombucha makes the extra SCOBY and there's no one waiting in line for a starter, peel off the layer of SCOBY.

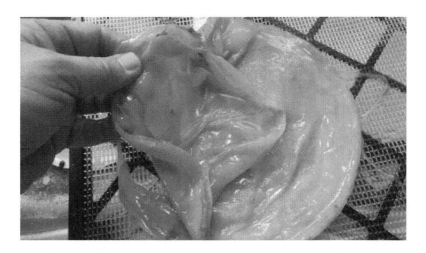

The thinner the SCOBY is, the more like stained-glass candy it will be; the thicker the SCOBY is, the more the end-product will be like taffy. Cut the SCOBY into rectangles with stainless steel scissors; then lay out on dehydrator trays. Drizzle a thin line of local honey and salt on the SCOBY strips and dehydrate on 115 degrees overnight or until it reaches your desired firmness.

These treats travel well for hikes and provide a probiotic boost.

Cheesy Kale Chips

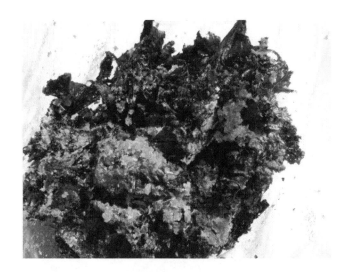

Kale chips are an easy go-to snack for any foodie; cheesy kale chips are the executive version of this tasty treat.

The easiest and fastest way to make kale chips is to do it in bulk. First, wash the kale leaves by filling a sink full of water, adding a splash of vinegar, and swishing the leaves around for a few seconds. Let them drain. Try to get as much water off the leaves as possible. If you buy your kale non-organic, it's most likely coated with corn starch. Be sure to wash all of the corn starch off as it feeds bad bacteria in the intestinal track. If you have a child on the spectrum or one who suffers from ADHD, it is vital to do a thorough job of washing off all the corn starch.

Rip all of the leaves into small, bite-sized pieces and throw them into an extra-large bowl or stock pot.

Pour good quality, cold-pressed, virgin olive oil onto all surface areas of the kale leaves. They should be fully saturated with oil. Olive oil is a good fat, and your body needs this fat to feed your brain and to prevent gallbladder issues.

Spread the leaves on dehydrator trays and sprinkle with mineral salt. These can also be made in the oven on 200 degrees until done.

Generously sprinkle nutritional yeast on top.

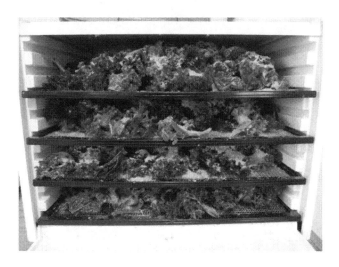

Stack the trays in the dehydrator and let it process at 125 degrees for 18-24 hours.

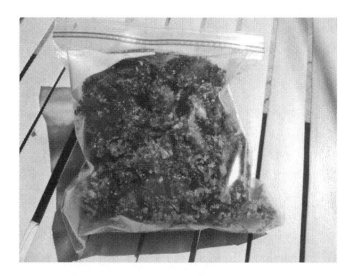

These are so amazingly delicious when eaten fresh out of the dehydrator when they're still warm. Store in zip-top bags.

Chapter 8:

Full GAPS

Full GAPS contains a lot of food choices and food cooking options. It is very easy to follow and leaves the person mentally satiated – not restricted. Many can just do Full GAPS and heal. Those who have a high level of toxicity or broken-down detox channels are recommended to stay on Full GAPS for three years before attempting the Introduction Diet. This is recommended for those with diseases such as fibromyalgia, ME, multiple sclerosis, lupus, schizophrenia, and the like.

Staying on Full GAPS while increasing probiotic foods is an excellent place to start. If you don't know what to do or if the protocol is overwhelming, Full GAPS is a good place to call home.

Full GAPS Foods

Full GAPS adds more foods and includes cooking the food in countless different methods.

• If not already added, Dr. Natasha says, "Put the peppers in on the Full."[cdlxxxiv] The harshness of the heat from peppers can cause disturbance of parasites which may not be ready to leave and could be too harsh on the sensitive microbiome while it repairs.

• Raw nightshades can be added.

• GAPS-approved beans, such as properly soaked navy beans, lentils, and lima beans, are added.

• Cocoa powder or cacao powder are added, as tolerated, giving variety to baked goods. These are not favored by Dr. Natasha – the protocol is best without it. She says, "Cocoa has some carbs in it which are not allowed on the diet. I recommend that it is avoided until main digestive symptoms are gone: diarrhea, pain, bloating, etc. In people with no digestive problems it can be used in small amounts."[cdlxxxv]

The problems with chocolate are something to monitor. Often, when we move through the protocol, we don't realize what is causing us upset – this is one to watch. Dr. Natasha says, "People with migraines should avoid it, as all chocolate products are notorious for causing migraines. This plant has substances in it (theobromines, theophyllines and other methylxanthines) which may cause an imbalance in neurotransmitters in the brain, which affect people with mental illness, epilepsy, tics and migraines. In my experience, nice as it is, all chocolate forms are better avoided."[cdlxxxvi]

The problem is, most folks cheat with chocolate. Making something clean is best, if needed.

The base recipe for making chocolate at home is equal parts cocoa powder and cocoa butter, with half that measure of local honey. This would mean 1/4 cup cocoa powder, 1/4 cup cocoa butter and 1/8 cup of local honey. The three should be melted slowly in a double boiler. Dr. Natasha says this recipe is fine – "sounds good" if chocolate is something the body craves.[cdlxxxvii]

• Bone broths are usually well tolerated, but for some, it is an advanced Full GAPS food.

• Aloe Vera is added.

• Seaweed is added.

• Foods can be cooked crispy, on the grill over charcoal (without using fire starters or chemically treated briquettes), in the oven, on the range top over any heat, over a fire, roasted, fried, steamed, sautéed, cooked in a sun oven, cooked in a pizza oven, or cooked in other ways. Foods should not ever be wrapped in silver, aluminum, tin metal foils, or cling wraps, and then cooked. Parchment paper can be used.

• On Full GAPS, dry red or white wine, vodka, gin, whiskey, and brandy can be added. Dr. Natasha says, "No more than one glass a day, with every dinner, if you tolerate it well. [The] problem with it is sulfates – because all wines nowadays are made with sulfates and many people get headaches. It is a nice digestive."[cdlxxxviii]

• Weak coffee can be added on Full GAPS. Due to the drain on the endocrine system, the coffee should be weak, meaning you can read a paper through it. Dr. Natasha says, "I love coffee! I drink one cup of coffee a day with cheese and honey and raw cream. If you put raw cream in your hot coffee, you're pasteurizing the cream. What's the point? If you put honey in the hot coffee, you're damaging the honey."[cdlxxxix] She consumes all of her ingredients separately, a sip of one, a sip of the other. "I have cream in one pot, coffee in another, honey in another. We always have cheeses on the table, French, Italian cheeses and honey. We just eat cheese with honey. I like my coffee black, with nothing mixed in it. But people mix it. They take it mixed."[cdxc]

• Raw vegetables can be a pleasing dish when marinated. Dr. Natasha says longer marinating times make food more digestible. Marinating for over 24 hours allows the marinade to permeate the food more thoroughly. She also recommends using fermented vegetable brine over vinegar or any other marinade ingredients.[cdxci]

• If not already introduced, winter squashes are added on Full GAPS. They should be served with the fibrous skin removed and deseeded. They include:

    Acorn squash
    Butternut squash
    Buttercup squash
    Delicata squash
    Spaghetti squash

• Dr. Natasha says that unfermented coconut water is "Full GAPS. It's very sweet, a lot of sugar in there."[cdxcii]

• Fermented coconut meat or coconut meat fall into the Full GAPS category due to the high fiber content.

• Topical essential oil use is introduced on Full GAPS. Making sure your source is reputable is important. Dr. Natasha says, "Start experimenting with these things on Full GAPS. With essential oils I'm still not sure whether they are a good idea internally because they work externally. They penetrate through the skin because they are fat soluble. They penetrate so well, just applying them to different parts of the body, and above acupuncture points I think works just as well, rather than taking them internally. I have people I tell take a tablespoon of coconut oil and mix the essential oil into it, and eat that – that's a good way of taking them. We didn't see any changes [internally]."[cdxciii]

• In recent years, products such as pastas made only from green peas or pastas made only from lentils, can be purchased in boxes from the store. Some people can tolerate these products, on a rare occasion, while on the advanced stages of Full GAPS; however, they are not a desired food since they are highly processed. The focus of the protocol should still be freshly made foods sourced from food found in its natural state. Dr. Natasha says they are "very fibrous and should be tried on the Full Diet quite a bit later. Also, it is too processed."[cdxciv]

• Apple cider is introduced if not already added.

• Fruit, in season, is introduced if it has not already been included. Fruit should not be purchased from a store, but instead from a farmer who doesn't spray. Outside of the previously introduced cooked apple and citrus, there is no order of introduction of fruit. Dr. Natasha says, "The fruit should be chosen from what is available locally in season from private gardens, not from supermarkets! It is always best to cook it first (and see if it is tolerated). With berries, the seeds should be removed by pushing the puree through a sieve in the initial stages. If that is tolerated, then we can start leaving the seeds in."[cdxcv]

• Cheeses are introduced, as tolerated, if not already introduced.

• Organic gelatin is introduced as a rare treat but should not be used as a substitute for Meat Stock. A better option for making gummies is to use ox tail or chicken feet Meat Stock. [cdxcvi] Organic gelatin can be used on rare occasions on earlier stages, such as for a birthday party.

The Full GAPS foods have boundless options.

Acorn squash
Almond butter (all nut butters are approved; raw organic nuts are best. Roasted nuts are not approved due to questionable processing practices).
Almond flour
Almond milk (without carrageenan, homemade is best).
Apple cider
Apple cider vinegar (with the mother)
Artichokes
Asiago cheese
Avocado
Avocado oil
Bacon
Baking soda
Beets
Beet tops
Bell peppers
Butter, grass-fed
Buttercup squash
Butternut squash
Blue cheese
Brazil nuts
Broccoli
Brussels sprouts
Cabbage
Camembert cheese
Cashews
Cashew butter
Cauliflower
Caviar
Celery

Cheese (good quality cheese should be in block form from small farm or small batches is best. Cheeses that are GAPS-approved, easier to digest, are asiago cheese, blue cheese, camembert cheese, cheddar cheese, Colby cheese, gorgonzola cheese, gouda cheese, Havarti cheese, limburger cheese, muenster cheese, Romano cheese, Roquefort cheese, stilton cheese, swiss cheese, and any other hard block quality cheese).
Cheddar cheese
Chicken (free ranging, not soy fed, NO injected solutions)
Chicken legs, wings, thighs, necks, feet, organs, and any other part of the chicken
Chicken Meat Stock made from carcass and meat
Chicken skin (schmaltz)
Chili peppers
Chives
Cocoa powder (sparingly, best if not at all).
Coconut butter
Coconut flour
Coconut oil
Coconut water
Coconut
Colby cheese
Collards
Cottage cheese (homemade, not from the store)
Cream cheese (homemade, not from the store)
Cubano peppers
Daikon radish
Dates (in moderation as they are high in sugars—NOT date sugar as it is too highly processed, medjool dates are optimal).
Delicata squash
Duck eggs (all fowl eggs are good)
Duck fat
Eggs – pastured eggs are best
Extracts (vanilla, lemon, almond, mint, etc.)
Figs (in moderation, watching that they do not feed yeast)
Fish (any wild-caught or wild-sourced fish is approved)
Flax seed
Flax seed oil
Fruit (eaten separately from other foods, on an empty stomach; the lower the sugar content, the better)
Garlic
Gelatin (organic and unflavored) from pastured animals. This is not a substitute for Meat Stock.

Ghee, homemade from pastured butter
Gizzards
Goose fat
Gorgonzola cheese
Gouda cheese
Green beans
Green onions
Havarti cheese
Hazelnuts
Hemp oil
Herbs
Honey, locally sourced and unheated is a sacred food
Jalapenos
Juice (juiced from your juicer)
Kale
Kefir (homemade)
Kimchi
Kombucha
Kraut juice
Lard (from pastured pork)
Leeks
Lemon
Lemon juice (without sodium benzoate, optimally from organic lemons)
Lentils
Lettuce
Lima beans
Limburger cheese
Meat (optimally, pastured meat that is not processed – preferably grass-fed, grass-finished. All meats are beneficial on GAPS. Meat from hunters is best).
Meat Stock (from any animal)
Mineral water
Muenster cheese
Mushrooms
Mustard
Mustard greens
Napa cabbage
Navy beans (properly prepared by soaking)
Nightshade vegetables
Nuts (all untouched with roasting or flavoring. Be watchful of roasting processes as the commercial industry cannot be trusted)
Nut butters (almond, peanut, sunflower, cashew, etc.)
Olive oil

Onions

Nut flours

Olives (all kinds, be careful of added ingredients that are not approved, such as canola oil, flavorings, and unapproved seasonings).

Patty pan squash

Pickles

Peanut butter

Peanuts

Peas

Peppers

Pickles (homemade or with compliant ingredients)

Pine nuts

Pork

Radishes

Romaine

Romano cheese

Roquefort cheese

Rum

Rutabaga

Salami and other dried meats with approved seasoning ingredients

Sardines

Sauerkraut

Seaweed (Dr. Natasha says, "On the Full Diet only, when digestive problems are gone."[cdxcvii])

Seeds

Sour cream (home-brewed at first)

Spaghetti squash

Spices (be sure there are no fillers like wheat, sodium ferrocyanide, yellow prussiate of soda, or any other anti-caking or free-flowing agents)

Spinach

Stevia (only green unprocessed stevia is GAPS-compliant)

Stilton cheese

Sugar snap peas

Swiss chard

Swiss cheese

Tallow (from grass-fed beef)

Tea, herbal (loose-leaf is optimal; bagged teas should not be used if they contain corn starch, baking soda, natural flavors, stevia, or other added ingredients)

Turnips

Turkey (not processed)

Vegetables (starches and GMO items are not beneficial to a damaged
    gut. This includes no: potato, sweet potato, corn, soy, or parsnips.
    All other vegetables are GAPS-approved)
Venison
Vinegar (vinegars are GAPS approved, as long as the ingredients are
    clean)
Vodka
Wine (dry)
White scallop squash
Yellow crookneck squash
Yogurt (full-fat, made at home from a quality starter yogurt from the
    store. Store-bought yogurt is an advanced Full GAPS food)
Zucchini

In a nutshell, if God made it, it's fine; if man altered it, it's not. If it was made in a manufacturing plant, it is best avoided. Think of products grown in nature and keep the end-product visibly viable to that original. Consider vegetable oil. If you took a basket of vegetables and squeezed out juice you wouldn't get vegetable oil. The processing has changed the molecular structure of the food. If it's not food, don't put it in your mouth. Butter, on the other hand, comes from cream and is stirred until it forms butter. Butter is GAPS-complaint; vegetable oil is not.

Food preparation is hard, and it takes a lot of work. We are currently paying the price for quick and easy processed food. Quick is not saving us time in the long run; it is negatively impacting our health. It is our job to feed our families healthy food. Processed food has directly risen with the rise of disease.

If it's not food, don't put it in your mouth.™

Adding in beans such as lentils, lima beans, or navy beans:

When we add foods like lentils, lima beans or navy beans, we are presented with the big question: to soak or not to soak. Soaking has to do with digestibility. Soaking causes phytic acid to be released. Phytic acid is classified as an antinutrient, meaning it takes more to digest the phytic acid than you get, so it leaves you depleted. Removing phytic acid through soaking makes the food easier to digest. Not everyone has to do this – it truly depends on the capabilities of your digestive tract.

Preparing beans or lentils is done in a progression, first making them very easy to digest while we advance to harder to digest methods. Some beans, like navy beans, may always need to be soaked; it depends on the person.

The harder the seed is, the longer it soaks. The general rule of thumb is to use three times as much water as seeds. If you use a sprouting jar lid, the job is easier as you just invert the jar to strain and then let it sit.

Let's take lentils as an example.

First, we start by (1) soaking the lentils in whey by covering lentils in a quart of water and a tablespoon to a quarter of a cup of home-brewed whey. Let that sit for 24 hours, strain, and enjoy.

Once that is tolerated, we move to (2) sprouting the lentils. This is done by placing a quarter cup of lentils in a Mason jar, filling it with two to three cups of water, and letting it sit on the countertop overnight or for eight hours. Drain the water and tilt the jar at a 45-degree angle, preferably upside down so that excess water drains (if you don't have a sprouting lid, a coffee filter with a rubber band will hold the sprouts in place while the water drains). Let this sit for a day or two or three, depending on the item. Twice a day, come back and fill the jar with fresh, cool water, and then rinse it out and let the jar sit inverted in the bowl again – repeat until the desired length of sprouts appear.

Once that is tolerated, we simply (3) let the lentils sit in water for a few hours.

Once that is tolerated, we (4) nothing; we try them by just cooking them with no prior prep.

The scale of 1 to 4 goes from easiest to digest to hardest to digest. Only your body can tell you how fast to move through the four stages.

GAPS Waffles

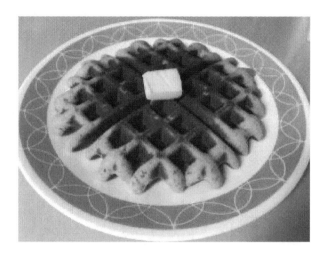

This recipe was created by Joshua, a single man who turned his life around with real food, using GAPS to support his body. Joshua started GAPS in April of 2018 due to acute colitis brought on by a *C. diff* infection. As a pro level Pickleball athlete, he was putting his training and competitions on hold due to his illness. He expected to be out of the game for a year or more, but instead, thanks to GAPS, he was playing in a matter of weeks. He is still on GAPS and doing very well. He is healthy and rebuilding lost gut flora wiped out by antibiotics. He makes many homemade probiotic foods. He tells others of the benefits of the protocol and is leaner and stronger than before.

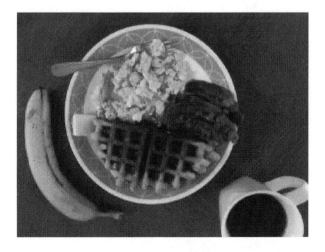

4 pastured eggs
3/4 cup almond flour
1/4 cup coconut flour
1/4 teaspoon Celtic sea salt
1/4 teaspoon baking soda
1-2 tablespoons honey
1 teaspoon vanilla extract
2 tablespoons melted pastured butter

Mix all ingredients well with a hand whisk. Heat and coat the waffle iron with butter, pour a scoop of batter into the waffle iron, and cook until done. Top with pastured butter and a drizzle of honey. Sprinkling cinnamon on top can add more variety.

This recipe, minus the vanilla and honey, makes a delicious savory bread.

Lentil Pancakes

By Christy Giambastiani who came to GAPS for her son Lachlan who was diagnosed with autism at age 3 and a half. On GAPS, he started with crazy behavior with the smallest speck of a salicylate—raging, destructive, hyperactive, 24-hour itching, hyper-sensory issues, and chronic constipation. He never moved his bowels outside the home. It was common for him to swipe a table clean of its contents, smashing everything onto the floor, run to every lightbulb he saw with an obsession to reach and crush it in the palm of his hand, put holes in the walls, and have such violent outbursts that the police were called by caring neighbors. He still experiences some minor ups and downs in comparison but plays peaceably with his brother, plays board games with friends, has intellectual conversations that bring tears to the eyes, and even wants to try a public restroom with excitement where he has bowel movements–often 3 to 4 times a day. Mom can now leave the house, for the first time ever, to go to the gym and have a well-earned moment of peace to herself.

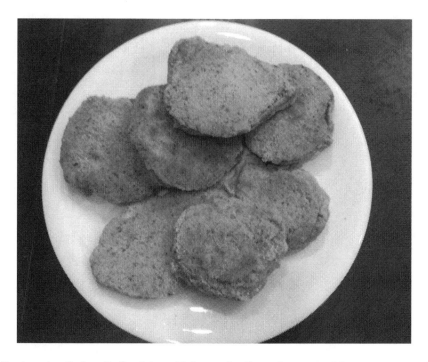

Soak red split lentils for 24 to 48 hours in filtered water with a teaspoon of whey added; then drain.

Put lentils in a food processor with enough water to make a watery paste. Add garlic, salt, pepper, and other desired spices.

Heat a frying pan to medium-low heat. Add a generous amount of animal fat; then scoop up paste and drop into rustic pancake shapes.

Fry pancakes until golden brown on each side. Add more animal fat as needed when frying for even cooking.

These are delicious warm, with avocado, butter, or sour cream, and can easily be frozen and reheated.

They can also be used as a crunchy salad crouton once cubed and reheated until golden brown on all sides.

Yum!

Chicken Nuggets

By Christie Giambastiani

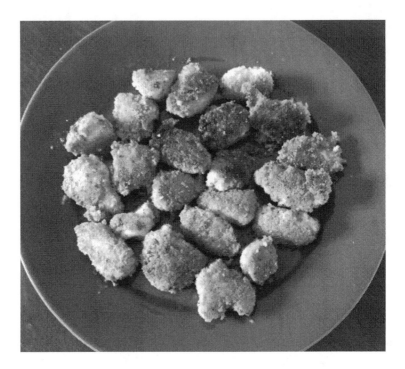

Dice chicken breasts into nugget-sized pieces; about one inch long.

Place approximately 6 thawed lentil pancakes (from the recipe above) into a food processor and process until crumbed.

Whisk two to three medium to large eggs to make an egg wash.

Dip chicken into egg wash to coat all sides.

Dip coated chicken into lentil pancake crumbs and cover all sides.

Heat two or three heaped tablespoons of tallow in a frying pan over medium heat.

Place chicken nuggets into the frying pan and cook on all sides until golden brown.

These can be served immediately or allowed to cool and freeze in batches for future use. Your GAPS child will love them!

Caramelized Pepper, Pork Belly, Onion, and Cheese

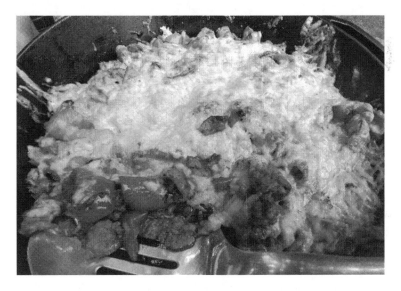

6 Cubanelle peppers, seeds and membrane removed
2 Onions
1 Pound pork belly or approved bacon
Mineral salt and pepper
2 Cups shredded cheese (optional)

Cut up pork belly or bacon and add to cast iron skillet; cook on medium until almost cooked. Add diced onion to the skillet; cook until caramelized. Add chopped peppers, salt, and pepper to taste and stir. Top with shredded cheese and place in the oven at 500 degrees. Cook for 12 minutes or until cheese is browned.

Baked Beans

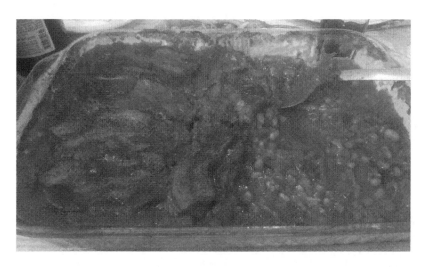

Baked beans are a staple for certain occasions; however, the high dose of sugar in them makes them not GAPS compliant—until now.

This recipe is tried and true with both GAPS and non-GAPS folks. If you tolerate navy beans, this one is worth a try.

First, place a one-pound bag of navy beans in a large bowl. The beans will expand, so the bowl needs to be 2/3 larger than the beans occupy. Fill the bowl with water and add 2 tablespoons of apple cider vinegar, with the mother. Let the beans soak in the bowl 16-24 hours, longer if needed.

Many people debate the need to soak beans. While on GAPS, beans should be soaked to remove phytic acid as well as other anti-nutrients.

Archivos Latinoamericanos de Nutrición reported a study entitled "The Domestic Processing of the Common Bean resulted in a reduction in the phytates and tannins antinutritional factors, in the starch content and in the raffinose, stachyose and verbascose flatulence factors" saying, "A decrease in the phytate content of the beans (85%) with use of soaking was observed."[cdxcviii]

The *Journal of Food Science and Technology* reported a study which found, "Soaking studied red beans before utilization will increase their nutritive value."[cdxcix]

Plant Food for Human Nutrition reported a study saying, "The removal of oligosaccharides was higher in legumes cooked in alkaline solution than in water."[d]

Toxins reported, "Phytate also has been shown to inhibit digestive enzymes such as trypsin, pepsin, α-amylase and ß-glucosidase. Therefore, ingestion of foods containing high amounts of phytate could theoretically cause mineral deficiencies or decrease protein and starch digestibility. Phytate is fairly heat stable but can be removed by soaking or fermentation."[di]

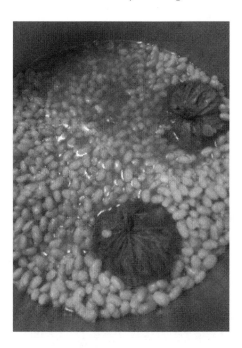

The key to adding sweetness to these baked beans is licorice root tea in the cooking stock. After the beans have soaked, put them in a Dutch oven with two quarts of previously prepared Meat Stock. To the top of the pot add 2 sachets of licorice root tea. A sachet is anything used to tie up herbal material. You can use a brown coffee filter, a piece of cheesecloth folded over many times or even an old piece of cloth. To make each sachet, fill an unbleached coffee filter with as much licorice root as will fit so that you can still tie the coffee filter closed. I simply gather the coffee filter together and wrap thread around the top, just wrapping it around and around, not even tying it together.

Cook on low for 2 hours or until beans are soft.

Remove the sachets and all other ingredients, minus one pound of pork belly, which is being saved to top the dish. Continue cooking for as long as you like. Some people prefer them immediately after adding the other ingredients; others prefer them cooked for many more hours.

Add four chopped onions to the beans cooking in the pot, one pound of sliced bacon, and one 16-ounce jar of organic tomato sauce. Heat until bacon is cooked.

Add one chopped green pepper and one chopped red pepper to the bean mix. Stir in 16 ounces of organic tomato sauce.

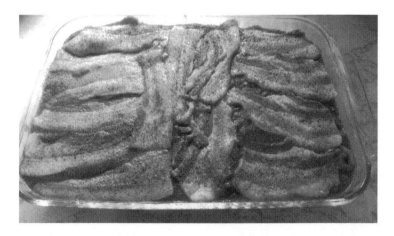

Pour the beans mixture into a 9×13 pan and top with the second pound of pork belly. Sprinkle salt and pepper on top of the port belly. Cook at 350 degrees for 45 minutes or until the bacon is cooked. The flavor of the beans is better the next day, after refrigeration.

Halloween Party Tray

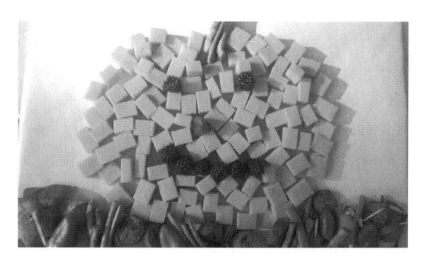

Going to a party with a restricted diet is daunting. Taking your own dish that looks fantastic and tastes delicious is not just beneficial to there being a food option for yourself – it's a memorable addition to the celebration.

Pumpkin: cheddar cheese cubes

Eyes and mouth: blackberries or olives

Nose: sweet red pepper

Pumpkin stem: green beans

Base: chicken wings, green beans, cherry tomatoes, chicken sausages, roast beef, and chicken rolls (be sure to check the ingredients to be sure they're clean).

Hash Browns

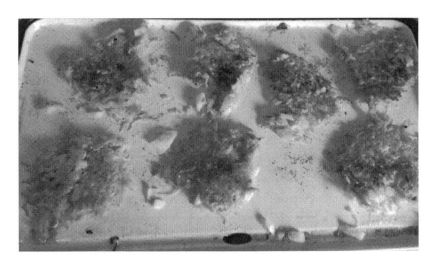

Hash browns can be made with any squash; this one is with buttercup squash, a low-starch, low-moisture squash. Butternut squash, spaghetti squash, and acorn squash also make good options. Remove the skin with a knife. Scrape the seeds out with a large serving spoon. Shred the squash with a cheese grater.

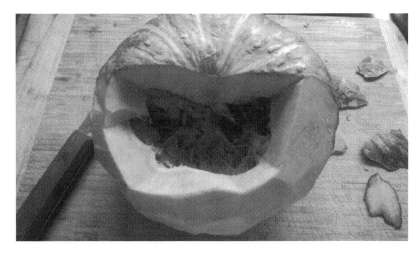

For every 2 cups of shredded squash, add one onion, finely chopped, two eggs, and 1/4 cup of almond flour. Mix until combined.

Spread circles of the mixture onto a buttered griddle heated to 350 degrees. Once they are browned on the bottoms, flip.

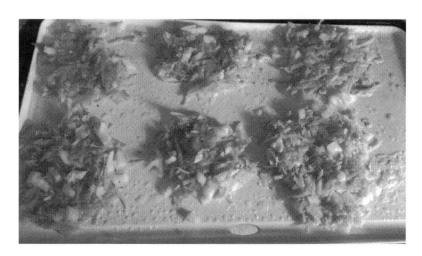

GAPS hash browns can be enjoyed with eggs and sausage or bacon. There are rarely leftovers. Once you start making them, it's hard to keep up with the demand.

Caramelized Curly Dock or other Caramelized Greens

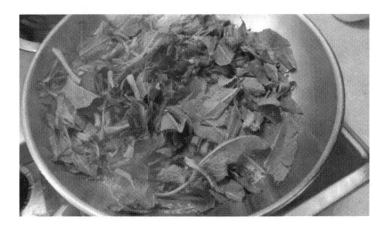

Caramelized curly dock is a side dish that enlightens your taste buds with a lemony butter flavor that makes the kids beg for more!

Gathering curly dock in the spring will provide ample amounts of fresh dock that is loaded with vitamin C, beta-carotene, and zinc.

Curly dock is often found in ditches, but grows everywhere. The specific leaves have an identifiable curl to the edges.

Springtime harvest of dock is best as the young leaves grow fast and are abundant. The optimum leaves for harvest are the youngest curled leaves in the center, the new growth.

All young leaves are delicious. Picking a variety of fresh new growth mixed in with some leaves a bit younger is good variety. You'll find which ones you like best.

Curly Dock, also called Yellow Dock, is a member of the buckwheat family and has a resemblance to spinach in the way it cooks and tastes. You can use curly dock: put the leaves in a pot of water and cook like you would spinach, drain, and then spritz with vinegar.

Sautéing them in a pan with butter is an easy way to caramelize them for a delicious side dish.

A mix of the youngest leaves, still unopened, and the ones just opened make a good blend.

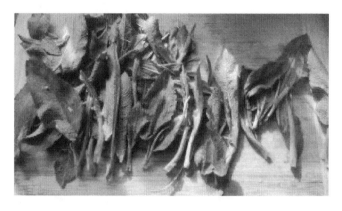

If you choose older leaves, they may have a bitter taste.

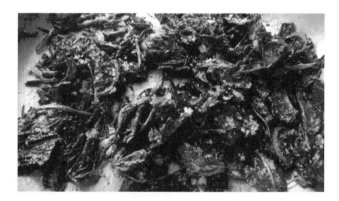

Caramelized curly dock tastes much like kale chips with a lemon zing.

Many vegetables can be cooked in this manner. Brussels sprouts, kale, chard, and collards are all especially good in this manner.

Blackberry Jam

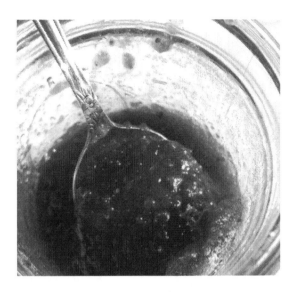

Leftover green tomatoes at the end of the season are a nuisance if you don't like fried green tomatoes. This blackberry jam recipe uses green tomatoes and tastes so good that you may just plant more tomato plants to get more green ones!

This recipe has a lot of forgiveness. If you have more tomatoes, the recipe can take it. The numbers are a rough guide. Adding twice as much honey is closer to the taste of jam found in the store. If sweet isn't your thing, go with less honey.

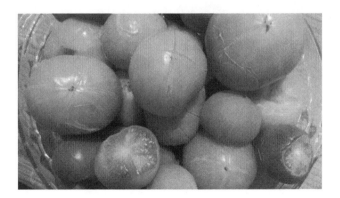

Score roughly six cups of green tomatoes on the bottoms and cut the core out of the tops. Place the tomatoes in boiling water until the skins tighten and pull apart as shown in the picture. Remove the tomatoes from the water, peel the skins, and chop, or not – your choice. We are only removing the skins; the seeds from the tomatoes give the jam a raspberry appearance, without the teeth capturing hard seeds.

Place the tomatoes in your Vitamix or food processor.

In a Dutch oven, over medium heat, place 54 ounces of blackberries. Mash the blackberries with a potato masher as they slowly heat.

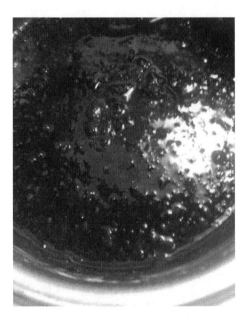

Continue mashing until the blackberries are in a liquid state.

Place the blackberry contents through a stainless-steel mesh strainer until all the hard seeds have been separated from the blackberries.

In the Vitamix or food processor, add tomatoes and strained, cooked blackberries; combine until the particles are mixed, but the seeds remain. The more you blend, the more the seeds disappear. Return the mixture to the Dutch oven and continue heating the strained mixture. Add 3 tablespoons of organic gelatin, sprinkled thin, stirring as you combine. Gelatin that is not organic is not part of the GAPS protocol. Add three cups local honey. Stir until combined.

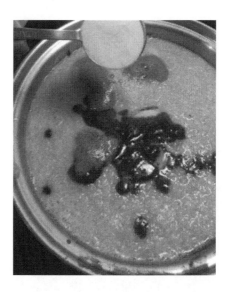

Once the mixture is combined, it can be poured into sterilized Mason jars. The easiest way to do this is to put the jars in the dishwasher on the hottest setting, having them finish when you are ready to pour the jam into the jars.

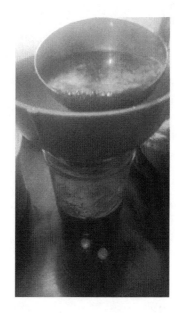

Pour the mixture into sterilized jars through a funnel, preferably one that is stainless steel.

Wipe the tops of the jars clean with a clean non-terry cloth towel.

This recipe makes a delicious sauce over Pumpkin Donuts.

Bone Broth

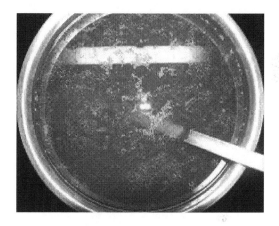

In the mid-1700s Royal Naval ships found a way to make extra money from one simple dish—bone broth.[dii]

Ships were out to sea for a long time, so the cook made soup. To make broth, they would take the large soup pot, fill it with water, add bones, and maybe add some bay leaves for flavor. The next step was simple: let it cook for hours. When the broth was rich with flavor, they made soup, kept the bones, and filled the pot with more water for the second, third, fourth, and fifth batch of broth from the same bones.[diii]

After the first batch was done, however, a thick layer of fat sat on top of the pot. It was too much for the soup, so the cook skimmed it off and saved the rich fat in empty beef or pork barrels.[div]

When the ship returned to port, the naval cook met individuals in the shipyard looking to purchase the rich fat skimmed from the top of the pot. This valuable ingredient was used for making candles and soap and for cooking. The money was the fund, the skimmed fat was the slush, historically giving us the origin of the phrase slush fund.[dv]

Today, rich bone broth is prized for healing ailing intestinal tracts as well as nourishing hungry bodies. The broth is rich in amino acids (specifically arginine, glycine, and proline) as well as gelatin which improves collagen and intestinal healing. Many people take a mixture of bones, broil them, and then make broth. Dumping a bag of frozen bones into a crock pot, filling it with filtered water, and adding some bay leaves and apple cider vinegar to extract nutrients from the bones is a fast and easy dish.

The rule of thumb is to keep cooking the bones in new water until the bones crumble between your fingers. Some cook one perpetual crock pot for five days solid, emptying the pot each day and refilling it with fresh filtered water. This one bag of soup bones will yield gallons upon gallons of bone broth— a new pot every day.

Please note: there is a difference between healing Meat Stock, which is used to heal the intestinal tract, and bone broth, which we are discussing here. Bone broth will not heal a Leaky Gut, but it is a nourishing food.

Variations of the recipe can include added onions, carrots, celery, and peppercorns to the pot while cooking.

Pineapple Lemon Bark

1 cup coconut butter
    (made from mixing 3 cups coconut flakes in Vitamix
    for 5 minutes on low)
1 cup coconut oil
1 cup almonds (presoaked and dried to remove the phytic acid)
2/3 cup dried pineapple
zest of 2 lemons
1 teaspoon vanilla
1/2 cup local honey

After the coconut butter is prepared, add coconut oil and almonds. Then blend until smooth. Add the remaining ingredients and blend lightly. Pour batter out onto a cookie sheet and freeze for 20-30 minutes. Remove from the freezer and slice. Store in the freezer.

Fermented foods that are more advanced for the digestive tract are added in Full GAPS.[dvi]

Fermented Ginger

Fermented ginger, otherwise known as gari, is a delicious, warming digestive aid. Ginger is a prokinetic, and fermentation assists in digestion, making this a perfect probiotic food for digestive health.

The International Journal of Food Sciences and Nutrition reported a study on lactic-fermented ginger using three different lactic acid bacteria. The tests include free radical scavenging, peroxide removal effects, and DPPH — a common test to help determine changes in antioxidant levels. The outcome was very encouraging.[dvii]

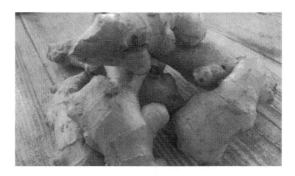

Select fresh, hydrated ginger. If it is sprouting eyes, it has a higher nutritional value. Slice ginger on a mandolin, using the thinnest setting possible. Thickly sliced ginger can take years to ferment. Ginger that is young will be more tender. If, while slicing, it is fibrous and feels like you are slicing rope, it will be fibrous and rope like after fermentation also. For five pounds of sliced ginger, add three tablespoons mineral salt.

Fermented ginger is fantastic with Asian-styled food dishes, but can be used with any meal.

Stir the ginger and salt mixture and allow it to sit for 30 minutes to a few hours. The salt will extract liquid from the ginger.

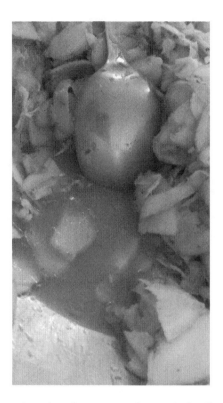

The sliced ginger can be stirred every so often to help distribute the salt and assist in the liquid extraction.

Stir in a half-cup of local honey. Pack ingredients into a Mason jar. Use a kitchen utensil to pack down the ginger, submerging all of the sliced ginger down below the brine.

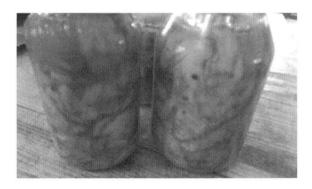

Kimchi

There is power in probiotic foods; kimchi ranks as one of the top most beneficial choices. When it comes to chemical toxicity, there is no contest.

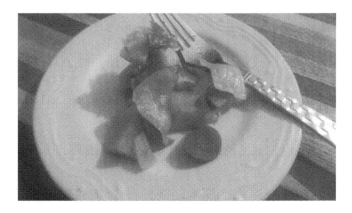

Using organic vegetables will yield a higher nutritional value, as well as a better flavor, to the kimchi. Using the freshest, most recently picked vegetables available is best.

Kimchi is a fermented food native to Korea. Koreans kimchi anything, including cucumbers, radishes, cabbage, and even octopus. Store-bought kimchi often has added maltitol, a sugar alcohol. The natural fermentation process will cause maltitol to be part of the resulting kimchi; however, adding maltitol, a synthetic chemical sugar alcohol, is not beneficial to the damaged intestinal tract.

1 small head of Napa cabbage, chopped
2 large daikon radishes, peeled and cubed
10 green onions, chopped
5 carrots, sliced
3 tablespoons freshly shredded ginger
5 large cloves garlic, chopped
3 teaspoons dried chili flakes or powder
1/2 cup fish sauce
2 tablespoons mineral salt

Mix all ingredients and add to crock or glass jar. Fill with water until the vegetables are covered. Put the lid on and allow to ferment for 12 days. Refrigerate and enjoy.

Finding clean fish sauce without corn syrup or other added processed ingredients is not easy. Usually, a good Korean grocery store will carry a clean one where the ingredients are just anchovies and salt.

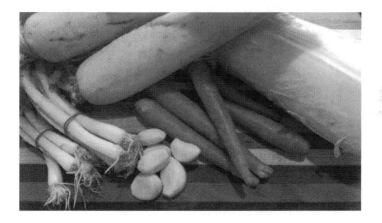

Keeping the vegetables submerged under the brine can be done with the weights in the crock, a crock rock, or even clean rocks from the yard.

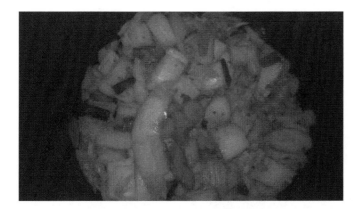

Serve kimchi as a garnish to any and every meal. Kimchi is such a staple to eating that Koreans often don't feel like they've eaten until they've had kimchi.

Strawberry Fruit Leather

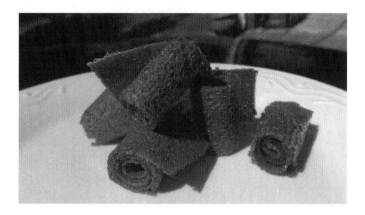

There are few better treats than a good, healthy fruit leather. Getting them to turn out right is difficult without chemicals and preservatives. This recipe wins every time.

Choose your strawberries straight from the farm or garden and process into leather the same day.

Since the magnesium load in these treats is high, a reasonable serving is necessary, which is hard to do because they are num, num, nummy. Too much may give you the high magnesium side effect of loose stools or overly calm for your personality.

These fruit leather roll-ups are pliable and roll easily, without parchment or wax to separate. Storage in a snack-pack, zip-top bag is sufficient.

Fill your Vitamix, blender, or food processor to the top with freshly picked, preferably organic, strawberries, washed with the tops on or removed, your choice. A lot of good nutrition is contained in the strawberry right next to the leaves and in the leaves themselves. For this reason, some people leave the stems on when blending – you'll never know they are there. The leaves are extremely high in vitamin C and other antioxidants and can be used fresh or dried for a medicinal tea. Strawberries tend to retain pesticide residue, so obtaining organic is best, if possible.

Herbalists use young strawberry leaves because they are antibacterial, antifungal, and astringent. They aid in bladder health, catarrh, diarrhea, digestion, liver health, rash control, lung support, joint paint, vascular issues, and weight loss.

Add 2 tablespoons of local honey, more if your strawberries need more sweetness, 1 teaspoon vanilla (home-brewed is best), 4 tablespoons unflavored magnesium citrate powder (such as Unflavored Natural Calm), and 1/2 teaspoon freshly squeezed lemon juice.

Blend the mixture smoothly. WARNING: this mixture will grow, foaming up from the magnesium powder, so once it is mixed, be sure to pour it right onto your dehydrator sheet. Dehydrate at 115 degrees for 8 hours or until dry to the touch. Cut into strips with scissors and roll.

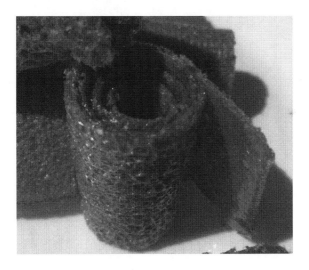

These fruit rolls store well in snack-pack, zip-top bags. If there is moisture left in them, mold will form.

Fermented Beans

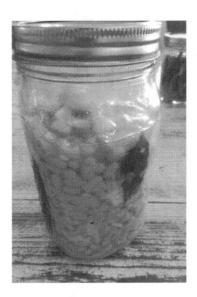

Fermented beans provide beneficial flora to the microbiome that cannot be provided from any other food. The benefits are numerous. Fermenting beans, specifically in the form of natto and tempeh, is a traditional practice in Asian countries. Different beans give different probiotic strains.

Frontiers in Microbiology says, "Functional properties of microorganisms in fermented foods include probiotics properties, antimicrobial properties, antioxidant, peptide production, fibrinolytic activity, poly-glutamic acid, degradation of antinutritive compounds."

Plant Foods for Human Nutrition says when fermenting beans, "Antinutrients, HCN, oxalate, and theobromine decreased with increasing duration of fermentation."

Some say that the way to tell if your body needs it is to try it. If you love it, are attracted to it, your body needs it. We are often attracted to what we need. This is not always the case.

When fermenting navy beans, Dr. Natasha says, "I add some whey. What I find with the beans, it's a good idea to cook them first. Parboil them first, and then ferment them. If you ferment them raw, they become so crunchy and no matter how much you cook them, they stay crunchy. They will not become soft and buttery."[dviii]

Fermented beans are usually referred to as bean paste. They are made by taking dry navy beans and soaking them in water with a tablespoon of apple cider vinegar, with the mother. After 24 hours, rinse; then repeat the soaking process for four days. After properly soaking and rinsing the beans, for every two and a half cups of prepared beans, mix three tablespoons of chopped onions and one tablespoon of chopped garlic together with three bay leaves and two teaspoons of mineral salt and two teaspoons of home-fermented and strained whey. Pack the ingredients into a quart Mason jar, leaving one inch of headroom. Put the lid on and let it sit tight on the counter or in a cabinet for three to five days, depending on the temperature in your kitchen.

This delicious treat goes fast!

Rosemary Watermelon Salad Dressing

Commercially prepared salad dressing is a difficult battle for those of us with food allergies. This gem is a family favorite. When watermelon is in season, store extras cubes in a freezer zip-top bag. When salad dressing is desired, drop a cup of watermelon in the Vitamix with a teaspoon of fresh rosemary. Add water and a tablespoon of apple cider vinegar to thin it out to your liking. This stores in refrigerator for up to a week.

1 cup watermelon
1 teaspoon rosemary
Apple cider vinegar to taste

Blend in blender until it reaches desired smoothness. Serve cold.

Cake—with Fermented Almond Flour

Monica Corrado, MA, CNC, CGP, is a teaching chef, Certified Nutrition Consultant, and Certified GAPS Practitioner who is passionate about illuminating the connection between food and well-being. She is a dynamic teacher, speaker, consultant, and author who loves to share the tools, knowledge, and inspiration to cook nourishing, traditional food. Monica has been teaching food as medicine for more than 12 years after 18 years in sustainable food sourcing and preparation, menu design, and management. She is a member of the Honorary Board of the Weston A. Price Foundation and started her own Cooking for Well-Being Teacher Training program in 2012. Monica has been teaching the cooking techniques for the *Gut and Psychology Syndrome* (GAPS) Diet in the online Certified GAPS Practitioner program with Dr. Natasha Campbell-McBride since its inception in 2018. For years, she has been known as the "GAPS Chef". For more information about Monica, her books, charts, traditional foods, and Teacher Training program, see www.simplybeingwell.com, monica@simplybeingwell.com. Her books include *Cooking Techniques for the Gut and Psychology Syndrome™ Diet: Part I: Meat Stock and Bone Broth, Part II: Culturing Dairy Part III: Lacto-fermentation*, along with Online Classes Meat Stock Why NOT Bone Broth.

Monica says:

One night, after dinner, my husband said he could "really go for a piece of chocolate cake". I said "Okay, give me about a half hour." He looked at me quite surprised; it wasn't something I had ever said before, and we were following the GAPS diet, so he thought cake was out of the question! I happened to have almond flour fermenting on the counter. Truth be told, I had "put it up" to ferment 2 days prior, intending to make muffins the day before. I had not had the chance to make the muffins, so I left the flour out to ferment for an additional day. (If I hadn't used it by the end of 48 hours fermentation time, I would have covered the bowl with plastic wrap and put it into the refrigerator to keep until I had time to bake with it). I got up and whipped this up. It was fluffy and DELICOUS! My husband loves grass-fed butter; he calls it "Nature's Frosting" and is always putting it on things...so of course, that is what he reached for when this cake came out of the oven. Since then, I have made it with yogurt cheese frosting or –the real hit— peanut butter frosting. You will find the recipes below. Enjoy!

"Chocolate" Cake—with Fermented Almond Flour and Raw Cacao can be made on Full GAPS by adding cocoa powder as shown below.

Makes one 9" round.

Recipe may be doubled for a layer cake.

> 2 1/4 cup almond flour
> 1/2 cup whey (from yogurt, kefir, or cheesemaking)
> 1/4 cup raw cacao powder (as a Full GAPS option)
> 1/2 teaspoon sea salt
> 1/2 teaspoon baking soda
> 1/3 cup raw honey
> 3 large pastured eggs
> 1 tablespoon organic vanilla extract
> Butter, coconut oil, ghee, or duck fat to grease the pan

This is a two-part process.

Instructions

First, ferment the almond flour: place almond flour in a medium bowl. Add in whey and mix well to combine. Cover bowl with a plate and place it on the counter out of the sun, at room temperature (68-72 degrees), for 48 hours. (Do not skip this step; it is what makes the cake fluffy).

After the flour is fermented, make the cake.

Preheat the oven to 350 degrees. Prepare one 9" round pan by cutting a round of parchment to fit. Place the parchment in the pan, and then grease the bottom and sides with butter, or another healthy fat (above), to keep it from sticking.

Gently warm the honey in a water bath until it is liquid. Meanwhile, in a small bowl, whisk 3 eggs with vanilla extract.

Mix the cacao, baking soda, and sea salt in a medium bowl. Place fermented almond flour into your standing mixer (or if you will be using a hand mixer, leave it in the bowl it is currently in) and add in the dry ingredients. Mix well. Add the egg and vanilla extract into the almond flour and mix well. Add the melted honey and mix well.

Pour the batter into the prepared pan. Be sure the batter is evenly distributed.

Bake for 25-30 minutes. The cake is done when a toothpick inserted into the center of the cake comes out clean.

Serve with grass-fed butter or yogurt cheese frosting (below) or peanut butter frosting (below).

Yogurt Cheese Frosting

makes about 2 ¼ cups

Ingredients

2 cups yogurt cheese
(strain 2 quarts of plain, organic, whole milk yogurt for 12-24 hours, and you will have 2 cups of yogurt cheese and 4 cups of whey)
¼ cup raw honey (optional)
2 tablespoons vanilla extract

Instructions

If using honey, gently warm the honey in a water bath until it is liquid. Combine all ingredients in a medium bowl and mix well.

Peanut Butter Frosting

makes about 2.5 cups

Ingredients

  1 cup unsalted peanut butter, organic, smooth, no fillers (or homemade)
  1 stick (4 oz.) grass-fed butter
  1 cup yogurt cheese
      (strain 1 quart, of plain, organic, whole milk yogurt for 12-24 hours
      for 1 cup of yogurt cheese and 2 cups of whey)
  1/4 cup raw honey
  1/2 teaspoon sea salt
  1 teaspoon vanilla extract
  1 teaspoon ground cinnamon

Instructions

In a large bowl, whip the peanut butter, butter, and yogurt cheese with a handheld mixer until smooth. Add in honey and blend well. Add remaining ingredients and blend until smooth. Use less honey if desired.

Chocolate Brownies

These chocolate brownies are amazingly healthy and disappear without a mama feeling the need to chase down sneaky children. There are two ways to make the recipe: gooey brownies or cake brownies. Gooey brownies are the same recipe as the cake brownies without the eggs and baking soda.

The whole recipe is made in the Vitamix. Add all ingredients and blend until smooth. Then, pour into a greased 8×8 pan and cook at 350 degrees for 35-40 minutes or until cooked in the center.

4 cups lentils properly soaked and cooked in Meat Stock
1 cup organic, grass-fed butter
1/2 cup local honey
1/2 cup cocoa
1 teaspoon baking soda
pinch of salt
1 tablespoon vanilla
6 eggs (preferably from a sun-soaking, bug-eating chickens)

Add all of the ingredients into a Vitamix or Cuisinart and blend until smooth. Pour into a greased 8×8 pan and cook at 350 degrees for 40 minutes, until done. Enjoy gooey brownies warm, but they are often best after being refrigerated. Use sugar-free, dairy-free, lecithin-free chocolate chips, or a homemade chocolate recipe as frosting, if desired.

Chocolate Chip Cookies

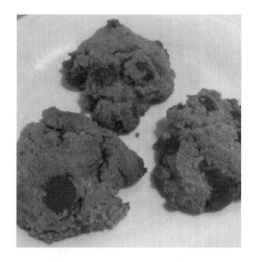

There are few treats that linger in your head like a fresh chocolate chip cookie.

The base recipe of blanched almond flour, local honey, vanilla, butter, and chocolate chips is not something a mama will sweat about and can be adapted to reduce sugar content if desired. Many people who are strict

GAPS have their favorite homemade chocolate chip recipe, while others can source clean chips already made.

    8 tablespoons grass-fed butter
    4 tablespoons local honey
    3 teaspoons vanilla, preferably homemade
    3 cups almond flour
    12 ounces GAPS-approved chocolate chips

Mix butter and honey on high until frothy, about 10 minutes. Add remaining ingredients and mix until smooth. Drop by teaspoon onto non-stick cooking sheet, pressing relatively flat if needed. Cookies with a thick middle and thin outer edge will burn at the edges before the middle is cooked. Bake at 350 degrees for 11-13 minutes. Cookies taste better not browned.

Dr. Natasha says sweet treats such as this "should be rare treats and not a staple."[dix]

Homemade Protein Bars

For each recipe, the ratio that works is one cup gummy stuff and one cup nuts. This recipe is a replica of Lara Bars on the store shelf.

This means that if you're making:

    Cherry Bars-
        1/2 cup dried cherries, 1/2 cup dates, 1 cup cashews.
    Peanut Bars-
        1 cup dates, 1 cup peanuts
    Blueberry Bars-
        1/2 cup dried blueberries, 1/2 cup dates, 1 cup cashews
    Cashew Cookie Bars-
        1 cup dates, 1 cup cashews

If there are issues with yeast, it's recommended to stick to just Peanut Bars or Cashew Cookie Bars, not the bars with dried fruits. Once your gut has healed a bit and you can tolerate small portions of sugar, then try other kinds.

Put nuts in a Vitamix or food processor and blend on low until they are a butter consistency. Add dates and cherries and lightly blend until combined. Fold out onto a flat surface and press into a rectangle.

Cut with a knife into bar sizes.

These bars keep in a drawer, but they keep fine in the refrigerator also. They are particularly favored for hiking on hot days as they contain no grains and no chocolate.

Dr. Natasha says sweet treats such as this "should be rare treats and not a staple."[dx]

Chocolate Pie

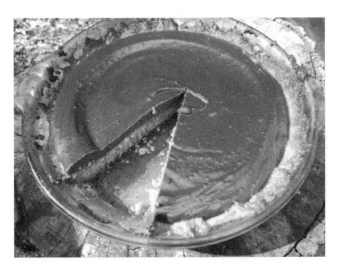

Chocolate pie with no guilt was impossible before this delicacy!

This pie shows well and is a treat that will disappear fast!

Crust

3 cups almond flour
1/2 cup organic, grass-fed butter
2 tablespoons local honey

Pie crust: combine almond flour and honey in mixer and blend until incorporated. Add butter and mix until combined. Press into pie pan. Cook at 350 degrees until lightly browned, roughly 20 minutes.

Filling

1/2 cup cocoa
1 cup kefir (preferably brewed from raw cream)
2 tablespoons organic grass-fed butter
1/2 cup local honey (add more if you like it sweeter)

For the filling, in a medium saucepan, add butter and heat on low until melted. Turn off the heat and add honey and kefir. Sprinkle in cocoa and let it sit for 5 minutes. Stir until velvety smooth. Pour into pie shell and refrigerate. Serve chilled.

Dr. Natasha says sweet treats such as this "should be rare treats and not a staple. Chocolate is not really allowed on the GAPS Diet, but for people whose digestive symptoms are gone and who feel well, they can be added safely."[dxi]

Italian Cream Cake

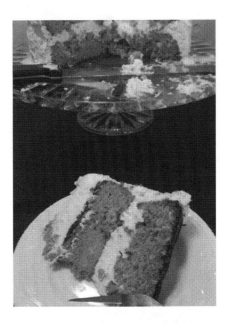

An Italian Cream Cake is a decadent, creamy addition to any celebration. This satiating treat can absolutely be made for a Ketogenic GAPS Protocol.

For the cake

> 2 sticks of pastured butter
> 16 ounces cream cheese
> 1/2 cup of local honey

Mix these ingredients in a mixer and beat for 20 minutes, until light and fluffy. Cream cheese is difficult to find without pathogen-feeding thickener gums, which are not for a damaged microbiome. Homemade cream cheese is easy to make and best for the protocol. Making cream cheese is easier than making yogurt or kefir.

Add:

> 1/2 cup home-brewed kefir
> 1 tablespoon vanilla

Mix until blended thoroughly.

Add:

- 1 teaspoon baking soda
- 2 teaspoons cinnamon
- 1 1/2 teaspoons nutmeg
- 1 pinch of salt
- 1 1/2 cups of chopped walnuts

Mix until combined thoroughly.

Add in:

3 cups of almond flour and 6 pastured eggs, alternating one egg then almond flour, then egg, then almond flour, etc.

Mix in 3 tablespoons of coconut flour.

Put the batter, split equally into circle pans that are buttered and dusted with almond flour, and bake at 350 degrees for 40 minutes. After the time is up, turn the oven off and leave the cake in the oven for an additional 30 minutes or until the center isn't jiggly.

Turn it out onto a cake serving tray and allow it to cool; then frost.

For the frosting

Mix together 16 ounces of cream cheese with one cup of pastured butter and a half-cup of local honey. Mix on high for roughly 20 minutes until fluffy. Frost.

Piña Colada Drops

Piña Colada Drops are a nourishing and satisfying treat made with coconut oil, pineapple, and local honey. They are fluffier than Lemon Drops or Mint Meltaways and create good variety in a healthy dietary plan.

Thoroughly blend one cup of organic pineapple until smooth—this will prevent stringy floaters in the end product candies. Add one cup of coconut oil and one tablespoon of local honey.

Drain off the small amount of pineapple juice so that it doesn't make the contents drippy. Fill a frosting bag with a large flower tip. Drop flowers onto parchment paper. Place in the freezer for 30 minutes. Scrape Piña Colada drops into a zip-top bag and store in the freezer until you are ready to eat.

Easter Bunny Candy Cups

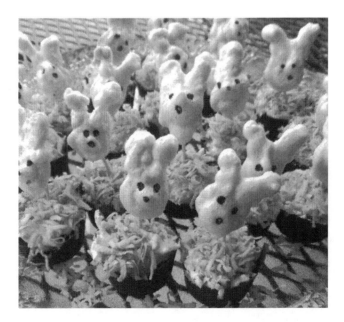

Easter treats can be healthy and tasty with these adorable, chocolate-filled cups with bunnies on top.

They make a great table decoration or centerpiece.

First, make chocolate from this recipe above using 1/2 cup of cocoa powder, 1/2 cup of cocoa butter, and 1/4 cup of local honey. Melt the ingredients together. Spread a cookie sheet with paper candy cup liners and fill with melted chocolate. Pick up each cup and roll the paper until the chocolate creeps up the sides of each cup. Chill in the refrigerator, remove paper cups, and line the cookie sheet with just the chocolate cups.

In a bowl, stir together:

   1/4 cup grass-fed butter
   1/2 cup home-brewed sour cream
   A small sprinkle of coconut flour can be added if the filling needs to be
       made firmer.

Fill the chocolate cups with the sour cream and butter mixture.

In a second bowl, mix together:

1/4 cup unsweetened coconut flakes with a small amount of freshly juiced kale for the desired green color. Too much kale juice for a darker "grass" makes it taste like kale, so less is more. Kale coconut—not cool.

Top each cup with the green "grass".

Bunny heads are made with the marshmallow fluff recipe, which makes it an off-GAPS treat. These cups can be filled with tiny carved and cooked pieces of butternut squash, beets, carrots, and small blueberries that look like Easter eggs. A toothpick will hold the bunny to the cup filling.

Dr. Natasha says, "Chocolate is not really allowed on the GAPS Diet, but for people whose digestive symptoms are gone and who feel well, they can be added safely."[dxii]

Chocolate Mousse Candies

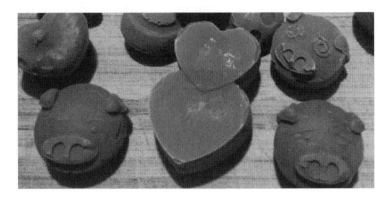

GAPS chocolates are often a craving; in fact, they are the most common cheat while on GAPS. This healthy chocolate will satiate and satisfy any sweet tooth.

In a Vitamix, food processor, or blender completely combine:

  5 or 6 ripe avocados
  2 cups home-brewed sour cream
  1/2 cup local honey
  1/2 cup cocoa powder
  1 teaspoon home-brewed vanilla

Blend until smooth. Pour the chocolate mixture in molds. Freeze. Enjoy. This mixture makes a hearty pudding.

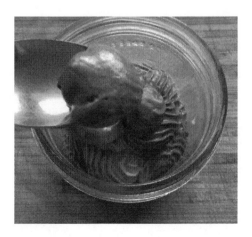

Dr. Natasha says, "Chocolate is not really allowed on the GAPS Diet, but for people whose digestive symptoms are gone and who feel well, they can be added safely."[dxiii]

Spice Cake

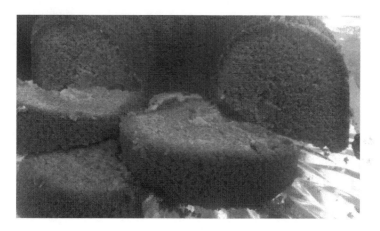

There's nothing better than a good old spice cake—this one for sure is a win!

1 cup pastured butter
1 cup medjool dates
1/2 cup local honey
2 cups pumpkin or any squash that is in season
2 teaspoons baking soda
4 teaspoons cinnamon
4 teaspoons ground nutmeg
3 teaspoons ground ginger
2 teaspoons allspice
1/4 teaspoon mace
1/3 teaspoon ground cloves
1 1/2 cups home-brewed kefir, preferably made from cream
    (home-brewed creme fraiche, yogurt, or sour cream also work well)
2 teaspoons vanilla
4 cups almond flour
2 tablespoons coconut flour
4 eggs from bug-eating chickens, free-ranging in the yard, preferred

Instructions

Cream the butter, dates, and honey until frothy, about 15-20 minutes.

Add squash, spices, baking soda, kefir, and vanilla, and mix until combined.

Alternate mixing in eggs and flours (almond flour and coconut flour), first adding one cup flour then one egg allowing a couple minutes for each to blend in before adding the next.

Pour batter into thoroughly buttered Bundt pan; spread to level to surface. Bake at 350 degrees for 50 minutes or until tester comes out clean.

Dr. Natasha says sweet treats such as this "should be rare treats and not a staple."[dxiv]

Birthday Cake

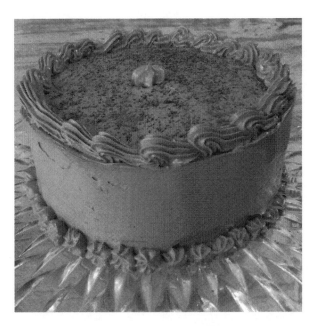

One of the roughest things to find is a clean and healthy birthday cake. After years of searching, this recipe satisfies every time. Now, making an extra cake every time your child is invited to a party isn't so bad since you can have a piece, too!

Cake

   1 cup pastured butter
   1/2 cup cocoa powder
   1/2-3/4 cup local honey
   2 teaspoons almond extract
   1/2 cup kefir (preferably kefir made from cream)
   1 teaspoon baking soda
   1 teaspoon ground cinnamon
   3 cups almond flour, preferably fine ground, blanched
   4 eggs, preferably from pastured chickens

Combine butter, cocoa powder, and honey in a stand-up mixer; beat until frothy, about 10 minutes. Add almond extract and kefir. Combine baking soda, cinnamon, and almond flour into a separate bowl. Alternate adding one egg and a little of the dry ingredients, mixing until fully combined. Pour batter into two greased, round cake pans. Bake at 350 degrees, 30 minutes or until tester comes out clean.

Better served cold.

* If you would like to use medjool dates as your sweetener, it is an option. Note that the use of dates will cause the cake to fall in the middle. The cake still tastes great though!

Frosting

   2 eggs
   2 teaspoons almond extract
   pinch of salt
   1 cup pastured butter
   1/2 cup honey (less if preferred)
   optionally a 1/4 cup cocoa powder

In stand-up mixer, add eggs, almond extract, and salt, and mix on low-medium until light and fluffy, a few minutes.

Pour egg mixture into a separate bowl and set aside.

Add butter, honey, and cocoa to mixer and beat until fluffy, about 15-20 minutes.

Pour the egg mixture slowly into the butter mixture and beat a few more minutes until well combined. Frost cake as desired.

*Dr. Natasha says sweet treats such as this "should be rare treats and not a staple. We also need to say that chocolate is not really allowed on the GAPS Diet, but for people whose digestive symptoms are gone and who feel well, they can be added safely."*dxv

Cocoa, Cacao, Carob, Alkalized vs Non-alkalized Cocoa Explained

For people with a damaged microbiome, choosing food options that are clean, with the least processing and additives, is vital. Cocoa is full of nutrition, including magnesium, iron, flavonoids, and antioxidants. The difference between alkalized, non-alkalized, cacao, cocoa, carob, cacao nibs, sweet chocolate, white chocolate, and chocolate liquor is where life gets confusing.

The most common food item used as a cheat while on GAPS is chocolate. Some practitioners say that this is because there is something in chocolate that the body needs for repair at that time. If the desire to eat chocolate is so high that you are controlled by it, or if you desperately want something so much you would kill someone for a piece, maybe there is something there that your body needs. It's wise during these times to make the right choice in feeding that craving so that you are not feeding the pathogens.

Dr. Natasha says sweet treats "should be rare treats and not a staple. Chocolate is not really allowed on the GAPS Diet, but for people whose digestive symptoms are gone and

who feel well, they can be added safely. "[dxvi] Since it is the most common cheat, if it something that you must have, choosing something healthier is best.

Just because a product says cocoa or cacao doesn't mean it's clean and healthy.

Chocolate comes from a pod grown on a cacao tree, a shade-loving tree, which thrives in the rain-forest region of West Africa. Each pod, when split open, contains roughly 50-60 seeds. The pods are picked from the tree and processed by hand; they will not open on their own. Each seed is so bitter that no animal will eat them.

The pods are scooped with the pulp and left to ferment in large vats, often wooden boxes, for around seven days. The beans are then spread flat to dry in the sun for another seven days.

The beans are then roasted and ground.

Two ingredients exit out of the grinding process at this point—cocoa solids, which are suspended in cocoa butter (a white, almost flavorless hard butter), and crumbly solids.[dxvii]

The FDA has guidelines that classify and name each step and resulting by-product.[dxviii]

The crumbly solids are cacao nibs.

These cacao nibs can be ground into powder, known as cacao powder or cocoa powder. There are no hard, definitive labels that distinguish between the two. According to the FDA, the terms "cocoa" and "cacao" can be used interchangeably.[dxix]

Non-alkalized cocoa is made from taking the cacao nibs and grinding them into powder. It is bittersweet with a slight fruity flavor. Generally, it has a light brown color and is often used for baking.[dxx]

Alkalized cocoa is treated with an alkalizing agent, processed with alkali. During alkalizing, the color turns slightly darker. This process raises the pH of the cocoa. Alkalizing makes cocoa dissolve in beverages and is often used in hot cocoa.[dxxi]

By law, alkali ingredients can be several options: "ammonium, potassium, or sodium bicarbonate, carbonate, or hydroxide, or magnesium carbonate or oxide, added as such, or in aqueous solution. For each 100 parts by weight of cacao nibs, used as such, or before shelling from the cacao beans, the total quantity of alkali ingredients used is not greater in neutralizing value (calculated from the respective combined weights of the alkali ingredients used) than the neutralizing value of 3 parts by weight of anhydrous potassium carbonate."[dxxii]

After alkalizing, neutralizing agents are used: "phosphoric acid, citric acid, and L-tartaric acid, added as such, or in aqueous solution."[dxxiii]

Obviously, sodium bicarbonate, also known as baking soda, is the cleanest option here, but there is no way of knowing which product is used without speaking to the processor himself. Even if baking soda is used, the neutralizing agent is still needed. The source of each ingredient used is chosen by the manufacturer seeking the highest profit, not what is most healthful, as is the case with citric acid.[dxxiv]

The FDA says, "Cacao nibs is the food prepared by removing the shell from cured, cleaned, dried, and cracked cacao beans. The cacao shell content is not more than 1.75 percent by weight, calculated on an alkali free basis."[dxxv]

More specifically, when the chocolate bean goes from the bean into cacao nibs, it is being processed. There is a certain level of processing for everyone that becomes unmanageable, indigestible. Each person needs to determine what his or her own system can tolerate. Cacao nibs, in their nib form, are very fibrous and difficult to digest for almost all people with a damaged microbiome.

In short, cocoa beans, when cracked open, contain cacao nibs inside.[dxxvi]

Finely ground cacao nibs are chocolate liquor, a paste like product.[dxxvii]

Chocolate liquor with added dairy, sweetener, and other ingredients, is called milk chocolate. Milk chocolate, by law, has to contain 10% or more actual chocolate in the product; the rest is sweeteners and other ingredients.[dxxviii]

Amano, Artisan Chocolate says that the average serving of milk chocolate has about the same amount of caffeine as a cup of decaf coffee.[dxxix]

The cacao fat is white – when dairy, sweetener, and other ingredients are added, this is called white chocolate.[dxxx]

Cocoa is cacao with the fat content between 10 percent and 22 percent.[dxxxi]

When defining cacao, "*Nomenclature*. The name of the food is 'cacao nibs', 'cocoa nibs', or 'cracked cocoa'."[dxxxii] These are all the same thing.

Carob comes from a completely different tree that also has pods; it is dried and ground into what we know as carob or carob powder. The carob tree, a small, evergreen, Arabian tree, grows in the Mediterranean region. Carob is used as a substitute for chocolate by some because it contains no caffeine and no theobromine, both of which are stimulants.

Scientific American says, "Caffeine works primarily on the central nervous system, theobromine stimulates the cardiovascular and pulmonary systems."[dxxxiii]

Caffeine is recommended by Dr. Natasha for low blood pressure. Caffeine is also used in the NICU to stimulate tiny bodies when they stop functioning. Caffeine is not part of the GAPS regimen for the great majority of people because it strips the endocrine system.

"Cocoa powder evolved in the chocolate industry as a by-product. The original purpose of pressing chocolate liquor was to obtain cocoa butter, which is utilized in the manufacture of chocolate coatings," says Bill Dyer from the Blommer Chocolate Company.dxxxiv

He goes on to say, "Not all cocoa powders are the same and no one cocoa powder meets the requirements for all applications."dxxxv

"% cacao" on a label refers to the weight of cocoa as a total percentage of ingredients. If milk chocolate contains 10 percent cocoa, then a product that contains 72 percent cocoa will obviously contain more cocoa and less sugar. This is why dark chocolate is always more nutritious – the higher the percentage, the more healthful the product.

Determining the cleanest and healthiest store-bought chocolate is not an easy task.

The problem with manufactured chocolate is that it still contains sugar. For every sugar molecule you eat, it takes 54 molecules of magnesium to process that sugar, robbing your body of magnesium. Local honey and dried fruit with no additives are the only approved sweeteners while on GAPS.

This leaves few options. Good quality chocolate is made with equal parts cocoa butter and cocoa powder and half that measure of local honey. This 1 to 1 to ½ mixture is delicious and can be used as chips, bars, or dipping chocolate. Variations such as adding another equal measure of peanut butter is divine. Adding another equal measure of grass-fed butter makes it even more smooth and creamy. Vanilla can be added for additional flavoring. Other flavorings such as peppermint extract or freshly grated lemon or orange zest are also good options.

Over the counter, Pure7 Chocolate is a fine choice for anyone whose digestive issues are gone and who cannot let go of wanting chocolate.

Pure7 Chocolate was started by two foodie friends, one of whom was on a strict GAPS protocol and looking for a GAPS-approved treat. Founder and CEO Julie MacQueen says, "I know how hard the GAPS diet is. I didn't pass Stage Four for over a year! And repeated intro 4x."[dxxxvi]

Julie says, "Nothing makes me happier than a GAPS customer!"[dxxxvii]

Raho says, "It needed to taste amazing because we are true foodies at heart. We made this chocolate for similar-minded folks."[dxxxviii]

All of that said, again, chocolate is the biggest cheat while on GAPS. Craving chocolate is a symptom of a magnesium deficiency and a sign that way more animal fat is needed in the protocol. GAPS folks are often magnesium deficient because the body uses great stores of magnesium to get better, as well as to push parasites and other pathogens out of the body.

It should be a rare treat, if used at all. The root cause of chocolate cravings, a magnesium and animal fat deficiency, should be addressed.

Chocolate Pudding

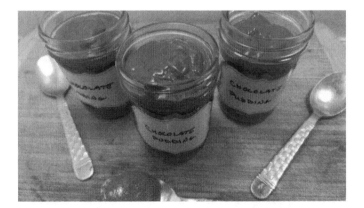

Pudding is a delicious treat that doesn't need to be forsaken; it can be made in a healthy manner.

Soak a half-cup of chia seeds in one and a half cups of home-brewed kefir for four hours.

Add:

2 heaping tablespoons organic cocoa
2 ripe bananas (with brown spots)
3 tablespoons local honey

Blend until smooth with a stick blender or food processor. Refrigerate and enjoy.

Dr. Natasha says, "Chocolate is not really allowed on the GAPS Diet, but for people whose digestive symptoms are gone and who feel well, they can be added safely."[dxxxix]

Gelatin

Processed gelatin powders can be added when the person is on Full GAPS – as a special treat, not as a staple. When asked if homemade gummies are approved for the GAPS Protocol, Dr. Natasha answered, "I don't think so. I'm not fond of hydrolyzed proteins, gelatins. It's much better to make fresh stock, fresh broth. You'll get plenty. That's where they get it from, it isn't processed. Too much processing. I don't use it. Too processed. Too processed. Too much processing."

After further discussion, the question was asked again, for clarity sake, "So, no gummies, no marshmallow fluff?"

Dr. Natasha answered, "No commercial gelatin. No commercial collagen. None of that. Only what you cook yourself."

Recipes made with gelatin, such as gummies, marshmallow fluff, and marshmallows, can be added after the person has completed the protocol but should not be favored or used heavily.

When Dr. Natasha was asked, "We've discussed organic gelatin - what stage would organic gelatin be?"

She said, "I would introduce it after the Intro Diet is completed (Full GAPS)."[dxl]

When asked, "If gelatin is made from chicken feet or ox tail stock, can it be Stage One? As in making gummies from ox tail thick stock on Stage One?"

She says, "On the full diet please."[dxli]

For parents on GAPS, it's hard. Using gelatin or collagen powders make their lives easier, especially with birthday parties or celebrations where a treat is needed. The mindset that we must eat treats is only a focus in recent years. Previously, traditionally, gatherings were to be with people; food was an accessory to the gathering. It's not a necessity. Focusing on the people you are with is important, not focusing on food. Since so many people are pulled towards collagen powders, it's been considered OK to use, but should not be a focus in any way; it is purely a rare treat. It falls into the same category as chocolate: something that folks use; but the real focus should be the real foods in their natural form. It's truly a treat.

Marshmallow Fluff

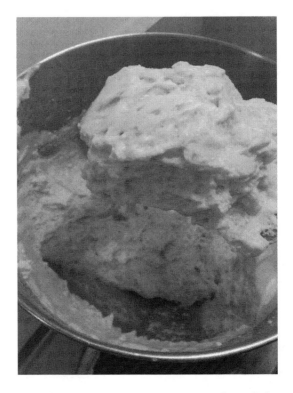

Marshmallow fluff is a treat that surpasses most others. It is a rare treat for those on GAPS and should not be consumed regularly. Rare treats are for things like a birthday.

Fluff uses local honey, water, and an organic gelatin. Collagen hydrolysate is designed to dissolve in cold water, does not gel, and is too highly processed.

Making fluff is easy.

Place 3 tablespoons of gelatin with 1/2 cup of filtered water in a mixer. Mix on med/low setting to stir. Be sure to scrape sides.

While the gelatin and water are mixing put another 1/2 cup of water with 1/2 cup of local honey into a medium saucepan, heat until roughly 240 degrees. When honey is heated, it loses valuable nutritional enzymes. This recipe works just fine if the honey and water is just warmed.

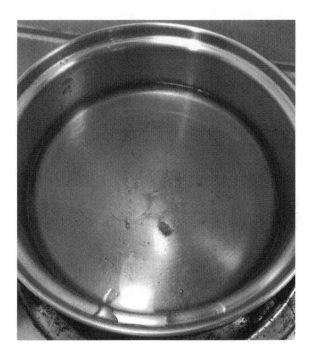

If it is heated to the full 240 degrees, the marshmallow fluff is perfect every single time, fluffy and airy. If it's not heated, the fluff is hit or miss, sometimes isn't fluffy, but is still good. The choice is yours.

Be sure to scrape the powder down into the mix or it will turn into a glue-like gummy structure along the side wall.

Check your gelatin and water mix. Be careful that it is all mixed thoroughly and that there are no gelatin globules, but rather that it is all mixed into granules. If there is a globule pillow stuck to the side of the bowl, be sure to break it up with a spoon.

Add the hot honey water to the gelatin water slowly with a slow steady stream while the mixer is still mixing. The product is hot, so adding it slowly will help keep a marshmallow fluff consistency.

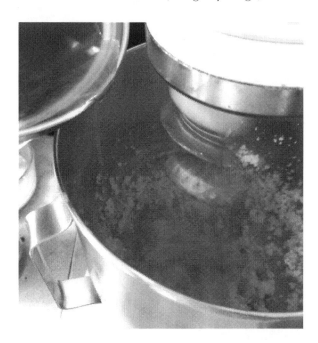

Once the honey water is all added to the water and gelatin mixture, turn the mixer to high and continue to mix for ten minutes. If you over-mix, you will have firm marshmallows that harden rather quickly. If you under-mix, the product will be more like a thin pudding consistency.

Store marshmallow fluff in jars or zip-top bags for camping.

Fluff Cupcakes

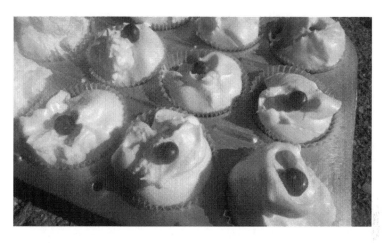

For those who stay on the Introduction Diet, different factors occur at different times. Birthday parties are one of the most common times where a child just wants to have something like what Standard American Diet kids consume. Marshmallow Fluff cupcakes fill this void.

This is a quick treat that looks just like a cupcake, especially when you need a clean birthday cake option for a trip to a friend's party. It's prepared, start to finish, in less than 14 minutes and keeps for days.

Simply fill cupcake liners with marshmallow fluff and top with a blueberry or other desired garnish.

Bunny Heads

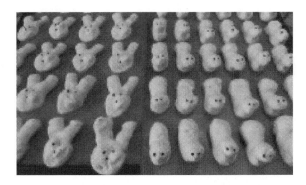

To make Easter Basket treats, first, make the marshmallow fluff recipe.

Immediately, when the fluff is done, scoop it into a zip-top bag. Snip the end of the bag with scissors – a small snip gives you smaller bunnies.

On a buttered piece of parchment paper, start with one ear.

Then, add a second ear.

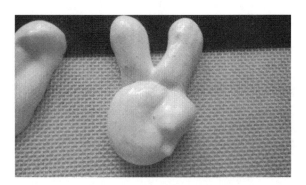

Then, draw a circle for the face. Although it looks like a hand making a peace sign, it's a little piece of bunny magic.

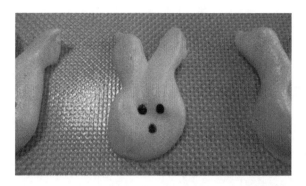

Once you have filled the whole sheet up with bunny heads, let them dry a bit. Then, put a few drops of water in a cup with a small amount of activated charcoal. Mix together. Cut off the cotton tip of a Q-tip and dip it into the charcoal. Blend and dab eyes and a nose on the bunny.

These make great Peeps, bunny heads, and hearts – perfect for a healthy Easter snack. This recipe makes 133 bunny heads.

These bunny heads hold well but do not stack well because of the sticky marshmallow factor. For later stages, you can dip these treats in cinnamon or cocoa powder. They can be put in the dehydrator to make a cookie; it's a different variety, more like shelf-stable taffy. Freezing them makes them like taffy, also.

They are always a crowd favorite and are quick to make. In addition, you can show up at an event with a whole tray-full for pennies, they present well, and all the kids love them!

We have made these with heating the honey to just before boiling point as well as just heating the honey with water to retain more enzymes. Both work well.

Snowman Heads

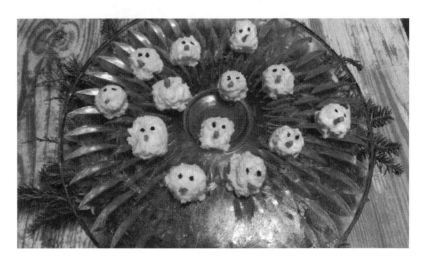

This festive snack is the easiest Christmas treat you'll make this season.

Make marshmallow fluff with the previously listed recipe.

Grease a non-stick baking sheet with pastured butter or ghee.

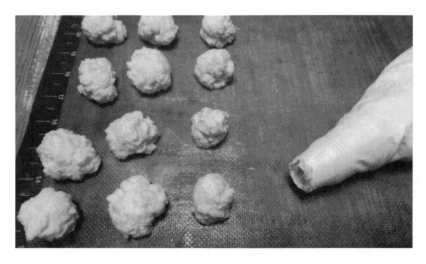

Pipe snowballs onto the greased cooking sheet using a piping bag with no tip. Snowballs are easiest made using an extra-large piping bag or gallon zip top bag with a large hole cut into the corner. These balls can be carved later to shape them into perfect balls so don't worry too much about the shape.

Insert cut carrot pieces and tap on eyes with activated charcoal mixed with a little water. This is easily done with a circular-shaped toothpick with a flat bottom.

Santa Hats

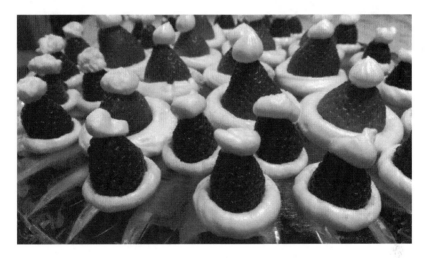

Three ingredients are all you need for mustering up these treats for Christmas. Sometimes, while on GAPS, holiday festivities are a challenge. These festive Santa Hats are the perfect taste combination, much like peas and carrots—they just go together.

Make marshmallow fluff; remember though, time is of the essence while making these treats. If things aren't properly prepped and making the hats isn't done swiftly, the fluff will dry and become difficult to use. It may be best to read the whole recipe first or even do some of the prep work like buttering the tray, cutting the stems off the strawberries and preparing the frosting bag before making the fluff, especially the first time the recipe is made.

While the marshmallow fluff is mixing, grease your tray with pastured butter or ghee. Prepare your piping bag so that when the fluff is done, you can work fast. Piping the fluff and adding the strawberries and raspberries need to be done quickly. The fluff dries and cracks quickly. If the fluff gets too dry while in the piping bag, it'll give the appearance of cellulite as it's squeezed out—which is great for making marshmallow bunny heads or snowman heads but doesn't look so great for Santa Hats.

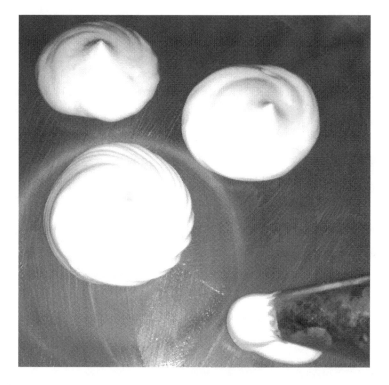

On the greased tray pipe out the bottom of the Santa Hats.

Then, working quickly, add the strawberries by firmly pressing them into the center of the hat bottoms.

Work in groups: pipe out the bottoms and then add the strawberries; then add the next grouping of hat bottoms. Move on to the red raspberries in the same manner.

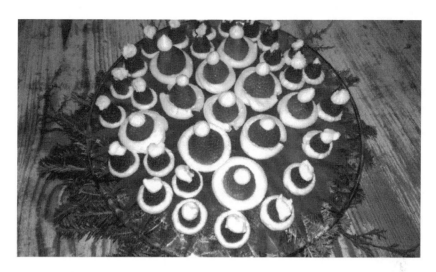

Place white dollops on the top of each hat. Since the red raspberries are wetter than the strawberries, it's harder to get the dollops to stick. You may need to scrape the dollop off the piping bag with a butter knife or toothpick.

These Santa Hats are quick and easy, 15 minutes from start to finish. They make an amazingly beautiful tray if you are bringing "Christmas Cookies" to a gathering, yet they are inexpensive. The taste of strawberries and fluff is a combination made in heaven; they go together, complementing and embellishing each other.

Saving Money While On GAPS

It doesn't take long to determine that switching to GAPS food is not a cheap route to health; however, it is the most thoroughly effective option for health. It may not be that switching to real food costs more; it may be a paradigm switch that inexpensive food costs so little because it's not real food. Regardless, nourishment is essential to rebuilding.

Washington State University published a report showing food expenditures and that found Americans spent 6.8 percent of their annual budget on food—shockingly lower than the rest of the world.[dxlii]

International Business Times wrote a descriptive explanation reporting, "The US Spends Less on Food Than Any Other Country In The World."^{dxliii}

Ironically, though, it doesn't have to be this way—the most healing foods are generally the cheapest cuts in the real food world. There are ways to save money while walking out healing when on GAPS. Following some simple tips can help save you money, but remember, your future health expenses will decrease as your body is healthier. So, you may be spending more on food, but you'll be spending less on future medical expenses. The steps to saving money are simple but take time.

First, find a farmer. When you find a local farmer who raises his animals on pasture, he is an asset. He is a real person, a neighbor in your community who relies on consistent customers. He probably sells his cattle by the head to people filling a freezer. These customers may not be using the cuts of meat or bones you desire. If you are a consistent customer of his, you can ask him to be on the lookout for you, asking his customers if they will need their bones, liver, and other organ meats. Many people who process a cow don't use their prepackaged fat, organ meats, and bones. These are valuable to a person healing with GAPS. Most farmers sell cattle to those filling their freezers in mid to late spring, after the cows have eaten their fill of the quick-growing, fresh spring grass. This makes the meat more tender. Ask your farmer during this time if he has any customers that may not be wanting their bones or organ meats when the animal goes for processing.

Find hunters. Hunters are valuable in so many ways. They are most often Christians, who believe in giving to those in need. These are salt of the earth people. In addition, they process their kill while throwing away their bones and organ meats. Hunters are often a network. Once you ask one hunter if he has access to the cuts you need, telling him the importance of these cuts for your child's health or your health, he will help—especially if you bake him cookies. Even more accessible is the processor. Many towns have a guy who processes the deer, as well as other animals, in his garage. If you ask the hunters where they take their animals for processing, you can pick up his bones and other cuts that he throws in the garbage.

Get your own laying chickens. In his book, *Folks, This Ain't Normal,* Joel Salatin says not to waste money on a pet when a chicken can give you food.[dxliv] Chickens can live inside, just like a dog, if your neighborhood has restrictions. Chicken diapers are available, as well as harnesses, if you would like to take them for a walk. Chicken diapers have a housing that secures a pantyliner to catch any output.

Go heavy on the organ meats, which are, generally, the least expensive cuts. Again, most processors and farmers are throwing these cuts away. Many give them to their dogs for a treat. These cuts are by far the most nutrient-dense parts of the animal. Dr. Natasha Campbell McBride recommends eating the amount of liver that would cover the size of your hand, not your palm—your hand. After eating liver for a few weeks, you will notice the dark circles from under your eyes recede and skin tone grow more vibrant.

Make your own ferments. Commercial probiotics are expensive – it's no secret. Making your own probiotics at home with fermented vegetables is just as effective, if not more effective. Recent tests show 2 ounces of home-fermented sauerkraut has more probiotics than a bottle of 100 count probiotic capsules.[dxlv] Other research showed that kefir has 150 billion colony forming units per tablespoon with 10 to 20 different types of beneficial bacteria and yeasts.[dxlvi] Research is showing that commercial yogurt has very little to no probiotics; home-brewed, however, is loaded with beneficial strains.[dxlvii] The same numbers are proving true for kvass, Kombucha, pickles, and all other home-brewed ferments. McBride says that she has many patients who cannot afford commercial probiotics and heal up just fine using home-brewed ferments.

It is best to get food from farmers, where you know the methods in which the food has been raised. In cases where that's not possible, join COSTCO instead of shopping at big-money, specialty health food stores. COSTCO has been carrying more and more organic foods, meeting the desires of their customers. GAPS folks can source many different foods from COSTCO, supplementing with their farmer and that's it. If you do not have a membership yet, go with a friend. If you sign up at customer service with a referring member with you, COSTCO will give you a $10 in-store gift card because someone referred you, and they will do the same to your referring friend. If your friend is a giving person, she'll give the gift card to you and you've just gotten your membership for a $20 discount. COSTCO also has amazing customer service and an incredible return policy.

Shop the sales and cook from the foods you have on hand. If you happen to hit a store, look for organic vegetables on sale. If organic cabbages are on sale for 99 cents a pound, buy as many as you can and make your sauerkraut in bulk. If the kraut is under the brine, it'll be shelf stable for many months without refrigeration.

Grow your own garden. This refreshing hobby can become addictive and really save with the budget. Vegetables can be grown in pots if you do not have yard space. When you grow your own garden, you control the pesticides and GMOs. You can sow seeds directly into the ground or start your own veggie starter trays to plant into the ground after your last frost.

Saving Time On GAPS

Big-batch stock is a lifesaver on GAPS. Meat Stock doesn't have to be made one bird at a time, every day. On a weekend day, or whatever day works best for you, an extra-large lobster pot can be used to make massive batches of stock. First, put in one cut up bird, layer salt and peppercorns over top; then, put another layer of another bird with salt and peppercorns, and another layer and another layer until the pot is full. Follow the directions for Meat Stock as usual. Since the pot is larger, it takes longer to heat up, but the rest of the directions are the same. This usually produces enough stock to last all week long.

Buy eggs from your farmer in bulk; they will often offer a discount with larger purchases.

Contact all of the farmers in your area to let them know you have a child with severe health issues who thrives on clean food. Make sure you let them know that your money is tight and, if they ever have an animal going to slaughter where a buyer backs out, to call you. It is not uncommon for folks to score a pastured pig for $2 a pound because a farmer is desperate. Stay in touch with these same farmers to access their organ meats, bones, or animal fat that they are not even putting on their kill sheet because they don't eat them.

Contact local processing houses near you frequently, and ask if they have unclaimed organ meats, bones, or animal fats.

Cut back on your obligations so that your time is simplified. Less to do means you have less to do. Cleaning up your lifestyle brings peace of mind.

Spinning your wheels is a waste of time. There are many things that cause us to spin our wheels; when it's involved in health-related issues, the waste is amplified. For example, if you are working on pulling metals out of the body through chelation, but the child is not moving his or her bowels every day, you're pulling out metals but reabsorbing them because the body can't get rid of them. This is spinning your wheels. Working with a good Certified GAPS Practitioner can help to make sure your methods are moving you along at the quickest pace.

Big-batch ferments, like big-batch Meat Stock, means you make it once but eat off the batch for much longer, which creates less work.

Tween and teenage helpers are extremely helpful. These kids are best source from neighbors as you don't have to drive to pick them up for "work." The goal is for them to work as an aide in the kitchen or house in general. They do simple tasks like dishes, picking up toys, and playing with children to keep them occupied so that Mom can cook or vacuum. Since they are still young, you can hire them for a lower price than you would an adult professional. Remember that you may also be getting a lower quality of work, which can be used in your favor as you can teach them exactly how it should be done. In cases like this, the more you use their help, the more valuable they are as you don't have to keep teaching them.

Chapter 9:
Coming Off GAPS

Coming Off GAPS is the last stage of the GAPS Protocol and is one that should not be taken lightly. While progressing through Coming Off GAPS, it is very important to watch for any regression in symptoms. If regression happens, go back to an earlier stage to allow more healing to take place. These symptoms often include the return of autistic symptoms, joint pain, ADHD behaviors, defiance, the desire for sugar-filled foods, incontinence, constipation, loose stools, trouble sleeping, headaches, bloating, or any other adverse symptoms.

These symptoms are not something to push through as in previous stages when introducing probiotic foods in certain cases.

More times than not, Certified GAPS Practitioners see GAPSters come off GAPS too early, and the symptoms return to be worse than what they were prior to GAPS.

This stage should not be rushed. It is very much a stage where the GAPS dance is still in effect: one step forward, one step back, one step forward, two steps back. Some people remain on Full GAPS for two years with no symptoms, then step off GAPS during a birthday, Easter Sunday or Thanksgiving Day or Christmas Day, and then resume with Full GAPS. If in doubt, this is a very safe place to camp.

Coming Off GAPS starts with young white potato. Young potatoes are small. Older potatoes are large. Potatoes should always be organic. Frequently, it is said that they are like sponges, sucking up pesticides. Potatoes are heavily sprayed, due to the potato bug, which is roughly the size of the palm of your hand and can decimate your crop quickly. Many potato farmers have their own plot of potatoes for their own family, far away from their commercial crop, due to this reason. Many GAPSters find that this is where they stop. They feel well on Full GAPS with the addition of occasional young white potato.

Fermented Porridge is a more advanced step. This is done by filling a bowl full of millet, quinoa, or other, and then covering it with milk kefir or whey and letting it sit overnight. This makes a lovely bowl of porridge in the morning. Add honey if desired and enjoy. Advancing more to fermented wheat is best by starting with Ancient Grains, grains that have not be altered since Biblical times.

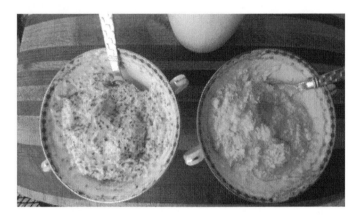

The texture of fermented porridge is up to you; the longer it is left to ferment, the softer the porridge will be. It can be warmed or left cold – the choice is yours. As stated in the book Probiotic Foods VS Commercial Probiotics, when kefir is heated, the beneficial probiotics are reduced in number.

Kefir Bread

Kefir bread is a recipe by Liliane Widmer, NTP, CGP, and mother of 9. After they progressed through GAPS and were ready to try more advanced foods, it was a real treat for them all.

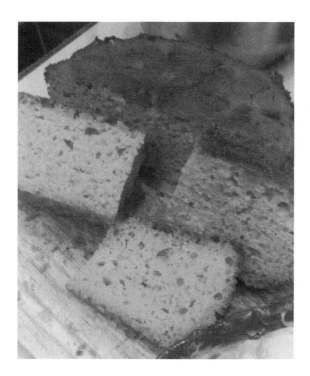

2 cups kefir
4 cups organic flour
1/2 teaspoon mineral salt
1 tablespoon local honey
1 tablespoon tallow or lard

Combine all the ingredients in a food processor.

Cover baking pan with additional tallow or lard. Fill the pan with dough, put the lid on, and leave it on the counter for 24 hours. The dough will double in size.

Bake at 350 degrees for 45 minutes with the lid on, then an additional 15 minutes with the lid off. Be sure your lid is oven safe.

Sourdough Bread That Slices

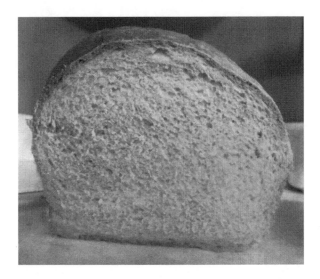

Creating a sourdough bread that slices can be daunting—but not with this amazing recipe by Ashlee Purdie, a good friend, foodie, and self-sustaining homesteader who slings babies while delivering calves and looks great the whole time. Ashlee uses real food to keep her family healthy.

First, make a sourdough starter or get one from a friend. To make a sourdough starter, mix one tablespoon of flour with one tablespoon of water twice a day until bubbly. If you are not using your starter, put it in the refrigerator.

Take your sourdough starter out of the refrigerator at around 7 or 8 pm. Dump about 3/4 cup of the active starter into a mixing bowl. Don't scrape the jar clean!

Combine your 3/4 cup of starter with 1 cup of water and 1 1/2 cups of whole wheat flour. It may be thinner or thicker, depending on the initial consistency of your starter.

Cover with a plate or plastic wrap and forget about it until morning.

Add 3/4 cup each of water and flour to your starter jar and mix well. Let sit on counter a couple of hours.

It may have swelled a little but should have some bubbles. It is quite active and happy, so stick it back in the fridge until you're ready to bake again.

Next morning—nice and bubbly. It is ready to bake.

Add the following:

> 1 1/2 cups white bread flour
> 1/2 cup whole wheat flour
> 2 teaspoons mineral salt
> About 1 tablespoon butter or lard
>   (coconut oil tends to make a heavier loaf)
> 1 egg
> 1-2 tablespoons of honey

This bread can be made with or without the egg – both work fine. If you have extra eggs, use one; otherwise, don't stress.

Mix with the paddle until the dough forms a loose ball.

Switch to the dough hook and knead on low-med until the dough is smooth and tacky, but not sticky. When you pinch the dough, it should not stick to your fingers. You may need to add a little more flour or water to get the right consistency. Add small amounts at a time, though, and let it mix for a few minutes before making any more changes. When it's ready, cover the bowl. Don't oil the bowl! Oiling the bowl can lead to large holes inside the loaf of bread. It causes the dough not to stick to itself when you shape it.

At this point, turn the dough out onto a sheet of parchment paper and place in the dehydrator at the lowest temperature, 95 degrees, or in a warm spot of the kitchen.

The dough will have doubled in size.

I prefer to let the dough sit and sour while it rises for 18 hours.

Bake until the internal temp is between 190 and 195. Brush with butter/oil while still hot. This is generally 350 degrees for 35 minutes.

Remove from pan and cover with damp tea towel until cool. Your crust will be soft and lovely.

We have used this dough and shaped it into garlic bread, shaped into hot dog buns, and shaped into hamburger buns. It's good for more than slicing bread.

As people phase off GAPS, one of the first foods desired is bread. The phasing off GAPS protocol has an order for a reason. Much like rebuilding on GAPS, Coming Off GAPS is a building protocol.

"The beauty of sourdough fermentation is lactobacillus does such a wonderful thing in bread. It cuts apart those bonds they get difficult to digest, the bacteria digest the sugar, and deactivates the phytic acid [*sic*]," said Min Kim[dxlviii] Kim is an Einkhorn sourdough specialist who phased her family off GAPS and onto a Weston A. Price food protocol.

Kim says that each sourdough bread is specific to each household in which it was made as the starter captures yeast from the air in your own environment.[dxlix]

"There is more than one way to make bread," she says.[dl]

Einkhorn is an unhybridized grain, meaning it hasn't been altered in any way. This is considered an Ancient Grain or Biblical wheat.

Einkhorn literally means one seed, Kim says. It grew in modern day Iraq and Syria, in the Fertile Crescent. It contains a strong root system, which enables it to take up more nutrition from the soil. It contains less starch and more protein.

Each grain has a protective husk, which adds another step in the processing. This husk protects the wheat berries from collecting mold.

Einkhorn is low in glutamines and has different gliadins, she says. Einkhorn has a favorable ratio of gliadins, making it easier to digest, even for those with non-symptomatic celiac and others with sensitive digestive systems.

In mass production, Einkhorn does not produce favorable results, so it is not chosen as a desired grain for commercial production. In addition, the price point is higher, leaving a smaller profit margin for commercial bread production.

"Phytic acid is found in the bran and interfere[s] with the body's ability to absorb calcium, iron, zinc, magnesium and copper," Kim says.[dli] Wheat bran has 4,873 mg of phytic acid per 100 grams. Sourdough whole wheat bread has 79 mg per 100 grams of weight.

Kim adds that ground Einkhorn should be stored in the refrigerator since the germ, once ground, becomes rancid fairly quickly.

Sourdough Hamburger Buns, Sourdough Hot Dog Buns

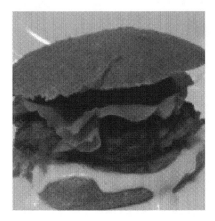

We've tried countless sourdough recipes for hamburger buns over the years, working the recipe and reworking the recipe, looking for a version that holds up to a quality burger. This recipe is the winner so far. It is the easiest and most consistent. It works amazingly well as a hot dog bun recipe, making the hardest part of hamburgers and hot dogs to be simply finding a clean dog without chemical additives and filler ingredients that aren't really food.

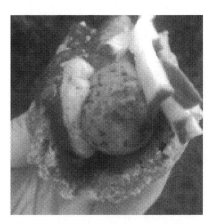

A sourdough starter can be easily made at home if you do not have a friend who already makes sourdough bread. To start a sourdough starter from scratch, take equal parts of organic wheat flour and water and mix them together in a glass bowl. Some people use one tablespoon of each; others use 1/4 cup of each or more, depending on the size of your family.

Make the quantity appropriate to the size of the starter you are already feeding. This means that if you have been feeding your starter twice a day for 2 weeks, it's going to be quite large. Feeding a large bowl filled with roughly 4 cups of starter with one tablespoon fresh flour/water isn't going to be enough to feed the whole bowl. Leave the starter covered and let it sit on the countertop.

Feed this starter with equal parts flour and water twice a day.

When it has bubbles rising to the top, it is active and ready for use. If you leave for vacation or need to slow down the starter activity, put it in the refrigerator until you need it again, and allow a couple of feedings to revive the starter.

When the starter is active and bubbly, you are ready to make bread. I usually make bread when the starter gets so big, I need to discard some to lessen the quantity in the bowl.

Add together:

    5 cups fresh-ground, organic Einkhorn wheat berries
    4 cups sourdough starter
    5 tablespoons grass fed butter
    4 teaspoons mineral salt
    2 pastured chicken eggs

Add all ingredients into a mixer with the bread paddle. Mix on medium until the edges pull away from the wall, sticking to itself but not the bowl. You may need to add a bit more flour, a little at a time, until the dough ball can be pinched between your fingers without sticking.

This recipe makes 2 loaves of bread, one loaf of bread and 6 hamburger/hot dog buns, or 12 hamburger/hot dog buns. We like to put half the mixture into a greased loaf pan and spoon the other half onto parchment paper in hamburger bun size rounds or hot dog sized buns. Set in the dehydrator overnight on lowest setting, around 95 degrees.

Some folks make their bread before going to bed so it can rise overnight. This way, when you wake up, you can put the bread in the oven, and breakfast is done in 30 minutes.

First thing in the morning (or after 8-10 hours of rise time), take the risen dough out of the dehydrator and put it in an unheated oven. The buns will do best if you place another cookie sheet upside down over top to keep the buns moist, cooking with steam. Turn the oven on 350 degrees and cook the hamburger buns for 14 minutes; cook the bread loaves for 30-40 minutes or until the top is browned and pulls away from the sides of the pan.

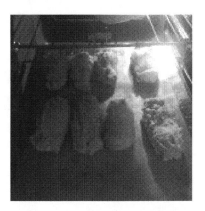

The hamburger buns will stay moist if you keep the 9×13 over the top of the buns as a lid while the buns are cooling.

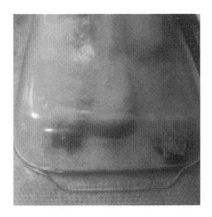

If you skip this step or eat the buns fresh out of the oven, they will not hold together very well.

Slice and enjoy. The hamburger buns hold together well warm or chilled.

When wheat is fresh-ground, it should always be eaten within 48 hours or frozen for the future. Once wheat berries are ground, they decline in nutrients. It is best to eat the bread while the nutrient content is highest. The further away from grinding it is, the more the nutrients degrade. Some say that after 72 hours, the nutrient level of the bread is non-existent, and it pulls nutrients from your body, specifically vitamin B12. Sourdough bread flour does not need to be soaked and sprouted – the sourdough itself does this step for you.

Chapter 10:

Off GAPS Foods

Many foods are Off GAPS Foods – too many to list. When stepping Off GAPS, it's important to remember that real food nourishes the body. The more a food is processed, the less natural it is, and the less the body can identify it. Things like coconut aminos, seltzer water, or soda water are common foods that are hit first when coming Off GAPS.

To get an idea of Dr. Natasha's thoughts on coconut aminos she says, "No, I don't like that, no – highly processed, definitely. There's MSG in it, which naturally occurs, apparently, and ingredients which might have not been listed. That's why. The more processed something is, the less we can trust it."[dlii]

What to Do When Progress Isn't Happening

Sometimes, people feel like they aren't making the progress they desire on GAPS. When people come to a position of great damage in the microbiome, it takes time. The older the person is, the more time it takes. The deeper the damage is, the more time it takes. The more intolerances there are, the more time it takes. The more toxic the environment is, the longer it takes.

Dr. Natasha says, "Just keep going. I'm sure there really are improvements. If they really sat down and add what they were like a few months before. When people are in the midst of it, they just focus on the negatives."

When we've been on the protocol for some time, at least a year, addressing metals or parasites is an option. Binders such as bentonite clay, activated charcoal, food-grade diatomaceous earth or the like can be added, but not within the first four stages.[dliii]

Dr. Natasha says, "I would say we don't touch any parasites or worms in the first four stages. We just work on the protocol." When the person is on Extended Stage Two for over a year, this can be addressed.[dliv]

The buildup of parasites in the body becomes more and more prominent as the microbiome declines in health. Dr. Natasha says, "I have no doubt the rise in these parasites are because our rise in toxicity. The more toxins there are in the body, the more parasites, the more parasites the body will invite and grow. The body actually cultivates them and then you get Lyme. Lyme is a result. I'm sure Glyphosate is going to lead to Lyme – EMFs too."[dlv]

The truth is, parasites have a job in body. If the body is not ready for them to go, they stay. The best way to approach them is to eat proper food, reduce inflammation, and rebuild the good flora that the balance can establish.

Dr. Natasha says, "Parasites are difficult to get rid of; that's, I think, a signal to people that the body's not ready to let go. It doesn't let go of them – there's too much toxicity. They're doing some good jobs there. And of course, they cause symptoms of their own which are uncomfortable. People want to get rid of them, but it's better to keep them in."[dlvi]

About the Author

Nourishing Plot is written by Becky Plotner, ND, traditional naturopath, CGP, D.PSc., who sees clients in Rossville, Georgia. She is a Board-Certified, Naturopathic Doctor who works as a Certified GAPS Practitioner who sees clients in her office, Skype, and phone. She has been published in Wise Traditions, spoken at two Weston A. Price Conferences, Certified GAPS Practitioner Trainings, has been on many radio shows and television shows, and writes for Nourishing Plot. Since her son was delivered from the effects of autism (Asperger's syndrome), ADHD, bipolar disorder/manic depression, hypoglycemia, and dyslexia through food, she continued her education, specializing in Leaky Gut and parasitology at Duke University, finishing with distinction. She is a Chapter Leader for The Weston A. Price Foundation.

"GAPS™ and Gut and Psychology Syndrome™ are the trademark and copyright of Dr. Natasha Campbell-McBride. The right of Dr. Natasha Campbell-McBride to be identified as the author of this work has been asserted by her in accordance with the Copyright, Patent and Designs Act 1988.

Also by Becky Plotner

Food Probiotics vs Commercial Probiotics
Joyous Song, The Proverbs 31 Woman
A Walking Tour of Lincoln Road, South Beach
Ocean Drive Guidebook, Ask a Local
The Fontainebleau, Miami & Los Vegas (Ask a Local)

Connect with Becky Plotner

Blog: https://nourishingplot.com
Website: https://gapsprotocolhelp.com
Facebook: https://www.facebook.com/nourishingplot

Recipe List

Recipe	Page	GAPS Stage
Adrenal support shake	196	2
Adrenal support stock	195	2
Almond Veggie Wrap	314	5
Bacon and Kale	337	6
Bacon Jerky	344	6
Bacon Mayonnaise	331	6
Bacon Mayonnaise Deviled Eggs	334	6
Bacon Wrapped Asparagus	265	4
Bacon Wrapped Hearts	268	4
Baked Beans	366	Full
Beef Meat Stock	58	1-5
Beet Gel-o	76	Full
Beet Kvass	102	1
Birthday Cake	402	Full
Blackberry Jam	374	Full
Bone Broth	377	Full
Bunny Heads	416	Full
Butter Cream Mints	228	3
Butter Honey Frosting	83	1
Cake-with fermented almond flour	388	Full
Caramelized Curly Dock or other Caramelized Greens	372	Full

Recipe	Page	GAPS Stage
Carrot Cake	339	6
Carrot juice	210	2
Cauliflower Cream Soup	77	1
Cheesy Kale Chips	349	6
Chicken Meat Stock	50	All
Chicken Nuggets	364	Full
Chicken Soup Variations	53	1-5
Chocolate Brownies	391	Full
Chocolate Chip Cookies	392	Full
Chocolate Mousse Candies	400	Full
Chocolate Pie	394	Full
Chocolate Pudding	409	Full
Chowder	201	2
Creamed Carrot Soup	72	1
Easter Bunny Candy Cups	398	Full
Eggnog	205	2
Electrolyte Drink	141	2
Fermented Beans	386	Full
Fermented Coconut water	127	1
Fermented Cranberry Sauce	321	5
Fermented Fish	207	2
Fermented Garlic	239	3
Fermented Ginger	380	Full
Fermented Nut Butter	217	3

Recipe	Page	GAPS Stage
Fermented Pineapple and Peppers	323	5
Fermented Porridge	428	Off GAPS
Fish stock	62	All
Fluff Cupcakes	415	Full
Fried Zucchini	329	6
GAPS Shake	190	2
GAPS Waffles	361	Full
Halloween Party Tray	369	Full
Hash Browns	370	4
Homemade Protein Bars	393	Full
Homestyle Chicken Casserole	272	4
Ice Cream-Eggnog	243	3
Ice Cream-Honey Vanilla	203	2
Italian Cream Cake	396	Full
Kefir Bread	428	Off GAPS
Key Lime Pie	302	4
Key Lime Pie Smoothie	206	2
Kimchi	382	Full
Kombucha	130	1
Kraut Juice	99	1
Lemon Drops	227	3
Lemon Extract	226	3
Lentil Pancakes	362	Full
Liver Pâté	92	1

Endnotes

[i] Campbell-McBride, Natasha. *Gut And Psychology Syndrome.* Cambridge: Medinform Publishing, 2012. Print.

[ii] Cambell-McBride, Natasha. "Re: Book." Message to Becky Plotner 1 May 2020. -E-mail.

[iii] Ibid.

[iv] Ibid.

[v] Ibid.

[vi] Ibid.

[vii] Ibid.

[viii] Campbell-McBride, Natasha. Personal interview. 15 November 2018.

[ix] Campbell-McBride, Natasha. (November, 2018). *Q & A.* Weston A. Price Annual Conference. Baltimore, Maryland.

[x] Campbell-McBride, Natasha. (November, 2017). *GAPS Practitioners Q & A.* Weston A. Price Annual Conference. Minneapolis, Minnesota.

[xi] Campbell-McBride, Natasha. Personal interview. 7 March 2017.

[xii] Campbell-McBride, Natasha. (November, 2017). *GAPS Practitioners Q & A.* Weston A. Price Annual Conference. Minneapolis, Minnesota.

[xiii] Ibid.

[xiv] Ibid.

[xv] Campbell-McBride, Natasha. "Re: Book." Message to Becky Plotner 27 March 2018. E-mail.

[xvi] Campbell-McBride, Natasha. "Re: Book." Message to Becky Plotner 27 March 2018. E-mail.

[xvii] Campbell-McBride, Natasha. "Re: Questions" Message to Becky Plotner 8 February 2018. E-mail.

[xviii] Campbell-McBride, Natasha. (November, 2017). *GAPS Practitioners Q & A.* Weston A. Price Annual Conference. Minneapolis, Minnesota.

[xix] Ibid.

[xx] Campbell-McBride, Natasha. "Re: Questions" Message to Becky Plotner 8 February 2018. E-mail.

[xxi] Ibid.

[xxii] Campbell-McBride, Natasha. Personal interview. 15 November 2018.

[xxiii] Campbell-McBride, Natasha. (November, 2017). *GAPS Practitioners Q & A.* Weston A. Price Annual Conference. Minneapolis, Minnesota.

[xxiv] Campbell-McBride, Natasha. "Re: Book Questions." Message to Becky Plotner 4 September 2018. E-mail.

[xxv] Campbell-McBride, Natasha. (November 2017). *GAPS Practitioners Q & A.* Weston A. Price Annual Conference. Minneapolis, Minnesota.

[xxvi] Campbell-McBride, Natasha. *Gut And Psychology Syndrome.* Cambridge: Medinform Publishing, 2012. Print. P 131.

[xxvii] Campbell-McBride, Natasha. Personal interview. Weston A. Price Conference. 12 November 2015.

[xxviii] Campbell-McBride, Natasha. "Re: Thank you" Message to Becky Plotner 2 June 2016. E-mail.

xxix Brownstein, David. *Iodine, Why You Need It, Why You Can't Live Without It*. Michigan: Medical Alternatives Press, 2008. Print.

xxx Farrow, Lynne. *The Iodine Crisis, What You Don't Know About Iodine Can Wreck Your Life*. USA: Devon Press, 2013. Print.

xxxi Campbell-McBride, Natasha. *Gut and Psychology Syndrome*. Cambridge: Medinform Publishing, 2012.

xxxii Campbell-McBride, Natasha. "Re: Thank you" Message to Becky Plotner 2 June 2016. E-mail.

xxxiii Ibid.

xxxiv Brownstein, David. *Iodine, Why You Need It, Why You Can't Live Without It*. Michigan: Medical Alternatives Press, 2008. Print.

xxxv Farrow, Lynne. The Iodine Crisis, What You Don't Know About Iodine Can Wreck Your Life. USA: Devon Press, 2013. Print.

xxxvi Brownstein, David. *Iodine, Why You Need It, Why You Can't Live Without It*. Michigan: Medical Alternatives Press, 2008. Print.

xxxvii Ibid.

xxxviii Farrow, Lynne. The Iodine Crisis, What You Don't Know About Iodine Can Wreck Your Life. USA: Devon Press, 2013. Print.

xxxix Brownstein, David. *Iodine, Why You Need It, Why You Can't Live Without It*. Michigan: Medical Alternatives Press, 2008. Print.

xl Ibid.

xli Campbell-McBride, Natasha. "Re: Book Questions, Case Study." Message to Becky Plotner 4 July 2018. E-mail.

xlii Arnold, Justin and Brent Morgan. Management of Lead Encephalopathy with DMSA After Exposure to Lead-Contaminated Moonshine. *Journal of Medical Toxicology*. August 6, 2015. Web. September 2018.

xliii Ibid.

xliv Baby teeth link autism and heavy metals, NIH study suggests. June 1, 2107. Web. September 2018.

xlv Campbell-McBride, Natasha. (November, 2015). *GAPS Practitioners Meeting*. Weston A. Price Annual Conference. Anaheim, California.

xlvi Ibid.

xlvii Campbell-McBride, Natasha. "GAPS FAQS". GAPS.me. Gut and Psychology Syndrome. March 2017. Web. March 2017.

xlviii Campbell-McBride, Natasha. Personal interview. 15 November 2018.

xlix Sears, Margaret. Chelation: Harnessing and Enhancing Heavy Metal Detoxification – A Review. 18 April 2013. Web. September 2018.

l Campbell-McBride, Natasha. Personal interview. 15 November 2018.

li Selenium. National Institute of Health. Web. September 2018.

lii About Dental Amalgam Fillings. U.S. Food and Drug Administration. Web. September 2018.

liii Ibid.

liv Chelation: Therapy or "Therapy". *Poison*. March 2011. Web. September 2018.

lv Ibid.

lvi Campbell-McBride, Natasha. "Re: from DR Natasha." Message to Becky Plotner 25 January 2019. E-mail.

lvii Campbell-McBride, Natasha. "Re: Clarifying." Message to Becky Plotner 23 September 2018. E-mail.

[lviii] Campbell-McBride, Natasha. "GAPS FAQS". GAPS.me. Gut and Psychology Syndrome. March 2017. Web. March 2017.

[lix] Ibid.

[lx] Ibid.

[lxi] Campbell-McBride, Natasha. (November, 2017). *GAPS Practitioners Q & A*. Weston A. Price Annual Conference. Minneapolis, Minnesota.

[lxii] Campbell-McBride, Natasha. *Gut And Psychology Syndrome*. Cambridge: Medinform Publishing, 2012. Print. P 96.

[lxiii] Ibid. P. 122.

[lxiv] Campbell-McBride, Natasha. "GAPS FAQS". GAPS.me. Gut And Psychology Syndrome. March 2017. Web. April 2018.

[lxv] Campbell-McBride, Natasha. "GAPS FAQS". GAPS.me. Gut And Psychology Syndrome. March 2017. Web. March 2017.

[lxvi] Ibid.

[lxvii] Ibid.

[lxviii] Ibid.

[lxix] Ibid.

[lxx] Campbell-McBride, Natasha. (November, 2017). *GAPS Practitioners Q & A*. Weston A. Price Annual Conference. Minneapolis, Minnesota.

[lxxi] Campbell-McBride, Natasha. "Re: Book Questions, Case Study." Message to Becky Plotner 4 July 2018. E-mail.

[lxxii] Ibid.

[lxxiii] Ibid.

[lxxiv] Ibid.

[lxxv] Campbell-McBride, Natasha. "Re: Book Questions, Case Study." Message to Becky Plotner 4 July 2018. E-mail.

[lxxvi] Campbell-McBride, Natasha. (November 2017). *GAPS Practitioners Q & A*. Weston A. Price Annual Conference. Minneapolis, Minnesota.

[lxxvii] Campbell-McBride, Natasha. Personal interview. 15 November 2018.

[lxxviii] Ibid.

[lxxix] Campbell-McBride, Natasha. Gut and Physiology Syndrome. Cambridge: Medinform Publishing, 2012. Print.

[lxxx] Campbell-McBride, Natasha. (November 2017). *GAPS Practitioners Q & A*. Weston A. Price Annual Conference. Minneapolis, Minnesota.

[lxxxi] Ibid.

[lxxxii] Campbell-McBride, Natasha. "Re: Book Questions." Message to Becky Plotner 4 September 2018. E-mail.

[lxxxiii] Campbell-McBride, Natasha. "Re: Questions" Message to Becky Plotner 8 February 2018. E-mail.

[lxxxiv] Campbell-McBride, Natasha. (November, 2017). *GAPS Practitioners Q & A*. Weston A. Price Annual Conference. Minneapolis, Minnesota.

[lxxxv] Ibid.

[lxxxvi] Brownstein, David. *Salt Your Way To Health*. Michigan: Medical Alternatives Press, 2006. Print.

[lxxxvii] Campbell-McBride, Natasha. (November, 2017). *GAPS Practitioners Q & A*. Weston A. Price Annual Conference. Minneapolis, Minnesota.

[lxxxviii] Ibid.

[lxxxix] Ibid.

[xc] Brownstein, David. *Salt Your Way To Health*. Michigan: Medical Alternatives Press, 2006. Print.

[xci] Campbell-McBride, Natasha. (November, 2015). *GAPS*. Certified GAPS Practitioner Meeting. Anaheim, California.

[xcii] Ibid.

[xciii] Campbell-McBride, Natasha. (November, 2017). *GAPS Practitioners Q & A*. Weston A. Price Annual Conference. Minneapolis, Minnesota.

[xciv] Campbell-McBride, Natasha. "Re: Moldy Ferments." Message to Becky Plotner 12 June 2018. E-mail.

[xcv] Campbell-McBride, Natasha. (November, 2015). *GAPS*. Weston A. Price Annual Conference. Anaheim, California.

[xcvi] Campbell-McBride, Natasha. *Gut And Psychology Syndrome*. Cambridge: Medinform Publishing, 2012. Print. P 179.

[xcvii] Campbell-McBride, Natasha. "Re: Book." Message to Becky Plotner 10 May 2018. E-mail.

[xcviii] Campbell-McBride, Natasha. (November, 2017). *GAPS Practitioners Q & A*. Weston A. Price Annual Conference. Minneapolis, Minnesota.

[xcix] Campbell-McBride, Natasha. *Gut And Psychology Syndrome*. Cambridge: Medinform Publishing, 2012. Print. P 145.

[c] Ibid.

[ci] Ibid.

[cii] Ibid. P 259.

[ciii] Ibid. P 178.

[civ] Campbell-McBride, Natasha. (November, 2017). *GAPS Practitioners Q & A*. Weston A. Price Annual Conference. Minneapolis, Minnesota.

[cv] Ibid.

[cvi] Ibid.

[cvii] Campbell-McBride, Natasha. *Gut And Psychology Syndrome*. Cambridge: Medinform Publishing, 2012. Print.

[cviii] Campbell-McBride, Natasha. (November, 2017). *GAPS Practitioners Q & A*. Weston A. Price Annual Conference. Minneapolis, Minnesota.

[cix] Ibid.

[cx] Ibid.

[cxi] Tapp, D. 2014, Grow Your Own Food Summit. July 4, 2014.

[cxii] Ibid.

[cxiii] Ibid.

[cxiv] Ibid.

[cxv] Ibid.

[cxvi] Ibid

[cxvii] Troxal, Tom. Grass-Fed Standards For Ruminants. AUEX. University Of Arkansas System, Division Of Agriculture Research And Extension. March 2017. Web. March 2017.

[cxviii] Grass-Fed Marketing Claim Standards. USDA. March 2017. Web. March 2017. http://www.ams.usda.gov/AMSv1.0/ams .fetchTemplateData.do?template=TemplateN &navID =GrassFedMarketingClaimStandards&rightNav1 =GrassFedMarketingClaimStandards&topNav =≤ftNav=GradingCertificationandVerification&page =GrassFedMarketingClaims&resultType=&acct=lss.

[cxix] Smith, Stephen. Grass-Fed Vs. Grain-Fed Ground Beef – No Difference In Healthfulness. *Beef Magazine*. March 2014. Web. March 2017.

[cxx] Does Chipotle Mexican Grill Have A Beef With Texas? AOL. Finance. June 2014. Web. March 2017.

[cxxi] Ells, Steve. Conventional Vs. Grass-Fed Beef. *HuffPost*. May 2014. Web. March 2017.

[cxxii] Ibid.

[cxxiii] Our Standards. American Grassfed. June 2014. Web. March 2017.

[cxxiv] Campbell-McBride, Natasha. (November, 2015). *GAPS.* Weston A. Price Annual Conference. Anaheim, California.

[cxxv] Ibid.

[cxxvi] Ibid.

[cxxvii] Ibid.

[cxxviii] Ibid.

[cxxix] Ibid.

[cxxx] Ibid.

[cxxxi] Ibid.

[cxxxii] Hallen-Adams, Heather and Mallory J. Suhr. Fungi in the healthy human gastrointestinal tract. *Virulence.* October 2017. Web. June 2018.

[cxxxiii] Plotner, Becky. Gut Damage Creates Drug Addict Behavior. *Nourishing Plot.* October 2013. Web. June 2018.

[cxxxiv] Kumamoto, Carol A., Inflammation and gastrointestinal *Candida* colonization. *Current Opinion in Microbiology.* August 2011. Web. June 2018.

[cxxxv] Harnett, Joanna, et al., Significantly higher fecal counts of the yeasts *candida* and *saccharomyces* identified in people with coeliac disease. *Gut Pathogens.* May 2017. Web. June 2018.

[cxxxvi] Siri-Tarino, Patty W., et al., Meta-analysis of prospective cohort studies evaluating the association of saturated fat with cardiovascular disease. *The American Journal of Clinical Nutrition.* March 2010. Web. June 2018.

[cxxxvii] Campbell-McBride, Natasha. "GAPS FAQS". GAPS.me. Gut And Psychology Syndrome. March 2017. Web. March 2017.

[cxxxviii] Ibid.

[cxxxix] Campbell-McBride, Natasha. "Re: Book." Message to Becky Plotner 10 May 2018. E-mail.

[cxl] *Oleomargarine Heir,* 2017. Web. October 2017. http://www.oleoheir.com/the-oleo-fortune/41-pink-margarine.

[cxli] Ibid.

[cxlii] Graefer, Deborah. How Did I Get Gallbladder Problems? Gallbladder Attack. September 2016. Web. September 2016

[cxliii] Newport, Mary. *Alzheimer's Disease, What If There Was A Cure? The Story Of Ketones.* Read HowYouWant, 2013. Print.

[cxliv] Alzheimer's Doctors Taking Note Of Coconut Oil. Health Science. *CBN News.* January 2013. Web. March 2014.

cxlv Paoli, A., et al. Beyond weight loss: a review of the therapeutic uses of very-low-carbohydrate (ketogenic) diets. European Journal of Clinical Nutrition. August 2013. Web. March 2014.

[cxlvi] Campbell-McBride, Natasha. *Gut And Psychology Syndrome.* Cambridge: Medinform Publishing, 2012. Print. P 122.

[cxlvii] Campbell-McBride, Natasha. "Re: Book" Message to Becky Plotner 6 March 2018. E-mail.

[cxlviii] Ibid.

[cxlix] Ibid.

[cl] Campbell-McBride, Natasha. "Re: Book" Message to Becky Plotner 7 March 2018. E-mail.

[cli] Campbell-McBride, Natasha. "Re: Book" Message to Becky Plotner 6 March 2018. E-mail.

[clii] Campbell-McBride, Natasha. *Gut And Psychology Syndrome.* Cambridge: Medinform Publishing, 2012. Print.

cliii Campbell-McBride, Natasha. (November, 2017). GAPS Practitioners Q & A. Weston A. Price Annual Conference. Minneapolis, Minnesota.

[cliv] Campbell-McBride, Natasha. "Re: Questions" Message to Becky Plotner 8 February 2018. E-mail.

[clv] Campbell-McBride, Natasha. "GAPS FAQS". GAPS.me. Gut And Psychology Syndrome. March 2017. Web. March 2017.

[clvi] Abenavoli, L, et al. Milk thistle in liver diseases: past, present, future *Phytotherapy Research.* October 24, 2010. Web. February, 2018.

[clvii] Marnewick, JL, et al. Modulation of hepatic drug metabolizing enzymes and oxidative status by rooibos (Aspalathus linearis) and Honeybush (Cyclopia intermedia), green and black (Camellia sinensis) teas in rats. *Journal of Agriculture and Food Chemistry.* December 31, 2003. Web. July 2017.

[clviii] Boim, MA, et al. Phyllanthus niruri as a promising alternative treatment for nephrolithiasis. *International Brazilian Journal of Urology.* November- December 2010. Web. January 2018.

[clix] Natural remedies for vaginal infections. *Sidahora.* Winter 1995. Web. July 2017.

[clx] Boss, Anna, et al. Evidence to Support the Anti-Cancer Effect of Olive Leaf Extract and Future Directions. *Nutrients.* August 8, 2016. Web. February 2018.

[clxi] Rahnama, Marjan, et al. The healing effect of licorice (Glycyrrhiza glabra) on Helicobacter pylori infected peptic ulcers. *Journal of Research in Medical Sciences.* June 18, 2013. Web. February 2018.

[clxii] Wimgo, Fonyuy E., et al. The Physiological Effects of Dandelion (Taraxacum Officinale) in Type 2 Diabetes. *The Review of Diabetic Studies.* August 10, 2016. Web. February 2018.

[clxiii] Viapiana, Agnieszka and Marek Wesolowki. The Phenolic Contents and Antioxidant Activities of Infusions of Sambucus nigra L. *Plant Foods For Human Nutrition.* January 13, 2017. Web. February 2018.

[clxiv] McKay, DL and JB Blumberg. A review of bioactivity and potential health benefits of peppermint tea (Mentha peperita L.). *Phytotherapy Research.* August 20, 2006. Web. February 2018.

[clxv] Khan, SS., et al. Chamomile tea: herbal hypoglycemic alternative for conventional medicine. *Pakistan Journal of Pharmaceuitical Science.* September 27, 2104. Web. February 2018.

[clxvi] Oprica, Lacramioara, et al. Ascorbic Acid Content of Rose Hip Fruit Depending on Altitude. *Iranian Journal of Public Health.* January 2015. Web. February 2018.

[clxvii] Durzan, Don J. Arginine, scurvy and Carier's "tree of life". *Journal of Ethnobiology and Ethnomedicine.* February 2, 2009. Web. February 2018.

[clxviii] Ghayur, Muhammad Nabeel and Anwarul Hassan Gilani, Species differences in the prokinetic effects of ginger, *International Journal of Food Sciences and Nutrition.* July 6, 2009. Web. August 2009.

[clxix] Hu, Ming-Luen, et. al. Effect of ginger of gastric motility and symptoms of functional dyspepsia. *World Journal of Gastroenterology.* January 7, 2011. Web. February 2011.

[clxx] Ibid.

clxxi Bhatia, Shobna Bhatia and Anumeet Singh Grover. Natural History of Functional Dyspepsia. *Journal of Association of Physicians of India.* March 2012. Web. May 2012.

clxxii Campbell-McBride, Natasha. *Gut And Psychology Syndrome.* Cambridge: Medinform Publishing, 2012. Print.

clxxiii Bhatia, Shobna Bhatia and Anumeet Singh Grover. Natural History of Functional Dyspepsia. *Journal of Association of Physicians of India.* March 2012. Web. May 2012.

clxxiv Klewicka, Elzbieta, et al. Effects of Lactofermented Beetroot Juice Alone or with N-nitroso-N-methylurea on Selected Metabolic Parameters, Composition of the Microbiota Adhering to the Gut Epithelium and Antioxidant Status of Rats. *Nutrients.* July 7, 2015. Web. February 2018.

clxxv Ibid.

clxxvi [Townsends]. (2015, August 31). Making Fresh Sauerkraut [Video File]. Retrieved from https://www.youtube.com/watch?v=ITpr3e_Ld3U.

clxxvii Katz, Sandor Ellix. The Art Of Fermentation. Vermont: Chelsea Green Publishing, 2012. Print. Pp 103-4.

clxxviii Ibid.

clxxix Ibid.

clxxx Ibid.

clxxxi Campbell-McBride, Natasha. (November, 2017). *GAPS Practitioners Q & A.* Weston A. Price Annual Conference. Minneapolis, Minnesota.

clxxxii Ibid.

clxxxiii Ibid.

clxxxiv Ibid.

clxxxv Ibid.

clxxxvi Ibid.

clxxxvii Ibid.

clxxxviii Ibid.

clxxxix Ibid.

cxc Ibid.

cxci Ibid.

cxcii Ibid

cxciii Ibid.

cxciv Ibid.

cxcv Ibid.

cxcvi Ibid.

cxcvii Ibid.

cxcviii Ibid.

cxcix Campbell-McBride, Natasha. "Re: Book." Message to Becky Plotner 27 March 2018. E-mail.

cc Campbell-McBride, Natasha. "Re: WAPF Conference" Message to Becky Plotner 18 November 2016. E-mail.

cci [Mercola]. (2011, September 8). Dr. Mercola Interviews Dr. Stephanie Seneff [Video File]. Retrieved from https://www.youtube.com/watch?v=5QUChSlUEH0.

ccii Ibid.

cciii Ibid.

cciv Campbell-McBride, Natasha. (November, 2017). *GAPS Practitioners Q & A.* Weston A. Price Annual Conference. Minneapolis, Minnesota.

ccv Nguyen, Nguyen Khoi, et al. Lactic acid bacteria: promising supplements for enhancing the biological activities of kombucha. *Springer Plus*. February 24, 2015. Web. July 217.

ccvi Ibid.

ccvii Walaszek, Z. Potential use of D-glucaric acid derivatives in cancer prevention. Cancer Letters. October 8, 1990. Web. July 2017.

ccviii Barati, Fardin, et al. Histopathological and clinical evaluation of Kombucha tea and Nitrofurazone on cutaneous full-thickness wounds in rats: and experimental study. *Diagnostic Pathology*. July 17, 2013. Web. July 2015.

ccix Ibid.

ccx Ibid.

ccxi Velićanski Aleksandra S., et al. Antimicrobial and antioxidant activity of lemon balm Kombucha. *Acta Periodica Technologica*. 2007. Web. July 2017.

ccxii Nhuyen Khoi Nhuyen, et al. Lactic acid bacteria: promising supplements for enhancing the biological activities of kombucha. *Springer Plus*. February 24, 2015. Web. July 2016.

ccxiii Niacin. *Medline Plus*. Web. July 2016.

ccxiv Bauer, Brent A. What is kombucha tea? Does it have any health benefits? Mayo Clinic. Web. July 2017.

ccxv Ibid.

ccxvi Thomson, Stuart. 'Kombucha' Green Tea Symbiont: A Scientific Health Literature Review. Gaia Research Institute. Web. July 2017.

ccxvii Campbell-McBride, Natasha. (November, 2017). *GAPS Practitioners Q & A*. Weston A. Price Annual Conference. Minneapolis, Minnesota.

ccxviii Crum, Hannah. Top 10 Questions About Sugar And Kombucha. *Kombucha Kamp*. Web. February 2018.

ccxix Ibid.

ccxx Campbell-McBride, Natasha. (November, 2017). *GAPS Practitioners Q & A*. Weston A. Price Annual Conference. Minneapolis, Minnesota.

ccxxi Campbell-McBride, Natasha. "GAPS FAQS". GAPS.me. Gut And Psychology Syndrome. March 2017. Web. March 2017.

ccxxii Wells, S.D. The flu shot is the most defective vaccine ever made – here's proof. *Natural News* January 2017. Web. January 2017.

ccxxiii Vincent J. Christiancy v. Secretary of Health and Human Services, No. 14-1285v (May 2, 2016)

ccxxiv Shilhavy, Brian. Vaccine Court Stats on Injuries and Deaths Betray Government's Position on Vaccine Safety. *Vaccine Impact*. December, 9 2017. Web. December 2017.

ccxxv Ibid.

ccxxvi De Serres, Gaston, et al. Influenza Vaccination of Healthcare Workers: Critical Analysis of the Evidence for Patient Benefit Underpinning Policies of Enforcement. *PLOS One*. January 27, 2017. Web. February 2017.

ccxxvii Yoon, KY, et al. Production of Probiotic Cabbage Juice by Lactic Acid Bacteria. *Bioresource Technology*. August 2006. Web. December 2006.

ccxxviii Swain, Manas Ranjan, et al. Fermented Fruits and Vegetables of Asia: A Potential Source of Probiotics. *Biotechnology Research International*. May 28, 2014. Web. December 20165

ccxxix Girraffa, G., et al. Importance of Lactobacilli in Food and Feed Biotechnology. *Research In Microbiology*. July-August 2010. Web. December 2011.

[ccxxx] Mitropoulou, Georgia, et al. Immobilization Technologies in Probiotic Food Production. *Journal of Nutrition and Metabolism.* October 2013. Web. December 2015.

[ccxxxi] Planas, Gladys Mazzei and Joseph Kuc. Contraceptive Properties of Stevia rebaudiana. *Science vol 162, Issue 3857.* November 29, 1968. Web. December 2015. pp.1007.

[ccxxxii] Ibid.

[ccxxxiii] Ibid.

[ccxxxiv] Carey, Elea. Truvia vs. Stevia: What's the Difference? *Healthline.* February 2015. Web. December 2015.

[ccxxxv] Sunwin International Neutraceuticals Has Received Purchase Orders of Stevia in Excess of $2 million. *Business Wire.* March 2005. Web. December 2015.

[ccxxxvi] Wisdom of the Ancients. Stevia: Sweetener of Choice for Future Generations. *Total Health Secrets.* Web. December 2015.

[ccxxxvii] All About Stevia. *Healthy Shopping Network.* Web. December 2015.

[ccxxxviii] Chan, Paul, et al. A double-blind placebo-controlled study of the effectiveness and tolerability of oral stevioside in human hypertension. *British Journal of Clinical Pharmacology.* September 2000. Web. December 2015.

[ccxxxix] Gasmalla, Mohammed Abdalbasit A., et al. Nutritional Composition of *Stevia rebaudiana* Bertoni Leaf: Effect of Drying Method. *Tropical Journal of Pharmaceutical Research.* 13(1):61-65. January 2014. Web. December 2015.

[ccxl] Stevia Herbal Properties and Actions. *Raintree.* Web. December 2015. http://www.rain-tree.com/stevia.htm#.WixBlUpKtPY

[ccxli] Yasukawa, Ken, et al. Inhibitory Effect of Stevioside on Tumor Promotion by 12-*o*-Tetraderanoylphorbol-13-Acetate in Two-Stage Carcinogenesis in Mouse Skin. *Pharmaceutical Society of Japan* 25(11) 1488-1490. July 23, 2002. Web. December 2015.

[ccxlii] Gould Soloway, Rose Ann. Using Skin Patch Medicines Safely. Poison Control. Web. December 2015.

[ccxliii] Dr. Michael Hansen. 2017. *Food Revolution Summit.* May 7, 2017.

[ccxliv] Vaesa, Janelle. Genetically Modified Organisms: Pros and Cons of GMO Food. *Decoded Science.* January 2013. Web. December 2015.

[ccxlv] Dr. Michael Hansen. 2017. *Food Revolution Summit.* May 7, 2017.

[ccxlvi] Ibid.

[ccxlvii] Ibid.

[ccxlviii] Ibid.

[ccxlix] Technical Consultation On Low Levels of Genetically Modified (GM) Crops in International Food and Feed Trade. FAO, Food and Agricultural Organization of the United Nations. March 2014. Web. December 2015.

[ccl] Dr. Michael Hansen. 2017. *Food Revolution Summit.* May 7, 2017.

[ccli] Ibid.

[cclii] Ibid.

[ccliii] Ibid.

[ccliv] Ibid.

[cclv] Ibid.

[cclvi] Ibid.

[cclvii] Ibid.

[cclviii] Resnik, David. Retracting Inconclusive Research: Lessons from the Séralini GM Maize Feeding Study. *Journal of Agricultural and Environmental Ethics.* August 2015. Web. December 2015.

cclix GMO Study Retracted – Censorship or Caution. *PRI, Public Radio International.* December 2013. Web. December 2104.

cclx Ibid.

cclxi Ibid.

cclxii Ibid.

cclxiii Lynn R. Goldman, M.D., M.S., M.P.H., Dean. Public Health Online, Milken Institute School of Public Health. Web. December 2017.

cclxiv Dr. Michael Hansen. 2017. *Food Revolution Summit.* May 7, 2017.

cclxv Graham, Karen. Alarming New Study by USDA Proves it was Wrong About Monsanto's GMO Alfalfa. *Food Democracy Now.* January 24, 2016. Web. February 2016.

cclxvi Hilbeck, Angelicka, et al. No scientific consensus on GMO safety. *Environmental Sciences Europe.* January 2015. Web. January 2015.

cclxvii Dark History of the Evil Monsanto Corporation. BestMeal.Info. Web. December 2017.

cclxviii Ibid.

cclxix Nickel, Rod. Canadian Wheat Board cautious about GM wheat. *Reuters.* May, 15, 2009. Web. December 2010.

cclxx Smith, Jeffrey. *Genetic Roulette: The Documented Health Risks of Genetically Engineered Foods.* Iowa: Yes! Books, 2007.

cclxxi Ibid.

cclxxii Ibid.

cclxxiii Smith, Jeffrey. Autism. Institute For Responsible Technology. Web. December 2015.

cclxxiv 'Roundup' Glyphosate Hormone Inhibitor Monsanto's toxic herbicide in Our Food Chain at "Extreme Levels". *Scoop, EcoWatch.* September 2015. Web. December 2015.

cclxxv Smith, Jeffrey. Autism, *The Institute for Responsible Technology,* Web. April, 2016.

cclxxvi Ibid.

cclxxvii Ibid.

cclxxviii Khan, AQ, et al. Keratin 8 expression in colon cancer associates with low fecal butyrate levels. *BMC Gastroenterology.* January 10, 2011. Web. March 2013.

cclxxix Smith, Jeffrey. *Genetic Roulette: The Documented Health Risks of Genetically Engineered Foods.* Iowa: Yes! Books, 2007.

cclxxx Ibid.

cclxxxi Plotner, Becky. Is Ice Making You Sick? Nourishing Plot. April 9, 2014. Web. April 2014.

cclxxxii Parker, Allen. Effective Cleaning and Sanitizing Procedures. JIFSAN Good Aquacultural Practices Program. 2007. Web. March 2013.

cclxxxiii Plotner, Becky. Is Ice Making You Sick? Nourishing Plot. April 9, 2014. Web. April 2014.

cclxxxiv Isomatic Technical Manual, B, EC and ECP Series. Mile High Equipment Company. August 2001. Web. November 2015.

cclxxxv Plotner, Becky. Is Ice Making You Sick? Nourishing Plot. April 9, 2014. Web. April 2014.

cclxxxvi Slime In The Ice Machine: How To Prevent Ice Contamination. Houston Department of Health and Human Services. 2005. Web. 2015.

cclxxxvii Ibid.

cclxxxviii Popken, Ben. Slime Slops Into Sodas, Manager Too Busy To Clean Ice Machines. *Consumerist.* November 5, 2010. Web. December 2010.

cclxxxix Idaho knew about mold in yogurt at Chobani factory before recall: FDA. *NY Daily News.* December 6, 2013. Web. December 2015.

[ccxc] Title 21 – Food and Drugs Chapter I – Food and Drug Administration. Department of Health and Human Services Subchapter E – Animal Drugs, Feeds, and Related Products. Part 589 – Substances Prohibited From Use In Animal Food or Feed. Subpart B – Listing of Specific Substances Prohibited From Use In Animal Food or Feed. US Food and Drug Administration. April 2017. Web. December 2017.

[ccxci] Formaldehyde In Food. Center For Food Safety, The Government Of The Hong Kong Special Administration Region. January 2006. Web. December 2017.

[ccxcii] Monte, C. Woodrow. *While Science Sleeps*. San Francisco: Amazon Create Space Publishing. 2011.

[ccxciii] Huff, James. Benzene-induced Cancers: Abridged History and Occupational Health Impact. International Journal of Occupational and Environmental Health. Volume 13. Issue 2. 2007.

[ccxciv] Benvenuti, Nicki Zevola. Do Vitamin C and Sodium Benzoate Together Form a Carcinogen? *FutureDerm*. September 2, 2012. Web. December 2013.

[ccxcv] Questions and Answers on the Occurrence of Benzene in Soft Drinks and Other Beverages. US Food and Drug Association. FDA. Web. December 2017.

[ccxcvi] McCann, Donna, et al. Food additives and hyperactive behavior in 3-year-old and 8/9-year-old children in the community: a randomized, double-blinded, placebo-controlled trial. *The Lancet*. November 2007. Web. December 2011.

[ccxcvii] Phillips, III, John A. et al. USPTO Patent Full-Text and Image Database. US Patent Number 6,362,226. December 2000. Web. December 2000.

[ccxcviii] Noyes, Dan. 'Meat glue' poses health risks for consumers. Eyewitness News ABC 7. April 30, 2012. Web. November 2012.

[ccxcix] Wolinsky, Howard and Kristofor Husted. Science for Food, Molecular biology contributes to the production and preparation of food. *EMBO Reports*. March 2015. Web. December 2015.

[ccc] Transglutaminase. C&P Additives. Web. July 2013.

[ccci] Norén, Nils. Transglutaminase, aka Meat Glue. Cooking Ideas. Web. December 2016.

[cccii] Ibid.

[ccciii] Ibid.

[ccciv] Transglutaminase. C&P Additives. Web. July 2013.

[cccv] Noyes, Dan. 'Meat glue' poses health risks for consumers. Eyewitness News ABC 7. April 30, 2012. Web. November 2012.

[cccvi] The Facts About Ammonia. New York State Department of Health. July 28, 2004. Web. July 2004.

[cccvii] Kamozawa, Aki and H. Alexander Talbot. *Ideas in Food: Great Recipes and Why They Work*. New York: Clarkson Potter/Publishers. 2010.

[cccviii] Anderson, Jane. "Meat Glue": A Threat Or Not? *Very Well*. April 30, 2016. Web. April 2016.

[cccix] Dermatitis herpetiformis. Medline Plus. Web. April 2016.

[cccx] A, Tursi, et al. Prevalence of antitissue transglutaminase antibodies in different degrees of intestinal damage in celiac disease. *Journal of Clinical Gastroenterology*. March 2003. Web. December 2016.

[cccxi] Anti-tissue Transglutaminase Antibody. University of Rochester Medical Center. 2017. Web. December 2016.

[cccxii] A, Tursi, et al. Prevalence of antitissue transglutaminase antibodies in different degrees of intestinal damage in celiac disease. *Journal of Clinical Gastroenterology*. March 2003. Web. December 2016.

[cccxiii] Ibid.

cccxiv Cortez, Joao, et al. Transglutaminase treatment of wool fabrics leads to resistance to detergent damage. *Journal of Biotechnology.* April 2005. Web. December 2016. pp 379-386.

cccxv Campbell-McBride, Natasha. "Re: Clarifying." Message to Becky Plotner 23 September 2018. E-mail.

cccxvi Ibid.

cccxvii Campbell-McBride, Natasha. (November, 2017). *GAPS Practitioners Q & A.* Weston A. Price Annual Conference. Minneapolis, Minnesota.

cccxviii Campbell-McBride, Natasha. "Re: Book." Message to Becky Plotner 6 March 2018. E-mail.

cccxix Campbell-McBride, Natasha. (November, 2017). *GAPS Practitioners Q & A.* Weston A. Price Annual Conference. Minneapolis, Minnesota.

cccxx Campbell-McBride, Natasha. "Re: Ginger." Message to Becky Plotner 24 January 2019. E-mail.

cccxxi Campbell-McBride, Natasha. "Re: Book." Message to Becky Plotner 27 March 2018. E-mail.

cccxxii Campbell-McBride, Natasha. "Re: Thank you for meeting with us!" Message to Becky Plotner 19 November 2017. E-mail.

cccxxiii Cortez, Joao, et al. Transglutaminase treatment of wool fabrics leads to resistance to detergent damage. *Journal of Biotechnology.* April 2005. Web. December 2016. pp 379-386.

cccxxiv Campbell-McBride, Natasha. "GAPS FAQS". GAPS.me. Gut And Psychology Syndrome. March 2017. Web. March 2017.

cccxxv Ibid.

cccxxvi Campbell-McBride, Natasha. (November, 2017). *GAPS Practitioners Q & A.* Weston A. Price Annual Conference. Minneapolis, Minnesota.

cccxxvii Ibid.

cccxxviii Morehead, Kenneth. (Speaker). (2917, January 27). *Energy, Health and Vitality* [Audio podcast]. Retrieved from https://www.westonaprice.org/podcast/60-energy-health-vitality/.

cccxxix [Silicon Valley Health Institute]. (June 6, 2015). The Human Detoxification System – Christopher Shade (May 2015) [Video File]. Retrieved from https://www.youtube.com/watch?v=gITuONNWWK8

cccxxx Ibid.

cccxxxi Ibid.

cccxxxii Ibid.

cccxxxiii Ibid.

cccxxxiv Ibid.

cccxxxv Ibid.

cccxxxvi Lererdi, Enzo, et al. Intestinal microbial metabolism of phosphatidylcholine: a novel insight in the cardiovascular risk scenario. *Hepatobiliary Surgery and Nutrition.* August 4, 2015. Web. December 2016. p 289-292.

cccxxxvii Ibid.

cccxxxviii Campbell-McBride, Natasha. Gut And Psychology Syndrome. Cambridge: Medinform Publishing, 2012. Print. P 279.

cccxxxix C. Plotner, personal communication, November – March 2015.

cccxl Ibid.

cccxli Ibid.

cccxlii Ibid.

[cccxliii] Liu, Y.Q., et al. B-Cryptoxanthin biofortified maize (*Zea mays*) increases B-cryptoxanthin concentration and enhances the color of chicken egg yolk. *Poultry Science.* February 2012. Web. March 2015. pp 432-438.

[cccxliv] Ibid.

[cccxlv] Ibid.

[cccxlvi] Ibid.

[cccxlvii] Ibid.

[cccxlviii] Barbosa, Vanessa Camarinha, et al. Stability of the pigmentation of egg yolks enriched with omega-3 and carophyll stored at room temperature and under refrigeration. *Revista Brasileira de Zootecnia, Brazilian Journal of Animal Science.* July 2011. Web. March 2015.

[cccxlix] Hammershoj, M, et al. Deposition of carotenoids in egg yolk by short-term supplement of colored carrot (Daucus carota) varieties as forage material for egg-laying hens. *Journal of the Science of Food and Agriculture.* May 2010. Web. March 2015.

[cccl] Altuntas, A and R. Aydin. Fatty Acid Composition of Egg Yolk from Chickens Fed a Diet including Marigold (Tagetes erecta L.). *Journal of Lipids.* 2014. Web. December 2014.

[cccli] Huaqiang, Li, et al. Effect of Red Pepper (*Capsicum frutescens*) Powder or Red Pepper Pigment on the Performance and Egg Yolk Color of Laying Hens. *Asian-Australasian Journal of Animal Sciences (AJAS).* 2012. Web. December 2012.

[ccclii] Leeson, S. and L. Caston. Enrichment of eggs with lutein. *Poultry Science.* October 2004. Web. December 2012.

[cccliii] Altuntas, A. and R. Aydin. Fatty Acid Composition of Egg Yolk from Chickens Fed a Diet including Marigold (Tagetes erecta L.). *Journal of Lipids.* December 22, 2014. Web. December 2015.

[cccliv] Campbell-McBride, Natasha. "GAPS FAQS". GAPS.me. Gut and Psychology Syndrome. March 2017. Web. March 2017.

[ccclv] Campbell-McBride, Natasha. Personal interview of Sally Fallon and Dr. Natasha Campbell-McBride. 15 November 2018.

[ccclvi] Campbell-McBride, Natasha. "GAPS FAQS". GAPS.me. Gut And Psychology Syndrome. March 2017. Web. March 2017.

[ccclvii] Campbell-McBride, Natasha. (November, 2017). *GAPS Practitioners Q & A.* Weston A. Price Annual Conference. Minneapolis, Minnesota.

[ccclviii] Pompa, Daniel. The Dangers of Glyphosate: An Interview with Dr. Stephanie Seneff. *Pompa.* January 5, 2016. Web. December 2015.

[ccclix] Ibid.

[ccclx] Cadegiani, Flavio and Claudio Kater. Adrenal fatigue does not exist: a systematic review. *BMC Endocrine Disorders.* August 24, 2016. Web. December 2016.

[ccclxi] Head, KA And GS Kelly. Nutrients and botanicals for treatment of stress: adrenal fatigue, neurotransmitter imbalance, anxiety, and restless sleep. *Alternative Medicine Review.* June 14, 2009. Web. December 2015.

[ccclxii] Allen, LV Jr. Adrenal Fatigue. *International Journal of Pharmaceutical Compounding.* January- February 2013. Web. December 2015.

[ccclxiii] Campbell-McBride, Natasha. *Gut And Psychology Syndrome.* Cambridge: Medinform Publishing, 2012. Print.

[ccclxiv] Campbell-McBride, Natasha. "GAPS FAQS". GAPS.me. Gut And Psychology Syndrome. March 2017. Web. March 2017.

ccclxv Plotner, B. (2016. March 21) Shift Work And Poor Light, Cancer And Sleepless Nights {blog post}. Retrieved from http://www.nourishingplot.com/2016/03/21/shift-work-and-poor-light-cancer-and-sleepless-nights/.

ccclxvi Chilton, Setphanie, et al. Inclusion of Fermented Foods in Food Guides Around the World. *Nutrients*. January 7, 2015. Web. June 2015.

ccclxvii Selhub, Eva, et al. Fermented Foods, Microbiota, and Mental Health: Ancient Practice Meets Nutritional Psychiatry. *Journal of Physiological Anthropology*. January 15, 2014. Web. June 2015.

ccclxviii Sornplang, Pairat and Sudthidol Piyadeatsoontorn. Probiotic Isolates from Unconventional Sources: A Review. *Journal of Animal Science and Technology*. July 19, 2016. Web. August 2016.

ccclxix Paludan-Muller, C, et al. Characterization of lactic acid bacteria isolated from a Thai low-salt fermented fish product and the role of garlic as substrate for fermentation. *International Journal of Food Microbiology*. February 18, 1999. Web. June 2015.

ccclxx Kim, Min-Jeong, et al. Selection and Characteristics of Fermented Salted Seafood (*jeotgal*)-Originated Strains with Excellent S-adenosyl-L-methionine (SAM) Production and Probiotics Efficacy. *Korean Journal For Food Sciences and Animal Resources*. February 28, 2014. Web. June 2015.

ccclxxi Campbell-McBride, Natasha. (November, 2017). *GAPS Practitioners Q & A*. Weston A. Price Annual Conference. Minneapolis, Minnesota.

ccclxxii Ibid.

ccclxxiii Ibid.

ccclxxiv Ibid.

ccclxxv Ibid.

ccclxxvi Ibid.

ccclxxvii Campbell-McBride, Natasha. "Re: Clarifying." Message to Becky Plotner 23 September 2018. E-mail.

ccclxxviii Campbell-McBride, Natasha. "Re: Book Questions, Case Study." Message to Becky Plotner 4 July 2018. E-mail.

ccclxxix Corrado, Monica. (November, 2017). *GAPS Practitioners Q & A*. Weston A. Price Annual Conference. Minneapolis, Minnesota.

ccclxxx Campbell-McBride, Natasha. "Re: Clarifying." Message to Becky Plotner 23 September 2018. E-mail.

ccclxxxi Campbell-McBride, Natasha. "Re: Book Questions, Case Study." Message to Becky Plotner 4 July 2018. E-mail.

ccclxxxii Campbell-McBride, Natasha. "Re: Book." Message to Becky Plotner 10 May 2018. E-mail.

ccclxxxiii Campbell-McBride, Natasha. "Re: Clarifying." Message to Becky Plotner 23 September 2018. E-mail.

ccclxxxiv Corrado, Monica. (November, 2017). *GAPS Practitioners Q & A*. Weston A. Price Annual Conference. Minneapolis, Minnesota.

ccclxxxv Campbell-McBride, Natasha. "GAPS FAQS". GAPS.me. Gut And Psychology Syndrome. March 2017. Web. March 2017.

ccclxxxvi Campbell-McBride, Natasha. (November, 2017). *GAPS Practitioners Q & A*. Weston A. Price Annual Conference. Minneapolis, Minnesota.

ccclxxxvii Ibid.

ccclxxxviii Campbell-McBride, Natasha. "Re: WAPF Conference" Message to Becky Plotner 18 November 2016. E-mail.

ccclxxxix Campbell-McBride, Natasha. (November, 2017). *GAPS Practitioners Q & A.* Weston A. Price Annual Conference. Minneapolis, Minnesota.

cccxc Ibid.

cccxci Ibid.

cccxcii Fulton, April. FDA Probes Link Between Food Dyes, Kids' Behavior. *NPR.* March 30, 2011. Web. April 2011.

cccxciii Aguilar, F., et al. Assessment of the results of the study by McCann et al. (2007) on the effect of some colours and sodium benzoate on children's behaviour [1] - Scientific Opinion of the Panel on Food Additives, Flavourings, Processing Aids and Food Contact Materials (AFC). *EFSA Journal.* March 2008. Web. October 2017.

cccxciv Campbell-McBride, Natasha. *Gut And Psychology Syndrome.* Cambridge: Medinform Publishing, 2012. Print. P 131.

cccxcv Campbell-McBride, Natasha. (November, 2015). *GAPS.* Weston A. Price Annual Conference. Anaheim, California.

cccxcvi [Mercola]. (2012, August 28). *Dr. Mercola Interviews Sandor Katz about Fermentation* [Video File]. Retrieved from https://www.youtube.com/watch?v=LkXT-XgyzkI.

cccxcvii Ibid.

cccxcviii Campbell-McBride, Natasha. (November, 2015). *GAPS.* Weston A. Price Annual Conference. Anaheim, California.

cccxcix Campbell-McBride, Natasha. 2013, *GAPS.* The Gluten Summit. November 13, 2013.

cd Sacks, Katherine. (2015, July). Why Does Garlic Turn Blue? *Epicurious.*https://www.epicurious.com/expert-advice/why-does-garlic-turn-blue-article.

cdi Jung, YM, et al. (2011, May). Fermented garlic protects diabetic, obese mice when fed a high-fat diet by antioxidant effects. *Nutrition Research, (5).* pp. 387-96.

cdii Sato, E. et al. (2006, December). Increased anti-oxidative potency of garlic by spontaneous short-term fermentation. *Plant Foods For Human Nutrition,* pp. 157-60.

cdiii Ibid.

cdiv Yan, L., et al. (2013, June). Effects of dietary supplementation of fermented garlic powder on growth performance, apparent total tract digestibility, blood characteristics and fecal microbial concentration in weanling pigs. *Journal of Animal Physiology and Animal Nutrition, (Volume 97, Issue 3).* pp. 457-464.

cdv De Castro, Antonio, et al. (1998, February). Lactic acid fermentation and storage of blanched garlic. *International Journal of Food Microbiology (vol 39, Issue 3).* pp. 205-211.

cdvi Sacks, Katherine. (2015, July). Why Does Garlic Turn Blue? *Epicurious.* https://www.epicurious.com/expert-advice/why-does-garlic-turn-blue-article.

cdvii Zang, Jiachen, et al. (2013, April). Mechanism of discoloration in processed garlic and onion. *Trends in Food Science And Technology.* pp. 162-173.

cdviii Ibid.

cdix Bai, B., et al. (2005, September). Mechanism of the greening color formation of "laba" garlic, a traditional homemade Chinese food Product. *Journal of Agricultural and Food Chemistry (53(18).* pp. 7103-7.

cdx Moore, Michelle. "Garlic – an ancient remedy with a modern twist". Staph Infections Resources. March 2017. Web. March 2017.

cdxi Cutler RR. and P. Wilson. (2004). Antibacterial activity of a new, stable, aqueous extract of allicin against methicillin-resistant Staphylococcus aureus. *British Journal of Biomedical Sciences (61(2)).* pp. 71-4.

cdxii Simopoulos, Artemis, P., Essential fatty acids in health and chronic disease. *The American Journal of clinical Nutrition* September 1999. Web. June 2018.

cdxiii McDaniel, Jodi C., et al., W-3 fatty acids effect on wound healing. *Wound Repair Regen* May-June 2008. Web. June 2018. https://www.ncbi.nlm.nih.gov/pmc/articles/PMC2967211/

cdxiv Ibid. https://www.ncbi.nlm.nih.gov/pmc/articles/PMC2967211/

cdxv Essential Fatty Acids and Skin Health. Micronutrient Information Center at Oregon State University. Web. July 2018. http://lpi.oregonstate.edu/mic/health-disease/skin-health/essential-fatty-acids

cdxvi Liu, yulan. Fatty acids, inflammation and intestinal health in pigs. *Journal of Animal Science and Biotechnology* September 2015. Web. July 2018. https://www.ncbi.nlm.nih.gov/pmc/articles/PMC4564983/

cdxvii Campbell-McBride, Natasha. "GAPS FAQS". GAPS.me. Gut And Psychology Syndrome. March 2017. Web. March 2017. http://www.gaps.me/faqs.php.

cdxviii Ibid.

cdxix [Mercola]. (2011, December 20). *Dr. Mercola Interviews Dr. Natasha Campbell-McBride* [Video File]. Retrieved from https://www.youtube.com/watch?v=bYJkS3ZBqos.

cdxx Ibid. https://www.youtube.com/watch?v=bYJkS3ZBqos.

cdxxi Campbell-McBride, Natasha. (November, 2015). *Gut and Psychology Syndrome* (Part 1) Weston A. Price Annual Conference. Anaheim, California. 10:40.

cdxxii Ibid. (12:51).

cdxxiii Campbell-McBride, Natasha. One Man's Meat is Another Man's Poison. GAPS.ME. August 8, 2014. Web. June 2015. http://www.doctor-natasha.com/one-mans-meat-another-mans-poison.php.

cdxxiv Campbell-McBride, Natasha. (November, 2015). *Gut and Psychology Syndrome (Part 1)* Weston A. Price Annual Conference. Anaheim, California. (14:20).

cdxxv Ibid. (16:30).

cdxxvi Ibid. (16:50).

cdxxvii Ibid. (17:00).

cdxxviii Ibid. (17:25).

cdxxix Campbell-McBride, Natasha. "GAPS FAQS". GAPS.me. Gut and Psychology Syndrome. March 2017. Web. March 2017. http://www.gaps.me/faqs.php.

cdxxx Ibid. http://www.gaps.me/faqs.php.

cdxxxi Romagnolo, Donato, F., and Ornella I. Selmin. Mediterranean Diet and Prevention of Chronic Diseases. *Nutrition Today.* September 2017. Web. January 2018. https://www.ncbi.nlm.nih.gov/pmc/articles/PMC5625964/.

cdxxxii Pandalai, PK, et al., The effects of omega-3 and omega-6 fatty acids on in vitro prostate cancer growth. *Anticancer Research.* March 1996. Web. January 2018. http://europepmc.org/abstract/med/8687134.

cdxxxiii Lim, WS., et al. Omega 3 fatty acid for the prevention of dementia. London School of Hygiene and Tropical Medicine. The Cochran Library. 2006. Web. January 2018. http://researchonline.lshtm.ac.uk/12034/1/Lim_et_al-2006-The_Cochrane_library.pdf.

cdxxxiv Campbell-McBride, Natasha. (November, 2017). *GAPS Practitioners Q & A.* Weston A. Price Annual Conference. Minneapolis, Minnesota.

cdxxxv Campbell-McBride, Natasha. "Re: Book Questions." Message to Becky Plotner 9 June 2018. E-mail.

cdxxxvi Ibid.

cdxxxvii Ibid.

cdxxxviii Campbell-McBride, Natasha. "GAPS-Diet". GAPS.me. Gut and Psychology Syndrome. September 2018. Web. September 2018. http://www.gaps.me/gaps-diet.php.

cdxxxix Campbell-McBride, Natasha. (November, 2017). *GAPS Practitioners Q & A*. Weston A. Price Annual Conference. Minneapolis, Minnesota.

cdxl Campbell-McBride, Natasha. "Re: Book Questions, Case Study." Message to Becky Plotner 4 July 2018. E-mail.

cdxli Campbell-McBride, Natasha. (November, 2017). *GAPS Practitioners Q & A*. Weston A. Price Annual Conference. Minneapolis, Minnesota.

cdxlii Campbell-McBride, Natasha. "Re: Thank you for meeting with us!" Message to Becky Plotner 19 November 2017. E-mail.

cdxliii Campbell-McBride, Natasha. "Re: Questions" Message to Becky Plotner 8 February 2018. E-mail.

cdxliv Campbell-McBride, Natasha. "Re: Book." Message to Becky Plotner 10 May 2018. E-mail.

cdxlv Campbell-McBride, Natasha. "Re: Thank you for meeting with us!" Message to Becky Plotner 19 November 2017. E-mail.

cdxlvi Campbell-McBride, Natasha. "GAPS-Diet". GAPS.me. Gut and Psychology Syndrome. September 2018. Web. September 2018. http://www.gaps.me/gaps-diet.php.

cdxlvii (2010). Myxedema Coma Induced by Ingestion of Raw Bok Choy. *The New England Journal of Medicine* (362:1945-1946). Web. October 2015.

cdxlviii Ibid.

cdxlix Ibid.

cdl Ibid.

cdli Ibid.

cdlii Adams, Duncan. (2011, May). Deliverance from exophthalmic goiter deaths. *The New Zealand Medical Journal* (Volume 124 Number 1334).

cdliii Ibid.

cdliv What does a palpable thyroid mean – Doctor Answers. *HealthTap* 2015. Web. October 2016. https://www.healthtap.com/topics/what-does-thyroid-not-palpable-mean.

cdlv Bajaj, Jagminder K, et al. (2016, January). Various Possible Toxicants Involved in Thyroid Dysfunction *Journal of Clinical and Diagnostic Research* 10(1). Web. October 2016.

cdlvi Razaitis, Lynn. The Liver Files. The Weston A. Price Foundation (2005, July). Web. November, 2017.

cdlvii Campbell-McBride, Natasha. (November, 2015). *GAPS*. Certified GAPS Practitioner Meeting. Anaheim, California.

cdlviii Butler, Julie. How Heat, Light and Oxygen Harm Olive Oil. *Olive Oil Times*. May 2012. Web. December 2015.

cdlix Ayton, Jamie, et al. The Effect of Storage Conditions on Extra Virgin Olive Oil Quality. Australian Government, Rural Industries Research and Development Corporation. April 2012. Web. December 2012.

cdlx Allouche, Y, et al. How heating affects extra virgin olive oil quality indexes and chemical composition. *Journal of Agriculture and Food Chemistry.* November 2007. Web. December 2007.

cdlxi Ibid.

cdlxii Sutherland, Wayne H.F., et al. Effect of meals rich in heated olive and safflower oils on oxidation of postprandial serum in healthy men. *Atherosclerosis*. January 2002. Web. December 2002.

cdlxiii Assy, Nimer, et al. Olive oil consumption and non-alcoholic fatty liver disease. *World Journal of Gastroenterology*. April 2009. Web. December 2009.

cdlxiv Vitamin D. MedlinePlus, Web. August 2017.

cdlxv Stamets, Paul. Place Mushrooms in Sunlight to Get Your Vitamin D. *Fungi Perfect*. August 6, 2012. Web. June 2012.

cdlxvi Ibid.

cdlxvii Ibid.

cdlxviii Campbell-McBride, Natasha. "Re: Book Questions." Message to Becky Plotner 9 June 2018. E-mail.

cdlxix Campbell-McBride, Natasha. (November, 2017). *GAPS Practitioners Q & A*. Weston A. Price Annual Conference. Minneapolis, Minnesota.

cdlxx Ibid.

cdlxxi Ibid.

cdlxxii Ibid.

cdlxxiii Ibid.

cdlxxiv Campbell-McBride, Natasha. "Re: Book Questions." Message to Becky Plotner 9 June 2018. E-mail.

cdlxxv Campbell-McBride, Natasha. "Re: Clarifying." Message to Becky Plotner 23 September 2018. E-mail.

cdlxxvi Campbell-McBride, Natasha. "Re: Book Questions, Case Study." Message to Becky Plotner 4 July 2018. E-mail.

cdlxxvii Campbell-McBride, Natasha. "GAPS-Diet". GAPS.me. Gut and Psychology Syndrome. September 2018. Web. September 2018. http://www.gaps.me/gaps-diet.php.

cdlxxviii Campbell-McBride, Natasha. (November, 2017). *GAPS Practitioners Q & A*. Weston A. Price Annual Conference. Minneapolis, Minnesota.

cdlxxix Ibid.

cdlxxx Ibid.

cdlxxxi Ibid.

cdlxxxii Campbell-McBride, Natasha. "Re: From Dr. Natasha." Message to Becky Plotner 24 January 2018. E-mail.

cdlxxxiii Campbell-McBride, Natasha. (November, 2017). *GAPS Practitioners Q & A*. Weston A. Price Annual Conference. Minneapolis, Minnesota.

cdlxxxiv Ibid.

cdlxxxv Campbell-McBride, Natasha. "Re: Book." Message to Becky Plotner 12 March 2018. E-mail.

cdlxxxvi Ibid.

cdlxxxvii Ibid.

cdlxxxviii Campbell-McBride, Natasha. (November, 2017). *GAPS Practitioners Q & A*. Weston A. Price Annual Conference. Minneapolis, Minnesota.

cdlxxxix Ibid.

cdxc Ibid.

cdxci Razaitis, Lynn. The Liver Files. Weston A. Price. July 29, 2005. Web. August 2005.

cdxcii Ibid.

cdxciii Campbell-McBride, Natasha. (November, 2017). *GAPS Practitioners Q & A*. Weston A. Price Annual Conference. Minneapolis, Minnesota.

cdxciv Ibid.

cdxcv Campbell-McBride, Natasha. "Re: Book." Message to Becky Plotner 3 March 2018. E-mail.

cdxcvi Campbell-McBride, Natasha. "Re: Book Questions." Message to Becky Plotner 31 May 2018. E-mail.

cdxcvii Ibid.

cdxcviii de Oliveira, A.C., et al. The domestic processing of the common bean resulted in a reduction in the phytates and tannins antinutritional factors, in the starch content and in the raffinose, stachyose and verbascose flatulence factors. *Archivos Latinoamericanos de Nutrición.* September 2001. Web. September 2001.

cdxcix Zamindar, Nafiseh, et al. Effect of line, soaking and cooking time on water absorption, texture and splitting of red kidney beans. *Journal of Food Science and Technology.* January 21, 2011. Web. February 2011.

d Ohoh, HA., et al. Effect of soaking, cooking and germination of the oligosaccharide content of selected Nigerian legume seeds. *Plant Foods For Human Nutrition.* 2000. Web. December 2011.

di Dolan, Laurie, C., et al. Naturally Occurring Food Toxins. *Toxins.* September 2010. Web. November 2010.

dii *America's Secret Slang.* History Channel, 2013.

diii Ibid.

div Martin, Gar. Slush fund. Phrase Finder. 2017. Web. 2017. https://www.phrases.org.uk/meanings/slush-fund.html.

dv *America's Secret Slang.* History Channel, 2013.

dvi Campbell-McBride, Natasha. "Re: Book Questions." Message to Becky Plotner 9 June 2018. E-mail.

dvii Chen, IN., et al. (2008, October). Lactic fermentation and antioxidant activity of Zingiberaceae plants in Taiwan. *International Journal of Food Science and Nutrition, (60 Suppl 2).* pp. 57-66.

dviii Campbell-McBride, Natasha. (November, 2017). *GAPS Practitioners Q & A.* Weston A. Price Annual Conference. Minneapolis, Minnesota.

dix Campbell-McBride, Natasha. "Re: From Dr. Natasha." Message to Becky Plotner 24 January 2019. E-mail.

dx Ibid.

dxi Ibid.

dxii Ibid.

dxiii Ibid.

dxiv Ibid.

dxv Ibid.

dxvi Ibid.

dxvii Sertich Velie. What's the Difference Between Dutch Process and Natural Cocoa Powder. *Serious Eats.* Web. October 2016.

dxviii Code of Federal Regulations [Title 21, Volume 2][CITE: 21CFR163.110]. Title 21 – Food and Drugs Chapter I – Food and Drug Administration Department of Health and Human Services Sub Chapter B – Food for Human Consumption. US Food and Drug Administration. Web. October 2015.

dxix Ibid.

dxx Ibid.

dxxi Ibid.

dxxii Ibid.

dxxiii Ibid.

dxxiv Dykes, Aaron. A Sour Deception: Citric Acid Comes from GMO Black Mold, Not Fruit. *Truth Stream Media.* April 14, 2014. Web. November 2014.

[dxxv] Code of Federal Regulations [Title 21, Volume 2][CITE: 21CFR163.110]. Title 21 – Food and Drugs Chapter I – Food and Drug Administration Department of Health and Human Services Sub Chapter B – Food for Human Consumption. US Food and Drug Administration. Web. October 2015.

[dxxvi] Ibid.

[dxxvii] Ibid.

[dxxviii] Ibid.

[dxxix] How Much Caffeine Is in Chocolate? Amano Artisan Chocolate. March 19, 2013. Web. October 2013.

[dxxx] Code of Federal Regulations [Title 21, Volume 2] [CITE: 21CFR163.110]. Title 21 – Food and Drugs Chapter I – Food and Drug Administration Department of Health and Human Services Sub Chapter B – Food for Human Consumption. US Food and Drug Administration. Web. October 2015.

[dxxxi] Ibid.

[dxxxii] Ibid.

[dxxxiii] Reinagel, Monica. Carob versus Chocolate. *Scientific American.* April 6, 2014. Web. December 2014.

[dxxxiv] Dyer, Bill. Alkalized Cocoa Powders. Bloomer Chocolate Company. 57th PMCA Production Conference, 2003. 2003. Web. November 2004.

[dxxxv] Ibid.

[dxxxvi] MacQueen, Julie. "Chocolate Ingredients." Message to Becky Plotner. 4 March, 2016. Email.

[dxxxvii] Ibid.

[dxxxviii] Ibid.

[dxxxix] Ibid.

[dxl] Campbell-McBride, Natasha. "Re: Book Questions." Message to Becky Plotner. 31 May, 2018. E-mail.

[dxli] Ibid.

[dxlii] Annual Income Spent On Food. *Washington State Magazine.* Web. January 2017.

[dxliii] Mahapatra, Lisa. The US Spends Less on Food Than Any Other Country in The World. *International Business Times.* January 23, 2014. Web. November 2015.

[dxliv] Salatin, Joel. *Folks, This Ain't Normal.* New York: Hachette Book Group, 2011. Print. Pg 40.

[dxlv] Plotner, Becky. Sauerkraut Test Divulges Shocking Probiotic Count. Nourishing Plot. June 2014. Web. June 2014.

[dxlvi] Plotner, Becky. Surprising Probiotic Count of Kefir Revealed. Nourishing Plot. October 2015. Web. October 2015.

[dxlvii] Plotner, Becky. Microbiology Studies Show the Difference Between Store Kefir And Home Brewed Kefir. Nourishing Plot. January 2016. Web. January 2016.

[dxlviii] Kim, Min. (November, 2015). *Redeeming Bread, How to Make Einkorn Sourdough.* Weston A. Price Annual Conference. Anaheim, California.

[dxlix] Ibid.

[dl] Ibid.

[dli] Ibid.

[dlii] Campbell-McBride, Natasha. (November, 2017). *GAPS Practitioners Q & A.* Weston A. Price Annual Conference. Minneapolis, Minnesota.

[dliii] Ibid.

[dliv] Ibid.

[dlv] Ibid.

[dlvi] Ibid.

Made in United States
Troutdale, OR
10/04/2023

13399726R00266